volume **1**

Contemporary Dental Hygiene Practice

Patricia A. Phagan-Schostok, R.D.H., B.S., M.Ed., Ed.D.
Professor and Director
Division of Continuing Education and
Coordinator for Faculty Development
Northwestern University Dental School
Chicago, Illinois

Karen L. Maloney, R.D.H., B.S., M.Ed.
Associate Professor and Chairman
Dental Hygiene and Auxiliary Programs
Northwestern University Dental School
Chicago, Illinois

quintessence
books

Quintessence Publishing Co., Inc. 1988
Chicago, Berlin, São Paulo, London, Tokyo, and Hong Kong

Library of Congress Cataloging-in-Publication Data

Phagan-Schostok, Patricia A.
  Contemporary dental hygiene practice.

  Bibliography: p.
  Includes index.
  1. Dental hygiene. I. Maloney, Karen L. II. Title.
[DNLM: 1. Dental Prophylaxis—methods. WU 113 P532c]
RK60.7.P47 1988   617.6'01   87-7329
ISBN 0-86715-169-2 (v. 1)

quintessence
books

Lithography: Industrie- und Presseklischee, Berlin
Composition: Graphic World, Inc., St. Louis, MO
Printing and binding: The Ovid Bell Press, Inc., Fulton, MO
Printed in U.S.A.

Contents

part 1 **Preliminary procedures**

chapter 1 **Control of health hazards and disease transmission** **12**

chapter 2 **Health assessment and documentation** **31**

chapter 3 **Preparation for emergencies** **70**

chapter 4 **Supplemental components of the examination** **88**

part 2 **The treatment plan: Formulation and implementation**

chapter 5 **Individualization of treatment** **108**

chapter 6 **Techniques for optimal efficiency** **118**

chapter 7 **Composition of dental deposits** **124**

chapter 8 **The periodontal co-therapist** **130**

chapter 9 **Treatment modalities for the postsurgical patient** **147**

chapter 10 **Polishing mechanisms** **153**

part 3 **Preventive dentistry and oral health maintenance**

chapter 11 **The control of dental disease** **160**

chapter 12 **Fluoride therapies** **190**

Glossary **206**

General references **213**

Index **217**

Dedication

A friend is a present we give ourselves. . . .
Robert Louis Stevenson

We dedicate this book to each other. To have as your professional colleague, your most honest critic, and your most undaunting supporter, your best friend, is truly a present we have given ourselves.

Foreword

A few decades ago, a dental hygiene education was characterized by indoctrination and discipline. A limited body of knowledge was imparted largely by part-time professor–practitioners who were both skilled and dedicated. But the knowledge explosion that has taken place within the past two decades has changed all that. Indeed, it is not an exaggeration to say that more knowledge has become available in the dental health field within the past 20 years than had been uncovered in the entire history of the profession. It is equally true that this trend will continue at virtually the same pace.

Patricia A. Phagan-Schostok and Karen L. Maloney are dental hygiene educators who genuinely respect the amount of already existent learning, but who have a lively sense of the truths to be attained. Without diminishing the permanent values of indoctrination and discipline, they have insisted upon a growth in learning, not merely the possession of it.

Both were among a pioneer group of dental educators who insisted upon the place of a full-time faculty that recognized the need to be academically sound educators as well as dental professionals, this in order to combine a thorough knowledge of the science with a clear methodology for imparting it. Both professors view learning as a language of discovery, not rote memorization. Both have continued their own education because they share the creed of Dr. Greene Vardiman Black, the acknowledged father of modern American dentistry, that a professional person has no right to be other than a continuous student.

Dentistry, more than any other health science, has successfully promoted the concept of preventive care. Thanks in great measure to the skill and dedication of the dental hygienist, the incidence of dental caries has dropped markedly in recent years. Currently, Americans have a contagious enthusiasm for self-improvement and health maintenance. As a consequence, the hygienist is needed more than ever.

Dentistry is not going the way of the blacksmith. The competent hygienist, equipped with the expanded skills and knowledge described in these volumes, can look forward to a satisfying and rewarding career as a dental professional now and in the future.

The appearance of these texts and the accompanying laboratory manual represents an answer to a vital need. It has been some time since books of this breadth and depth have appeared. It is my hope that their adoption will not be confined to schools where dental hygiene is taught. These texts are basic references. They belong in the library of any dental hygiene practitioner who wishes to remain current.

Norman H. Olsen, D.D.S., M.S.D.
Dean, Northwestern University

Preface

The scope of dental hygiene practice has broadened dramatically over the past 70 years. With (1) growth in the various modes of dental health care delivery systems, (2) changes in the patterns of dental diseases and dental patient population groups, and (3) expansion of the educational preparation available to dental hygienists, significant options beyond the traditional private dental setting have evolved. The profession is a vital, dynamic one that will continue to grow well into the next century.

In today's dental care arena, command of background information and mastery of the technical skills of dental hygiene must be combined with a sound foundation in the basic and dental sciences; it is only with such a complete background that the dental hygienist can operate as a true professional. This text presupposes that the student will have a basic background in anatomy, physiology, microbiology, and biology. Because these areas are not covered in our text, we advise that, prior to studying the section on local anesthesia and pain control, the reader review material in head and neck anatomy. Prior to utilizing the section on temporization and restoration finishing and polishing, tooth morphology and biological materials should be reviewed; prior to working with the nutritional counseling chapter, biochemistry should be reviewed; and so on.

Dentistry is constantly generating new research, and for this reason we have chosen to include the most up-to-date information available on remineralization, chemical plaque inhibition, and sexually transmitted diseases. However, as educators, we charge you to remember one thing: all knowledge is subject to revision. Professionals must continually update their information.

We know that providers of dental hygiene therapy assume differing dental care roles among the different jurisdictions within the United States; this text will therefore present material related to the professional functioning of dental hygienists in most jurisdictions.

In order to correlate with dental hygiene curricula, the text is divided into two volumes; we hope that this presents a convenient approach for both faculty and students. The accompanying manual to Volume 1 is meant to be used for laboratory exercises for skill development. The evaluation sheets included for each section of the manual are designed to facilitate feedback from the instructor to the beginning dental hygiene student.

In a work of this size the contributions of many individuals are appreciated beyond words. Our thanks, of course, to our Dean, Dr. Norman Olsen, whose encouragement and support regarding all our projects for the advancement of the dental hygiene profession never waivers. Contributors to Volume 1 whom we wish to thank include: Connie Marshall, R.D.H., M.B.A.; Nancy Osburn, R.D.H., B.S., Northwestern University Dental School; Stephen Marshall, M.D. (Medical Emergencies); Ulana Kostiw-Cirincione, R.D.H., M.P.H., Northwestern University Dental School; Jean Wolff, R.D.H., B.S., and Paul Baker, B.S., Northwestern University Dental School and Kascot Media Inc. (intraoral photography); Dr. Peter Hurst and Wendy Wils, R.D.H., B.S., of Northwestern Memorial Hospital's Dental Center (oral cancer); Dr. Harold T. Perry and Dr. Roger Kallal, Orthodontics Department, Northwestern University Dental School; Dr. Anthony Gargiulo, Chairman, Periodontics Department, Loyola University; Dr. Leon Silverstone, Associate Dean of Research, University of Colorado; Cynthia Noonan and Robert Perry of Oral-B Laboratories; the Hu-Friedy Instrument Manufacturing Company; Diane Roberto, R.D.H., Margaret Daniell, R.D.H., B.S., Nancy Nichols, R.D.H., B.S., and Mary Gina Dicera, R.D.H., B.S., graduates of our dental hygiene programs.

A special thanks to our models for the many hours of photographic sessions: James Maloney, D.D.S., Susan Argondizzo-Marshall, R.D.H., and Nancy Osburn, R.D.H., B.S. We know that our readers will benefit from their clear, demonstrative poses. A heartfelt thanks to our office staff, Ms. Deborah Garnigan and Ms. Maria Pulido, for the hours devoted to assembling the manuscript, and to the faculty of the Dental Hygiene Department of Northwestern University Dental School for their patience, understanding, and support during this project.

To each other, a great salute! In the dedication of this book are expressed our feelings for each other. To our great surprise, even after this project, we are not only still speaking, but as ever, the best of colleagues and friends!

part 1

Preliminary procedures

chapter 1

Control of health hazards and disease transmission

The dental hygienist, as a primary health care provider, is responsible for taking an active part in preventing the occurrence and spread of disease, both among patients and to herself or himself and other dental office personnel. Because the oral cavity has a substantial population of microorganisms, the dental appointment presents an ideal opportunity for the transmission of disease. Infection may be disseminated via aerosols, dust, air, and by direct contact between one person and another. This chapter will explain the various means the dental hygienist may employ to control the spread of disease. It also includes descriptive explanations of certain disease states that present particular transmission hazards for dental personnel.

Preparation of the operatory

Before a patient is seated, the environment in which the patient is to be treated must be prepared.[1–5] All equipment, countertops, and other items used during the dental appointment should be thoroughly dusted and wiped with a chemical disinfectant solution at the beginning of each appointment (Fig. 1-1). In addition, items that are frequently touched or used during patient treatment should be disinfected and wrapped before and after each patient is treated. These include pens, pencils, light switches, chair-operating buttons, and patient-education materials. The bracket tray or work surface and headrest portion of the dental chair should be covered with disposable paper covers that can be discarded after each patient appointment. All metal instruments, prophylaxis angle, and handpiece should be sterilized prior to use. All water lines should be flushed daily, and evacuation systems should be flushed with a disinfectant solution. If the dental unit includes a cuspidor, it should be scrubbed with a cleaning agent and wiped

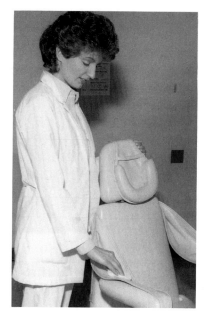

Fig. 1-1   Disinfect all contact surfaces prior to patient treatment.

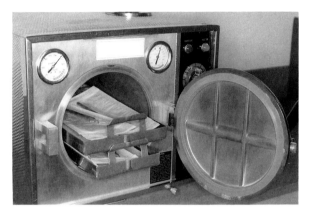

Fig. 1-2   Materials ready to be autoclaved.

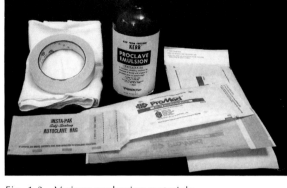

Fig. 1-3   Various packaging materials.

with disinfectant solution. All bracket tray attachments such as the air/water syringe, saliva ejector hose, and handpiece hookup should be wiped with disinfectant.

A wide variety of chemical agents are available for use in preparation of the operatory, including an aqueous formaldehyde, glutaraldehyde, chlorine compounds, and iodophors. Among the agents that are *not* recommended for surface disinfection are alcohols (both isopropanol and ethanol), phenolics, and quaternary ammonium compounds. Although many surfaces and materials used routinely in the dental office can only be sanitized or protected prior to use, other items can and should be sterilized for optimum control of disease transmission, and barriers and coverings applied when appropriate.

Sterilization methods

The destruction of all microbial life forms, including spores and viruses, is achieved by the sterilization process.[6-27] In the dental office, it is extremely important that all instruments be completely free of microorganisms in order to inhibit the spread of disease. This can be accomplished only through one of the available methods of sterilization: (1) steam under pressure, (2) dry heat, or (3) chemical agents. An additional method using ethylene oxide gas is reserved primarily for use in hospitals and for sterilizing commercial products. Recent developments indicate that microwave ovens may become a practical, timesaving sterilization method in the future.

Steam under pressure

The most reliable and efficient means to achieve sterilization of the majority of dental instruments is steam under pressure, commonly referred to as autoclaving.[28-31] Ten minutes' direct exposure to saturated steam at 121°C (250°F) under 15 pounds of pressure will destroy all living organisms. This destruction is achieved by the moist heat, not the pressure itself. Increasing the temperature and the pressure reduces sterilizing time.

A number of factors must be considered when using steam under pressure as a sterilization mechanism. First, *both* pressure and internal temperature must be relied on, not just the pressure itself. Second, the timing should begin only *after* the desired temperature is reached; this usually is accomplished within 10 minutes and depends on the number and arrangement of articles in the chamber of the autoclave. Third, articles to be sterilized must be packaged in materials that allow easy penetration of the steam: paper, muslin, or cheesecloth. Materials that do not allow easy penetration of the steam include cellophane, plastic cloth, aluminum foil, canvas, and closed metal containers.

When articles are placed in the autoclave, care should be taken so that the arrangement allows complete access of steam to all parts of the articles (Fig. 1-2). Packages should be separated from each other and should be wrapped so that metal-to-metal contact is avoided. Beakers, jars, and other glass containers should be placed on their sides or tilted, but not left in an upright position. Cloth bundles such as towels

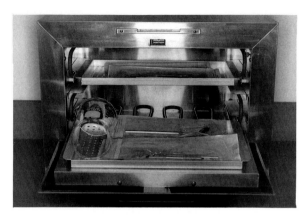

Fig. 1-4   Materials ready to be Dri-Claved.

or dressings should be packed loosely to allow even penetration of the steam.

Prior to packaging, all instruments and other items should be completely scrubbed or should be cleaned in an ultrasonic cleaner and dried. Any foreign matter remaining, including soap, may act as a barrier to steam penetration. Linens should be laundered and dried. Instruments made of carbon steel may be immersed in an anticorrosion liquid such as sodium nitrite to prevent rusting, and dried. Wrapping may then proceed, using paper, muslin, or cheesecloth. Bundles may be tied or sealed with autoclave tape that develops colored stripes at 121°C (250°F). Such tape aids in identifying packages that have been exposed to the appropriate heat. Alternatively, paper and cellophane bags designed to accommodate instruments or other items are available in various sizes. They have stripes or other color indicators that darken or change color upon exposure to heat (Fig. 1-3).

Once the autoclave is loaded, the manufacturer's directions should be followed. Generally, one of the following temperature/pressure/time formulas may be used: either 121°C (250°F) at 15 pounds pressure for 10 to 15 minutes *or* 134°C (270°F) at 30 pounds pressure for 3 to 7 minutes. Longer times may be required if many items are being sterilized.

The advantages of using steam under pressure to sterilize articles in the dental office are:

1. All microbial forms of life are destroyed.
2. The methodology is efficient and quick.
3. It is the most economical method available.

4. Many different types of materials may be sterilized in this manner.

The disadvantages of steam under pressure include:

1. Corrosion of carbon steel instruments occurs unless antirust agents are utilized.
2. Some dulling of cutting edges of instruments may occur.
3. Certain products are unsuitable for moist heat sterilization. Oils, powders, waxes, petroleum, plastics, and rubber products may deteriorate after numerous exposures.

Several indicators are available to check the efficiency of the autoclave and ultrasonic cleaners being used. Ampules or strips containing live spores may be purchased to test the sterilizing capability; aluminum foil strips in beakers may also be purchased to test ultrasonic functioning. Tests may be conducted on a weekly or monthly schedule, depending on the volume of the practice.

Dry heat

For items that cannot be sterilized by moist heat under pressure, dry heat is an acceptable substitute. It is the method of choice for thermostable powders and oils and for metal instruments that may be rusted by moisture. As with steam under pressure, all instruments and objects should be thoroughly cleaned and dried before packaging or wrapping. Paper, aluminum trays or foil, and muslin may be used to package the items to be sterilized. Packages should be small in size and distributed in the oven so as to permit even penetration of the heat (Fig. 1-4).

Once the oven has been loaded, the recommended temperature must be reached before the timing cycle begins. Generally, a temperature of 160°C to 170°C (320°F to 340°F) should be attained and held for 1 to 2 hours, depending on the number and type items to be sterilized. Items should be arranged to allow air to circulate freely around them.

Dry heat sterilization has the following advantages:

1. It is an acceptable method for materials that cannot be exposed to moist steam.
2. It will not cause rusting of metal instruments.
3. Sharp cutting edges are maintained longer when the appropriate temperature is used.

Disadvantages of dry heat include:

1. A long time is required for sterilization.
2. Some materials may not easily withstand high temperatures (e.g., cotton, paper, and solder).
3. Penetration of the heat is slow and uneven.

Chemical vapor

Sterilization may be achieved by the use of chemical vapor, which is a gas composed of water, acetone, ketone, formaldehyde, and alcohols. This compound, when heated under pressure, is capable of sterilizing instruments and other materials that are not affected by the heat of the vapor or by the vapor itself.

The device used in this method resembles an autoclave in its design and basic operation. A temperature/pressure/time formula is likewise employed: 127°C to 132°C (260°F to 270°F) at 20 to 40 pounds pressure for 20 minutes. If the number of items to be sterilized is substantial, the time element should be increased. Spore testing on a regular basis is recommended to assure adequate sterilizing capability.

Chemical vapor sterilization eliminates the occurrence of rusting of instruments, is a relatively simple procedure, and is accomplished in a short period of time. It does require adequate ventilation, however, and is therefore less desirable in a small, enclosed area.

Ethylene oxide

The least likely method of sterilization in a dental office employs ethylene oxide gas.[32] This mode is used most often by hospitals and large clinics, when large quantities of materials are to be sterilized. Although smaller units have become available for dental office use, the length of the sterilization cycle (4 to 5 hours) and the potential toxic properties of the gas, which can be retained by rubber and plastic items, make it the least favorable method. If ethylene oxide is used, aeration of plastic and rubber materials is necessary prior to use. Metal instruments do not require aeration. Adequate ventilation and removal of the gas is of the utmost importance.

Microwave sterilization[33]

Preliminary research has indicated that microwave ovens, when properly adapted, can readily kill representative viruses, fungi, and aerobic and anaerobic bacteria, including spore formers, in relatively short periods of time. A significant advantage of this method over existing modes of sterilization is its ability to leave the objects completely undamaged, regardless of the number of times they are sterilized.

The exact mechanism(s) by which microwaves destroy the microbes is still uncertain. Uniform sterility cannot be achieved unless the objects are rotated in both horizontal and vertical planes to avoid the oven's "cold spots." A three-dimensional rotation device has been designed for this purpose, for which a patent has been filed by the University of Oklahoma. Although substantial research studies have yet to be conducted on microwaves as a sterilization modality, with modifications the microwave oven may soon become a component of the dental office armamentarium.

Glutaraldehyde

At this time, the only chemical agent capable of achieving sterilization is glutaraldehyde at a 2% alkaline aqueous concentration.[34] This preparation will destroy bacteria (including *Mycobacterium tuberculosis*), viruses, and fungi after a 10-minute immersion cycle. Following a longer immersion time (6¾ to 10 hours), the more resistant bacterial spores are eliminated. Glutaraldehyde has not yet been demonstrated to destroy the hepatitis virus, primarily because the virus has not yet been cultured. As a result, any instruments or materials used to treat patients with known or suspected histories of hepatitis should be sterilized in a more conventional manner. Although the cycle length of 10 hours may make it an impractical method for routine use in the dental office, glutaraldehyde is ideal for materials that cannot withstand high temperatures.

The Council on Dental Therapeutics of the American Dental Association currently recognizes some glutaraldehyde products as accepted preparations. Two are Sporicidin* and Cidex 7.† Both of these agents require the addition of a buffer for activation. The manufacturers' directions for preparation, use, and recommended immersion times prior to use must be carefully read and followed (Fig. 1-5).

---

*Sporicidin Co., Washington, D.C.
†Johnson & Johnson Dental Products, East Windsor, N.J.

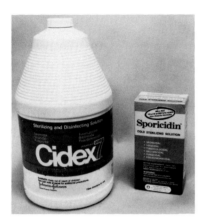

Fig. 1-5   Glutaraldehyde products accepted by American Dental Association Council on Dental Therapeutics.

Disinfection methods

Disinfection is any process by which disease-causing microorganisms can be destroyed. Disinfectants will *not* ordinarily eliminate viruses, spores, or tubercle bacilli. Disinfectant solutions are therefore generally unsuitable for routine decontamination of dental instruments and other articles used intraorally; heat sterilization is the preferred method for these items. Some materials and instruments, however, cannot withstand the temperatures that heat sterilization requires.

Chemical agents

A number of chemical solutions are currently available for disinfecting dental instruments, equipment, and surface areas of the operatory. These agents vary in the degree of bactericidal effects they convey; some lack sporicidal capability, and some are bacteriostatic only. The Council on Dental Therapeutics classifies high, intermediate, or low activity levels in terms of biocidal activity. The degree of biocidal activity is greatly influenced by many elements, including the situation of use of the product, the number of microorganisms present initially, the amount and type of organic material contaminants, and the physical properties of the objects to be disinfected. The concentration of the agent is another factor of importance, because a given solution can be either bactericidal or bacteriostatic or can actually enhance or stimulate microbial growth at various concentrations.

Surfaces and instruments to be disinfected must be

exposed to the preparation for a specific length of time. Prior to immersion, instruments must be dried to prevent dilution of the agent. Once the instruments have been placed in the solution, they must remain for at least the minimum amount of time specified by the manufacturer. If additional items are added before the timing has elapsed, the cycle must be started again, because the items already in the solution will be contaminated. The solutions must be replaced on a regular basis, because their ability to destroy microorganisms lasts for fixed periods of time.

Syringes and instruments that are hinged or have deep notches, crevices, or serrations are not effectively disinfected by most chemical agents. They should be sterilized by one of the other methods. Hypodermic needles should *never* be reused; rather, they should be disposed of appropriately after use.

High activity level disinfectants   These include formaldehyde and glutaraldehyde.

Formaldehyde in either an 8% aqueous solution or 8% in 70% alcohol is considered a good disinfectant when items are immersed for ten hours. The length of immersion makes it less than ideal for routine use in the dental office. Formaldehyde is a gas that dissolves easily in water and reacts with the protein component of microorganisms. The vapor is quite irritating to mucous membranes and skin and, as a result, its use is minimal.

Glutaraldehyde in a 2% alkaline aqueous solution for 7 to 10 hours is bactericidal for many microbial forms of life. At this point it cannot be considered a true form of sterilization, because of its uncertain capacity to destroy the hepatitis B virus, but would be classified in the high-activity level of disinfection.

Intermediate level disinfectants   These include formaldehyde at a 3% aqueous concentration for at least 30 minutes, chlorine compounds, and iodophors.

Chlorine compounds are used at a 1% solution of available chlorine (1:5 dilution of commercial bleach) for a minimum of 30 minutes. Corrosion of metal instruments, irritation to skin and eyes, and short shelf life are disadvantages. In addition, organic debris quickly deactivates the solution's disinfecting capacity. All items should be clean and dry prior to immersion.

Iodophors are used at a 1% solution of available iodine for at least 30 minutes. Instrument corrosion is a side effect, as is occasional potential allergic reaction of patients to the iodine component.

Not recommended Because of their low level of biocidal activity, quaternary ammonium compounds are not acceptable for disinfecting purposes. Examples include: benzalkonium chloride, dibenzalkonium chloride, and cetyldimethylethyl-ammonium bromide. Because they evaporate rapidly, isopropanol (90%) and ethanol (70%) alcohols are not acceptable. Because of sporadic virucidal capabilities, phenolic compounds are not acceptable. They include cresol, saponated cresol solution, and sodium pentachlorophenate.

Boiling water

When other methods of disinfection are unavailable, boiling distilled water may be used for glassware, metal instruments, and other objects that can be exposed to water. Items must be completely submerged, and the water kept boiling (100°C; 212°F) for at least 30 minutes. Although the amount of time required to disinfect with this method is relatively short, the method is less than ideal because of corrosion of instruments, decrease in instrument sharpness, and the ability of certain microbes to resist the disinfecting action of the heat of the water.

Hot oils

Hydrocarbon or silicon oils have been used as disinfectants, especially for handpieces and prophylaxis angles. Special units are available to achieve this type of disinfection. Timing for disinfection is 150°C (300°F) for 15 minutes or 125°C (260°F) for 30 minutes. Sterilization can be achieved if the oil is heated to 160°C (320°F) for at least 1 hour. Timing begins when the recommended temperature has been attained and, as with other methods, if additional instruments are added the timing cycle must begin again. All instruments and items must be dry when placed into the hot oil to avoid spattering. Corrosion and instrument dullness are *not* experienced with this method, but the oil may produce a disagreeable odor.

Occupational health hazards

One of the primary reasons for employing stringent sterilization and disinfection procedures is to protect the health of the operator and the patient from the inadvertant spread of disease. In addition, the health of future patients will be shielded from potential infection. While it is true that some dentally transferred diseases such as common colds may not be life threatening, the attitude of health care providers should be such that all efforts are made to safeguard the patient's health status. More important, however, several serious and potentially severe diseases are at an increased risk of being transmitted via the instruments, techniques, and personal habits of dental personnel unless appropriate precautions are employed. Because of the nature of treatment being rendered and the environment in which it is provided—that is, the oral cavity—diseases such as hepatitis, tuberculosis, herpes, and AIDS pose exceptional problems for the dental hygienist.

Hepatitis

In the strictest interpretation, hepatitis is inflammation of the liver.[38-46] Hepatitis may occur for numerous reasons, most of which are not of an infectious nature, such as cancer, obstructed jaundice, and reactions to anesthetic agents, chemotherapy, or antibiotic drugs. These types of hepatitis are not of concern to the dental hygienist from the point of view of transmittable disease. The infectious forms of viral hepatitis (Type A, Type B, and Type non-A, non-B) are of great concern to all dental personnel because they may easily be spread via routine procedures unless care is taken.

All forms of viral hepatitis are infectious in nature and are spread by a variety of types of intimate contact. Once an individual becomes ill, the only means of combatting the disease is through the body's immune system. Length of the illness may range from several weeks to 6 months or more, and long-lasting effects may include becoming a chronic carrier of the virus, as may occur following a case of hepatitis B. This is of particular significance because a practitioner who is a known carrier of the hepatitis B virus (HBV) may be forbidden by law to continue to practice. The concept of prevention is vital when treating patients with a past history of hepatitis.

Hepatitis A The hepatitis A virus (HAV) is transmitted through the fecal–oral route, meaning that the virus is excreted via the feces, and the individual who then contracts the virus does so by oral contact with something contaminated with the virus. Common sources of infection are shellfish from polluted waters, contaminated milk or drinking water, and communities or areas with poor sanitation facilities. Outbreaks of the disease are more likely to occur in institutions for the handicapped, military bases, schools, and child-care centers. Of primary importance is the fact that poor personal hygiene and unsanitary conditions provide ideal circumstances for transmission of the virus. Direct contact is not always necessary in order to become infected with HAV.

Incubation time for hepatitis A is approximately 4 weeks after exposure to the virus, although the time may vary from 2 to 6 weeks. The disease may occur in two stages, characterized by the presence or absence of jaundice. Symptoms of the *preicteric* (prior to onset of jaundice) stage are fever, nausea, vomiting, abdominal pain, fatigue, headache, muscle ache, darkened urine, and light-colored stools. The liver itself may enlarge and become sensitive when palpated. One of the major difficulties is an accurate diagnosis, because the symptoms are similar to those of influenza. If the patient progresses to the *icteric* phase, the onset of jaundice will aid in diagnosis. Jaundice refers to a yellowing of the skin and whites of the eyes and is caused by the release of a liver secretion called bilirubin into the blood and skin. Jaundice does not always occur in adults and is rare in children and infants. When it does manifest itself, it usually does so in the second week of the illness. The patient is infectious, however, even without the appearance of jaundice.

Laboratory tests are available to identify the antibody to the hepatitis A virus (anti-HAV), usually within 2 weeks of onset. High titers may remain for a number of years following the illness. Once the patient recovers, immunity to the disease is conferred. At the present time, no drugs or therapy is available to treat hepatitis A; the only means of combatting the illness is through bed rest and a light but nourishing diet. Alcoholic beverages are strictly forbidden. Precautions must be employed by those caring for the patient to avoid transmitting the disease to others. Personal hygiene measures, especially thorough handwashing, of both the patient and those caring for him or her are important to control the spread of hepatitis A. Immunoglobulin (IG), given within the first week following exposure, may be employed to prevent or modify the extent of the disease.

In the dental office visited by a patient with hep-

atitis A, all instruments should be sterilized and disposable supplies should be used. All surfaces and items that may have been touched by the patient should be disinfected with a solution of hot water and household bleach (2 cups water to ¼ cup bleach). Gloves should always be worn by the dental hygienist during patient treatment and posttreatment cleaning and disinfection procedures.

Hepatitis B   Although the name is similar, the hepatitis B virus (HBV) is quite different from the HAV, and the resulting disease is significantly dissimilar in all of its aspects. Immunity to hepatitis A does *not* confer immunity to either hepatitis B or to the non-A, non-B virus.

HBV may be transmitted both by patients with active cases of the disease and by chronic asymptomatic carriers. Blood, blood products, and other body fluids are the typical means by which the virus travels. The virus is usually transferred by a mechanism known as parenteral inoculation, meaning it is injected or finds its way into the body through an opening in the skin. Some examples of the parenteral route include transfusion of infected blood, contaminated needles (particularly needles reused by drug abusers), use of contaminated medical and/or dental instruments, and accidental self-inoculation.

The HBV may also be transferred by oral and sexual routes and by other types of close physical contact. The oral route is of particular significance in dentistry because the virus has been found in saliva, in low but still infectious concentrations, and may be transferred by both aerosols and the operator's hands. Salivary transmission is one of the major sources of hepatitis B for dental personnel and is more likely to produce a longer incubation time.

It is extremely important to identify not only patients who have had the disease and may be carriers but also individuals who fall into the high-risk groups of people who have been exposed to the disease and who may or *may not* have experienced an active case, and are more likely to be carriers. They include:

1. Persons who have been institutionalized, especially those with mental handicaps who have not lived in the familial home.
2. Patients who report a past history of either hepatitis or jaundice.
3. Self-injected drug abusers.
4. Male homosexuals and prostitutes.

5. Patients with histories of frequent blood transfusions, blood disorders, renal dialysis, immunosuppressive treatment, or radiation therapy.
6. Refugees, residents, or military personnel who have been stationed in countries where hepatitis is endemic, that is, some parts of Latin America, Haiti, the Mediterranean area, underdeveloped countries in Africa, and the Far East.
7. Families of hepatitis patients.
8. Medical and dental personnel, especially those who provide care to any of the above groups.

Transmission of the HBV from mother to infant during the birth process (termed perinatal transmission) is very rare in developed countries such as Europe and the United States. In some areas of underdeveloped countries, however, the disease is epidemic among newborn babies, and a high percentage can become chronic carriers. Children who are recent immigrants from such countries are more likely to be carriers, and precautions should be taken in order to prevent the spread of the disease.

The incubation period for hepatitis B is much longer than that for hepatitis A, lasting between 2 to 6 months, when the symptoms begin to appear. This lengthy incubation phase is a major reason for the difficulty in the control of hepatitis B because, by the time the symptoms appear, the patient may not be able to recall any of the circumstances surrounding his or her exposure to the virus.

Symptoms of hepatitis B are similar both to intestinal virus infections and to hepatitis A. The difference between the A and B infections lies with the degree of onset: hepatitis A is more often an acute infection, whereas the onset is slow and insidious with hepatitis B. Typical symptoms include fatigue, fever of a mild nature, loss of appetite, muscle soreness, joint pain, skin rash, itching, upset stomach (nausea may or may not occur), darkened urine, light-colored stools, and abdominal pain. These symptoms will usually become more severe as time passes. As with hepatitis A, jaundice (if it occurs) will manifest during the second week. A high percentage (an estimated 50% to 60%) of hepatitis B infections that occur are of a subclinical nature, with mild symptoms and no jaundice. These cases that may remain undiagnosed as hepatitis tend to become chronic carriers. These patients present the greatest risk, since they are unaware of their carrier state.

The treatment for hepatitis B is the same as for hepatitis A—bed rest. No drugs or other forms of therapy are available at this time to cure the disease. For those individuals who know or suspect they have been exposed to or infected with the HBV, Hepatitis B Immune Globulin (HBIG) or standard immune globulin should be administered by injection as soon as possible. Additional protection is available in the form of the Heptavax vaccine.

The hepatitis B virus presents a unique challenge to health care professionals in that it tends to be a very resilient microbial organism. It can withstand an extensive range of chemical agents and temperatures; in blood serum, the virus has been shown to retain its infectious nature for 15 years at $-20°C$, 6 months at room temperature, and 4 hours at 60°C. The immediate ramifications for the dental office are clear. Any surfaces that have been splashed with infected blood are potential sources of disease transmission unless they are thoroughly cleaned with a chlorine bleach mixture. Items such as air–water syringes, evacuation hoses, handpieces, prophylaxis angles, cuspidors, and instruments are easily contaminated and require specific attention during disinfection and sterilization procedures. Surfaces and items that appear to be devoid of blood are not to be considered uncontaminated; complete disinfection, sterilization and coverage, and proper sterilization and disposal of discardable items are essential habits to form with every patient treated.

Prevention of hepatitis transmission is dependent upon routine employment of aseptic techniques. All instruments and sterilizable items should be routinely sterilized. Disposable needles and syringes should be used only once and never reused for subsequent patients. Needles should be cut or broken by equipment specifically designed for that purpose; they should never be bent or broken by hand. If metal syringes are used, they should be completely cleaned, rinsed, and bagged or wrapped for sterilization. Instruments and other items that have been used while treating a hepatitis patient should be marked "hepatitis" somewhere on the package so that particular attention is drawn to them.

Any gauze, cotton rolls, patient napkins, or other disposable supplies that have been used with hepatitis patients should be wrapped and autoclaved prior to disposal to protect janitorial personnel who will empty trash receptacles. All environmental surfaces should be disinfected with a household bleach solution. Whenever possible, use of aerosol-producing ultrasonic devices and handpieces should be eliminated or reduced as much as is feasible. The clinician should wear safety glasses, a face mask, disposable gloves, and a gown to cover all clothing.

Serological testing of patients who fall into any of the high-risk groups should be performed prior to treatment. Dental personnel should also be tested routinely.

Serologic Terminology—Hepatitis B

HBsAg:

Hepatitis B surface antigen; found on the surface of the virus; indicates active case of the disease (either acute or chronic) or carrier state; formerly referred to as the Australia antigen.

HBcAg:

Hepatitis B core antigen; found inside the core of the virus.

HBeAg:

Hepatitis B "e" antigen; linked with contagious state.

anti-HBs:

Antibody to HBsAg.

anti-HBc:

Antibody to HBcAg.

anti-HBe:

Antibody to HBeAg.

Prior to 1970, the only serological test available for hepatitis B was the Australia Antigen Test, which measured the presence of the surface antigen. Since then a more advanced battery of tests has been devised. It is now possible to determine the presence or absence of all three antigens and each of their antibodies.

Early in the 1980s a vaccine became available to protect at-risk individuals from contracting hepatitis B. Heptavax-B* consists of hepatitis B surface antigen taken from the plasma of human carriers. The antigen is subsequently inactivated, purified, and placed in sterile suspension for intramuscular injection. Three doses of the vaccine are given over a 6-month period. The first two injections are given one month apart, with the third booster dose given 6 months after the

*Merck, Sharp and Dohme, Rahway, N.J.

first dose. The duration of immunity is not presently known; however, available data suggest a 5-year period for persons who have received all three injections. At that time, a booster dose may be necessary to preserve the immune state. A new synthetic vaccine, Recombivax-HB, is now available. Produced by a recombinant strain of yeast, this vaccine has the same immunization schedule as Heptavax-B, and appears to confer similar immunity to hepatitis B.

Side effects that have occurred with administration of the vaccine include injection-site soreness, swelling, warmth, erythema, or induration. They usually subside within 48 hours of the vaccination. Other reported side effects (fever, malaise, fatigue, headache, nausea, vomiting, dizziness, muscle pain, and joint pain) have been infrequent or occasional in occurrence.

Persons who are at an increased risk of contracting hepatitis B should seriously consider receiving the vaccine. Not only is hepatitis B a lengthy and potentially debilitating disease, but it can also cause a number of serious complications such as cirrhosis of the liver, chronic active hepatitis, chronic persistent hepatitis, liver cancer (carriers have a risk factor 273 times greater than noncarriers), and the chronic carrier state. Any health care professional who becomes a carrier may be restricted from patient contact because such a person, while not ill, is always infectious to others. The reported incidence of hepatitis among dentists is 14%. (Serological evidence suggests the actual incidence is closer to 28%, with a yearly increase of 3% to 5% among dentists who have never had hepatitis B.) The risk of exposure is thus fairly high. Dental hygienists are likely to be in a similar if not greater risk category, given the nature of treatment they routinely perform.

Heptavax B confers immunity *only* to the hepatitis B virus. The vaccine will *not* prevent either hepatitis A, hepatitis non-A, non-B, or any other virus known to infect the liver.

Hepatitis non-A, non-B   Hepatitis can occur even as a result of transfusions using blood that is free of hepatitis B contamination. Consequently, other viruses appear to be implicated in such disease; these agents are currently referred to as non-A, non-B viruses.

The means of transmission of this disease have not been identified completely, but it appears that intimate contact of the types that lead to hepatitis B are

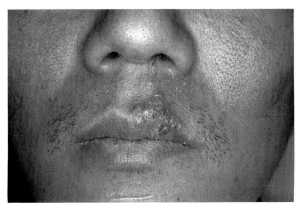

Fig. 1-6 Initial herpes lesion. (Courtesy of Dr. E. Steven Smith, Northwestern University, Chicago, Ill.)

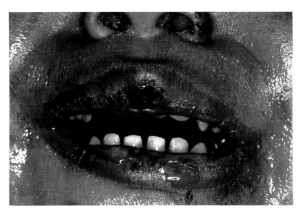

Fig. 1-7 Acute herpetic gingivostomatitis. (Courtesy of Dr. Mark Cannon, Northwestern University, Chicago, Ill.)

likely to result in the non-A, non-B disease. The incubation period ranges from 2 to 35 weeks, with an average of 7 to 8 weeks. Symptoms are similar to those of hepatitis B but of a milder nature. Few cases exhibit jaundice. Diagnosis is usually made by eliminating other forms of hepatitis. A carrier state can develop and may be more frequent in occurrence than with hepatitis B. In fact, the non-A, non-B disease may develop into a chronic illness and may be responsible for incidence of cirrhosis of the liver in people without histories of either alcohol abuse or hepatitis.

As yet no specific blood tests exist to identify a non-A, non-B infection. As with both A and B, no treatment exists other than bed rest. No vaccine is available to protect against non-A, non-B, and immunity to either A or B does not provide immunity to the non-A, non-B variety.

Herpes simplex diseases

Herpes simplex is a virus that produces either Type I or Type II infections, identifiable by clusters of vesicles on the skin. Although not a recent phenomenon, herpetic infections have commanded substantial attention recently as a disease that may be transmitted during dental therapy (Type I virus), as well as the single most frequently transmitted disease in the United States today (Type II, or genital herpes). Approximately 50 million people in the United States are estimated to be victims of herpes, with about half a million new cases reported each year. Because the

prevalence of herpes in the population makes it likely that health care personnel will have contact with patients with the disease, dental hygienists must know how to prevent both contracting it personally and spreading it to other patients.

Type I—oral herpes Childhood is usually the time that initial exposure to Type I herpes occurs. It appears as one or more white-colored blisters in the oral cavity or pharynx (Fig. 1-6). These may go unnoticed, and frequently no other symptoms occur. Occasionally a more severe case will manifest with fever of 101° F to 102° F, increased salivation, fetid breath, anorexia, swollen lymph nodes in the neck area, and a general feeling of illness. An even more virulent form of the disease is known as acute herpetic gingivostomatitis, which demonstrates, in addition to the previous symptoms, multiple lesions on the tongue, palate, pharynx, and other soft tissue of the oral cavity (Fig. 1-7). This acute form of the disease is extremely painful once the blisters break and form open ulcers.

The series of small blisters typically run together after formation, collapse into a flat lesion, and then appear red around the edges and covered with a yellowish material resembling a scab. The blisters will usually appear approximately 12 to 36 hours after exposure, which takes the form of direct contact (kissing or touching being the most common means of transmitting Type I herpes). Of primary importance is the realization that *any* contact with the fluid from the lesion causes spreading of the infection. Aerosols can mix with the fluid from lesions in a patient's mouth and deposit on environmental surfaces, remain suspended in the air, or be inhaled by the clinician. The scab itself is not a protective barrier; the virus is vital and easily oozes from beneath the scab.

Prior to the appearance of any blisters, a burning or tingling sensation is often felt at the site of eruption. As soon as this sensation occurs, the individual becomes contagious. The blisters then form and rupture, sometimes with slight bleeding. The yellow-like scab will turn reddish and then sometimes black after several days. The scab dries and cracks easily, causing pain. A patient with such lesions on the labial or oral mucosa should never be examined unless the operator is wearing gloves and a face mask.

The herpes virus, following the initial attack, migrates to the trigeminal nerve, where it lies dormant until stimulated to cause further attacks. It never leaves the body permanently, and no cure exists for the infection.

Type I herpes sores (also commonly referred to as fever blisters) typically recur when the individual's physical resistance is decreased. Lesions will reappear, usually on the lip, nose, or elsewhere intraorally, in response to one or more of the following: (1) emotional stress, (2) illness (especially upper respiratory), (3) fever, (4) trauma to the face or oral cavity, (5) dental treatment, or (6) overexposure to ultraviolet rays of the sun.

Another type of oral lesion that may occur is the aphthous ulcer, or "canker sore." Indecision exists as to whether the canker sore is actually a form of herpes or is caused by some other agent. The ulcer that forms the canker sore is round, with a red edge and grayish covering. Fever is rare, and the infection is not considered contagious. Aphthous ulcers may appear in response to stress, trauma, or food allergies. Healing time is about 14 days, regardless of any treatment rendered. Whether or not these ulcers are considered contagious, precautions such as gloves and face mask should always be employed when examining patients with any lesions.

Although frequently occurring on oropharyngeal mucous membranes, herpes simplex infections are *not* restricted to these locations. Herpes lesions may occur anywhere on the skin. Herpetic whitlow, a painful infection occurring on the fingers, is of great significance to dental personnel, especially because cases of herpes virus transmission have been traced to a dental hygienist treating patients prior to the ap-

pearance of lesions on her or his finger. The contagious stage begins *before visible lesions can be detected*. The dental hygienist is not only at risk, then, of contracting the infection by treating herpes-afflicted patients without gloves and face mask but also may inadvertently transmit the disease to others.

Other sites where herpes infections may occur are the eyes (herpetic keratitis, or ocular herpes), esophagus, brain (herpetic meningitis, herpetic encephalitis), and, of increasing frequency, the genital area (Type II, or venereal, herpes).

Type II—venereal herpes The difference between the two types of herpes viruses is subtle, with location on the body and means of transmission the major factors for determining which virus is present. Because the usual mechanism of transfer is sexual contact, Type II herpes is considered to be a form of venereal disease.

As with the Type I virus, venereal herpes is spread by direct contact with the lesions themselves or by surfaces or items contaminated with the microorganism. The primary occurrence usually begins 2 to 12 days after exposure; symptoms include enlargement of lymph nodes near the groin area, soreness, fever, and constant headache. Lesions may be multiple or sparse. They appear, ulcerate, and may cause extreme pain. The ulcers usually form scabs after the lesions begin to dry. Healing then progresses, usually without scarring, unless the infection has been very severe.

Following the initial attack, the virus withdraws to the cauda equina nerve in the spinal cord, where it stays until it is triggered to reactivate another outbreak. Usually the first attack is the most severe, lasting about 21 days from the initial outbreak to healing. Further occurrences range widely in frequency, duration, and severity. Circumstances that may cause recurrence of a Type II infection are:

1. Stress (probably one of the most significant factors).
2. Foods with high content of the amino acid arginine, which seems to promote outbreaks of herpes: peanuts, peanut butter, nuts, coconut, seeds, onion, carob, cocoa, and cabbage. Marijuana also seems to trigger outbreaks of herpes.
3. Smoking.
4. Overexposure to ultraviolet radiation.
5. Prolonged athletic activity, especially competition with accompanying stress.

6. Hormonal changes accompanying menstruation and the use of birth control pills.
7. Trauma.
8. Sexual activity.

Prevention of either type of herpes is largely a matter of avoiding direct contact with persons exhibiting obvious lesions. Personal items, such as makeup, lipstick, toothbrushes, dishes and glassware, towels, washcloths, eating utensils, and clothing should not be shared or used by others. Care should be taken to avoid touching another part of the body (especially the eyes) following contact with an herpetic lesion. If afflicted personally with a case of oral herpes, the dental hygienist must be particularly careful not to touch her or his mouth before treating a patient. Hands should always be washed thoroughly before and after each patient is treated. Gloves, face mask, and safety glasses should always be worn during patient care.

The virus is likely to be contained in the saliva of a herpes victim with lesions present, and the use of aerosol-producing instruments may transmit the virus to the operator. Moist heat sterilization of instruments, proper disposal of supplies, and complete disinfection of operatory surfaces with a chlorine bleach solution should be employed. Thorough medical histories are necessary to identify patients with histories of herpes infections.

Preventing the recurrence of herpes requires the maintaining of general health by regular exercise and a well-balanced diet and the decreasing of stress as much as possible. Foods containing large amounts of arginine should be avoided. Some experts in nutrition and medicine have identified the amino acid lysine as being helpful in fighting herpes outbreaks. Foods containing high amounts of lysine are beef, flour, fish, tomatoes, Chinese bean sprouts, figs, peaches, cow's milk and milk products, and goat's milk. Nonprescription lysine tablets or capsules (500 mg) are available, and one or two of these on a daily basis provide sufficient intake of the amino acid. During an active case of herpes, the regimen may be increased to one to two tablets or capsules three times per day. Vitamin C (100 mg two times per day) and bioflavonoids (500 mg two times per day) may also aid during an active outbreak.

Although herpes is currently not curable, several treatment modalities can provide some relief of discomfort suffered by victims. For oral herpes, aspirin or acetaminophen can be employed to reduce fever. Ibuprofen can be used to manage mild to moderate pain. Topical anesthetics such as viscous lidocaine hydrochloride or xylocaine ointment or spray can aid in temporary reduction of pain. Zinc sulfate mouthrinses (0.010 to 0.025%, for 1 to 3 minutes) or compresses (lukewarm, 0.25 to 0.05%) may also provide some relief. Other treatments include Burow's solution, witch hazel, ether, alcohol (which tends to burn upon application), and milk of magnesia, which may be applied directly to the lesions.

Several previously used remedies for herpes are no longer recommended, because they are ineffective, are hazardous to the patient's health, or can make the herpetic infection worse. These include dyes in combination with photoinactivation, x-radiation and ultraviolet light radiation therapy, smallpox vaccinations, and cortisone and hydrocortisone. Individuals who suffer from herpes should avoid these forms of treatment and seek more appropriate and valid means of combatting the virus.

Aside from the physical discomforts associated with oral herpes attacks, and the physical and emotional distress that frequently accompany genital herpes, evidence now links the herpes viruses with certain types of cancer. One form of cancer of the throat and a type of lymphoma associated with Hodgkin's disease are examples. In addition, women who experience genital herpes are at a higher risk of developing cervical, vulval, or external genital cancer.

A number of drugs being developed and experimented with may prove to be of value in the future. Antiviral drugs such as acyclovir (ACV, Zovirax*) and bromovinyldeoxyuridine (BVDU) are of special interest because they are activated only by enzymes produced by the herpes virus and thus have a specific site of action. Such drugs are therefore less toxic and more easily tolerated systemically. Toxicity is a major difficulty with many viricidal drugs.

Acyclovir in particular appears to show a great deal of promise in treating genital herpes. Some research is showing an ability to prevent recurrence of attacks for as long as 8 months, as well as a shortening of the contagious period when the virus sheds.

Other antiviral drugs being examined are idoxuridine (IDU) and the arabinosides. Idoxuridine has been used most commonly to treat herpetic eye in-

*Wellcome Laboratories, Research Triangle Park, N.C.

fections but appears to be ineffective when placed in a medium suitable to treat genital or skin lesions.

The drug interferon may at some point provide a type of treatment for herpes but in a manner different from ACV, BVDU, IDU or other drugs. Interferon is an immunopotentiator, which acts by increasing the body's own immune system. It is a glycoprotein released by cells that have been invaded by bacteria, viruses, and certain other infectious agents. Interferon acts as a stimulant to noninfected cells by causing them to synthesize another protein substance that has anti-infection characteristics (i.e., antiviral, antibacterial). The drug also functions to regulate cell growth and affects the immune system by activating or suppressing certain aspects of the system itself. It has therefore been of considerable interest in the treatment of cancer and other disorders of the immune system. Its value in the treatment of herpes may be related to its ability to prompt healthy cells to provide the antiviral protein material.

Acquired immune deficiency syndrome

Acquired immune deficiency syndrome, commonly referred to as AIDS, is a severe disease caused by the human immunodeficiency virus.[52-56] The natural immunity to disease is defective in some manner, which renders the patient susceptible to multiple opportunistic infections and neoplasms. These diseases are usually not found in patients with normal immune systems; if found, they are somewhat mild in nature.

In the late 1970s, the syndrome now known as AIDS was first noticed in several patients with a relatively rare form of cancer known as Kaposi's sarcoma (KS). Typically, KS occurs rarely in the United States, is very slow acting, and usually affects elderly men of Mediterranean heritage. These patients, however, were young homosexual men, in whom the disease spread very rapidly. Most of them died less than 2 years after the initial diagnosis.

Following the appearance of the KS cases, another unusual illness was noted with increasing frequency. *Pneumocystis carinii* pneumonia is an unusual infection of the lungs, typically seen in patients who are highly immunosuppressed (i.e., patients with kidney transplants) or people with severe malnutrition. This particular type of pneumonia is highly resistant to antibiotic treatment and quickly kills its victims.

The appearance of these two diseases, especially the virulent form of KS, led to the identification of the syndrome now known as AIDS. The number of reported cases has increased steadily since the late 1970s and is now doubling every 10 months.

The highest incidence of AIDS had been among sexually active homosexual and bisexual men, intravenous drug users, hemophiliacs, blood transfusion recipients, children of AIDS mothers, and individuals born in places where AIDS is pandemic. The incidence is rapidly increasing in the heterosexual population. Intravenous drug users and persons who engage in sexual activities with potential virus carriers are specifically at great risk.

Exactly how and why the disease developed and spread so rapidly, and why some population groups were at high risk of contracting AIDS, was not fully understood until recently. Initial theories included the possibility that sperm introduced into the bloodstream via repeated anal intercourse caused suppression of the immune system. The immune-overload theory held that repeated occurrences of infections over a number of years caused the immune system to cease functioning.

These theories lost ground as evidence accumulated showing that the infectious agent could be transmitted through body fluids or sexual contact. As the number of intravenous drug users, hemophiliacs, and blood-transfused patients who contracted the disease grew, it became increasingly clear that the transmission pattern resembled that of hepatitis B. AIDS is now known to be caused by a virus that is borne in blood and other body fluids.

Current research shows that the virus acts by directly attacking T-lymphocytes (also known as helper T cells) and invading them in a manner similar to the way in which the hepatitis virus attacks liver cells. Once the AIDS virus occupies the T cell, these lymphocytes are then unable to initiate the immune system's response to ward off disease-provoking organisms. The T cells then become AIDS-virus "factories" and the viruses replicate at an astonishing rate, approximately a thousand times as fast as other viruses. During the replication process, the AIDS viruses destroy the T cells, leaving the patient virtually helpless without a functioning immune system, highly susceptible to infections, and usually beyond recovery. No cure for AIDS has been found.

Interestingly, not all persons infected with the AIDS virus develop the syndrome. Most individuals have either mild symptoms or no symptoms, but suffer from persistent infections and are likely to be continuously infectious to others. Another group exhibits a mild version of depression of the immune system, with signs and symptoms including weight loss, malaise, fever, and swollen lymph nodes. This syndrome is known as AIDS-related complex (ARC) and may or may not develop into AIDS.

The Centers for Disease Control estimates that for each reported case of AIDS at least five to ten cases of ARC occur. Through sample studies of blood tests it is further estimated that, for each reported case of AIDS, 50 to 100 Americans are symptomless carriers of the virus and that a percentage of them may develop AIDS within 5 years. Of those who have ARC, the chances of developing AIDS within 3 years may be quite high.

As to why some individuals manifest AIDS while others simply carry the virus, it is thought that other viral infections may trigger or assist in the development of the syndrome. So far, the cytomegalovirus, Epstein-Barr virus, and hepatitis B virus have been implicated. Whether these viruses are actively involved in AIDS or are simply accompanying infections has yet to be determined.

Symptoms of AIDS   One of the major difficulties in the treatment of AIDS patients is the wide variation in the severity of their symptoms. The most severe cases occur in only about 10% to 20% of AIDS victims; the remaining 80% to 90% experience a milder occurrence (ARC). Some victims have no specific symptoms of any form of disease until the appearance of *Pneumocystis carinii* pneumonia, cryptococcal meningitis, or the skin or mucous membrane lesions of Kaposi's sarcoma.

When preliminary symptoms do manifest themselves, the patient may experience nonspecific weakness, fever, diarrhea, weight loss, malaise, and generalized lymphadenopathy. Localized herpes zoster may also develop, and, of primary significance for the dental hygienist, oral candidiasis is frequently detected. Unless a patient had been taking some form of antibiotic or steroid, oral candidiasis would be a rare occurrence in an otherwise healthy individual. These symptoms, known as the prodromal syndrome or symptoms, may last for several months or even years before further problems become apparent. Other oral manifestations that may occur in AIDS patients include hairy leukoplakia, intraoral Kaposi's sarcoma lesions, and premature and advanced periodontal disease.[56]

Infections of the herpes simplex virus are also common in almost all AIDS victims. While lesions may occur anywhere on the body, typical sites are on the oral mucosa and genital areas.

Precautions   It is now definitely known that the causative agent(s) of AIDS travels in blood and other body fluids. Because blood and saliva are easily mixed during dental hygiene therapy, the appropriate precautionary measures are necessary for all patients. AIDS patients may present a number of oral manifestations of the syndrome: herpes simplex, oral candidiasis, and mucous membrane lesions of Kaposi's sarcoma, which appear as bruises or ulcerations. A thorough medical history and oral examination are essential to prevent potential inadvertent spread of this or any disease.

If an AIDS patient or a person in a high-risk category requires dental treatment, precautions should include:

1. Wearing disposable gloves, mask, protective gown, and safety glasses.
2. Avoiding accidental wounds from sharp instruments and needles.
3. Thoroughly washing hands after removing mask, gloves, gown, and other items that may potentially be contaminated with blood or other body fluids.
4. Cleaning any blood on equipment or other surface areas of the operatory with chlorine bleach. The person who cleans the blood should wear gloves.

Tuberculosis

Tuberculosis is an infection, usually of the lungs, although other body organs may be affected as well, caused by the bacterial agent *Mycobacterium tuberculosis*. The bacilli are spread from infected persons by coughing, sneezing, or talking; susceptible individuals may then contract the disease by inhaling airborne droplets. This route of transmission, which presents a potentially significant hazard for dental personnel, requires careful screening of patients who may be at risk, prior to providing dental treatment. An estimated 30,000 new cases of tuberculosis are reported each year in the United States, making the disease a fairly considerable one in terms of prevalence.

The primary form of pulmonary tuberculosis is typ-

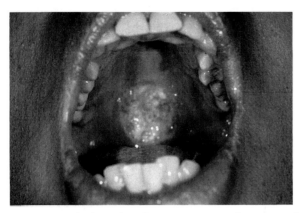

Fig. 1-8   Oral tuberculosis lesion. (Courtesy of Dr. Bernard Pecaro, Northwestern University, Chicago, Ill.)

ically mild, with general symptoms of chills, fever, cough, and production of sputum. Once the primary phase has resolved, the bacilli may remain dormant in the body for varying lengths of time. The infection may spread throughout the body and affect other organs, such as cervical and hilar lymph nodes, pericardium, peritoneum, liver, kidneys, and meninges. Oral manifestations may occur, either as a result of infection from the pulmonary lesions or from disseminated tuberculosis (i.e., seeding from the blood).

Tuberculosis is most often diagnosed following known exposure to the disease, through a positive TB skin test, or when evidence of lung scarring is seen on a chest radiograph. Because the disease is spread by close contact, family members who have tuberculosis provide increased risk to noninfected members. When obtaining medical histories, care should be taken to elicit information relative to any history of exposure to tuberculosis.

Laboratory skin tests, such as the Mantoux and tine tests, are very sensitive to detecting TB infection. Although active disease may not be diagnosed with a positive test result, the fact that infection has occurred can be determined. Both false positive and false negative results may also occur.

Treatment of tuberculosis has changed with the advent of effective chemotherapeutic agents. Prolonged periods of bed rest, isolation, institutionalization, and extensive surgery are no longer necessary to control the disease. Drug therapy, however, can be quite extensive in terms of the timeframe required to eradicate the infective microorganisms. The most commonly used drugs in the treatment of TB are isoniazid (INH), rifampin, streptomycin, and ethambutol hydrochloride.

Although oral manifestations are infrequent, according to most studies, the dental hygienist should be aware of and alert to the possibility of oral lesions during the oral examination. The infection is believed to result from microorganisms in the sputum affecting traumatized mucous membranes of the oral cavity. Seeding from the blood may also be responsible for oral TB lesions.

The base of the tongue is the most common site for oral TB. Other sites include the lip, gingiva, soft palate, tonsils, and tooth sockets. The secondarily spread lesions are ulcerative and painless and may have suppurated centers (Fig. 1-8). Lesions occurring at the corners of the mouth, called *cutis orificialis,* are shallow granulating ulcers. It is not possible to determine the diagnosis of oral tuberculosis lesions clinically, because they resemble oral cancer lesions. A definitive diagnosis can only be made by biopsy.

Gonorrhea

Gonorrhea, classified as a venereal disease, is a common infectious disease in the United States, with the number of cases each year estimated at more than 3 million. Because many patients who contract the disease are asymptomatic, the actual number of cases is probably much higher.

The causative organism is a gram-negative coccus known as *Neisseria gonorrhoeae*. The most common site for infection is the urethra, but the oral cavity may serve as a primary site for individuals who engage in oral sexual practices. The clinical appearance of the lesions resembles acute necrotizing ulcerative gingivitis (ANUG), including the presence of a necrotic pseudomembrane that covers the ulcers. The lesions are usually asymptomatic. Although ANUG is typically confined to the gingiva, the oral gonococcal infection usually affects other areas of the oral mucous membranes. However, extensive redness of the mucosa may be the only oral findings present.

Syphilis

Syphilis, perhaps the most well known of the venereal diseases, is caused by a spirochete called *Treponema pallidum*. The disease may either be acquired through sexual or close personal contact or may be congenitally transmitted to a newborn infant from the infected mother.

Primary, secondary, and tertiary stages of acquired syphilis are identified. In the primary phase, a chancre occurs where the spirochete enters the body. The chancre begins as a papule, which then develops into a painless, indurated ulcer. Although the chancre frequently occurs on the genitalia, it may be found intraorally on the lip, tongue, or tonsils. The lesion will typically heal after approximately 4 weeks. Lymph node enlargement is often found in the region of the body where the chancre occurs.

In the secondary phase, the number of spirochetes increases throughout the body, making it a systemic disease. This stage manifests itself 6 to 8 weeks after the patient has been exposed to the microorganism. Generalized lymph node enlargement and flu-like symptoms are often experienced. Oral manifestations are common in this stage. Mucous patches can be observed throughout the mouth and pharynx and typically are painless lesions. The patient may also exhibit generalized inflammation of the mucosa and may complain of a sore throat. The mucous patch lesions are highly contagious; the patient in the secondary stage of syphilis may also suffer from lesions at the corners of the mouth, resembling cheilitis. Because the disease is highly contagious, any patient with possible syphilitic lesions should be examined with great care. Gloves should be worn, particularly if the clinician has open wounds on the fingers or hands.

The third and final stage is known as tertiary syphilis. Oral lesions in this phase are quite common; the gumma and atrophic glossitis of the tongue are the manifestations noted most frequently. The gumma, typically found on the hard palate, is a necrotic, ulcerated painless lesion that may affect and destroy the underlying bone (Fig. 1-9). Because the gumma is clinically difficult to differentiate from a malignancy, biopsy is required to obtain a definitive diagnosis.

The tongue lesions associated with tertiary syphilis are significant in the potential for future development of squamous cell carcinoma and leukoplakia. Particularly during the secondary phase, the tongue becomes severely infected, with impairment of blood circulation and resultant atrophy of the fungiform and filiform papillae.

The drug of choice for the treatment of syphilis is penicillin. Patients who are allergic to this antibiotic

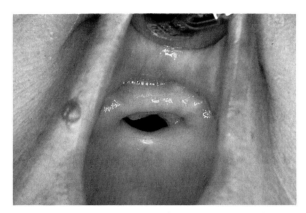

Fig. 1-9 Gumma. (Courtesy of Dr. E. Steven Smith.)

may be treated with either erythromycin or tetracycline.

Radiation exposure

Occupational hazards to dental personnel are not confined solely to those that involve interaction with patients who have histories or active cases of disease. Within the dental office itself, circumstances exist that provide opportunity for further potential problems. Responsibility for exposure of radiographs is often delegated to the dental hygienist, for example. With more conclusive evidence available on the effects of radiation on the body tissues, and increased awareness on the part of the consumer, the dental hygienist must be well informed, and must adhere to stringent radiation safety practices. Radiation safety will be dealt with more fully in Volume 2.

Mercury poisoning

The use of mercury in amalgam preparation has been identified as a possible biohazard.[61] Although the dental hygienist in the typical environment is not likely to be directly involved with the manipulation of the material on a regular basis, occasions will arise when it becomes necessary to do so. The dental hygienist with expanded functions will frequently be involved.

Because mercury is a liquid at room temperature and flows easily into corners and crevices, it is a difficult material to control if spilled. It also readily vaporizes at room temperature and is absorbed into materials such as carpeting, wood, tile, and other common materials in dental offices. Mercury poison-

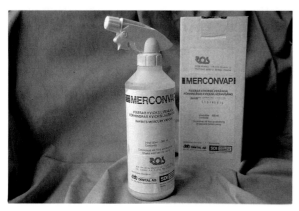

Fig. 1-10   Merconvap.

ing usually occurs as a result of absorption of the vapors through the lungs, although skin and gastrointestinal absorption are also possible. Upon entry into the body, mercury is stored primarily in the kidneys, although other body organs and sites are also involved (brain, heart, liver, spleen, thyroid, salivary glands, testes, skeletal muscle, and mucous membranes of the gastrointestinal tract).

Mercury poisoning may be either acute or chronic in nature. Once mercury has accumulated in body tissues, a number of signs and symptoms will occur, but diagnosis is often difficult because of the general or unusual nature of the symptoms. Some of the indications of mercury intoxication include:

1. Local dermatitis.
2. Tremor (observed in handwriting).
3. Loss of appetite.
4. Nausea and diarrhea.
5. Depression or fatigue.
6. Birth defects in offspring.
7. Pneumonitis.
8. Nephritis.
9. Insomnia.
10. Excitability.
11. Headache.
12. Swollen lymph nodes and tongue.
13. Ulceration of oral mucosa.

A number of measures may be employed to control the possibility of mercury toxicity. Most important is the education of all members of the office staff. Personnel should be keenly aware of the hazards of mer-

cury and routinely employ techniques to minimize the dangers to themselves and patients.

Mercury should be handled only in a well ventilated area. Air filtration devices are available that can be used to reduce inhalation hazards. Heating and air conditioning units should be operated so that air is not recirculated through the office.

Adequate cleaning after spills is difficult when floors are carpeted or tiled. The most appropriate floor covering in areas where mercury is used is a seamless nonporous material such as polyvinylchloride. It should be well sealed and extend several inches up the walls.

Amalgam triturators should be placed on special trays with replaceable sponge filters that absorb mercury spills and can be safely discarded. Like air filters, they reduce inhalation hazards. The area in which the mercury is manipulated should be free of crevices, cracks, and other minute spaces where the spilled material is difficult or impossible to clean completely.

Mercury is particularly sensitive to heat, and even small temperature increases can markedly affect its ability to vaporize. Mercury should never be handled near space heaters, heating ducts, sterilizing units, or other heat production devices.

Storage of mercury is another important aspect of control of the hazard. Plastic containers with well-fitting lids should be used to store the material. Excess scrap amalgam and squeeze cloths should be detoxified prior to disposal. Ideally, this is accomplished through the use of Merconvap* (Fig. 1-10), into which the amalgam may be placed. This special liquid may also be used to clean mercury spills. If it is not available, a bath of water or fixer solution for radiographs may be used, but the container must have a lid to avoid release of mercury vapor. Another option is to store scrap amalgam in glycerin, using an inch of glycerin for every inch of amalgam.

Mercury that is spilled must be cleaned immediately. Until the spill is cleaned with Merconvap or special devices for low-volume vacuuming, other personnel and patients should avoid the area. The individual cleaning the mercury should wear gloves during the procedure. Other protective devices such as a face mask may also be required, depending on the volume of the spill. Once a spill has occurred, it may not be possible to completely decontaminate carpeting.

*Mercury Protection Systems, Inc., Surrey, B.C., Canada.

When amalgam is prepared for use as a restorative material, it should never be touched with the bare hands. Trituration capsules should be routinely tested for potential leakage. Amalgam carriers should be thoroughly cleaned after each use. Water spray and suction should be employed during drilling, grinding, and polishing of amalgam materials. Manual or mechanical condensation is recommended, while the use of ultrasonic devices is discouraged.

Food, drinks, and other consumable items should never be kept near mercury or mercury compounds. Clothing should be inspected routinely for any mercury contamination. Face masks that are designed specifically to filter mercury are available. Anyone who works with mercury should remove all hand jewelry, as mercury combines easily with gold and silver and can destroy the jewelry. Careful handwashing is another important aspect in the control of potential mercury contamination.

References

1. Harvey, W.L., and Scrabeck, J.G. Current sterilization and disinfection procedures in dental practice. J. Colo. Dent. Assoc. 62(2):4–6, 1983.
2. Reingold, A.L., Kane, M.A., and Hightower, A.W. Disinfection procedures and infection control in the outpatient oral surgery practice. J. Oral Maxillofac. Surg. 42(9):568–572, 1984.
3. Singer, R.S., and Sisk, A.L. A simple means of maintaining light handle sterility. J. Oral Maxillofac. Surg. 42(4):269, 1984.
4. Hedtke, M. An introduction to microbiology and sterilization in the dental office. Dent. Assist. 52(5):25–30, 1983.
5. Beard, J.R. Upgrading office sterility. S. C. Dent. J. 41(1):55–58, 1983.
6. Palenik, C.J., and Miller, C.H. Monitoring the use of the office sterilizer. J. Wis. Dent. Assoc. 59(5):397–401, 1983.
7. Parkes, R.B., and Kolstad, R.A. Effects of sterilization on periodontal instruments. J. Periodontol. 53(7):434–438, 1982.
8. Eames, W.B., Boyington, S.Q., and Suway, N.B. A comparison of eight ultrasonic cleaners. Gen. Dent. 30(3):242–245, 1982.
9. Hung, C., and Annichiarico, J. Sterilization, disinfection asepsis and chemotherapy in dental practice. J. Bergen Co. Dent. Soc. 48(1):20–22, 1981.
10. Schaefer, M.E. Sterilization procedures for the dental office. Cert. Dent. Assist. J. 9(4):61–64, 1981.
11. ADA Council on Dental Materials, Instruments and Equipment. Current status of sterilization instruments, devices, and methods for the dental office. J. Am. Dent. Assoc. 102(5):683–689, 1981.
12. Kleier, D.J., and Barr, E.S. Alternative method of steam sterilization. J. Am. Dent. Assoc. 103(2):248–249, 1981.
13. Miller, C.H., and Palenick, C.J. Infection control and sterilization of dental instruments. J. Ind. Dent. Assoc. 59(6):15–20, 1980.
14. Suggested guidelines for asepsis in the dental office environment. N. C. Dent. J. 63(1):4, 1980.
15. Walsh, M.M. The effect of various sterilizing wraps on the corrosion of instruments during autoclaving. Dent. Hyg. 53(11):504–506, 1979.
16. MacFarlane, T.W. Sterilization in general dental practice. J. Dent. 8(1):13–19, 1980.
17. Matlack, R.E. Instrument sterilization in orthodontic offices. Angle Orthod. 49(3):205–211, 1979.
18. Ernst, R. Biohazards in dentistry. II. Procedures for clean vs. contaminated cases. Dent. Assist. 48(3):31–32, 52, 1979.
19. Ernst, R. Biohazards in dentistry. IV. Sterilization. Dent. Assist. 48(4):39–41, 1979.
20. Crawford, J.J. Office sterilization and asepsis procedures in endodontics. Dent. Clin. N. Am. 23(4):717–735, 1979.
21. Salerno, D. Cold sterilization—is it as effective as it should be? Dent. Hyg. 53(7):320–321, 1979.
22. Eccles, J.D. The management of sterilization in dental teaching hospitals. J. Dent. 8(1):3–7, 1980.
23. Gillespie, J., and Eisenbud, L. Disinfection and sterilization of dental instruments in a hospital dental clinic. J. Hosp. Dent. Pract. 13(3):96–97, 1979.
24. Hume, W.R., and Makinson, D.F. Sterilizing dental instruments: evaluation of lubricating oils and microwave radiation. Oper. Dent. 3(3):93–96, 1978.
25. Sterilization of dental instruments. J. Oreg. Dent. Assoc. 47(3):32–35, 1978.
26. Parker, R. Sterilization of instruments. J. Oreg. Dent. Assoc. 47(1):47–53, 1977.
27. MacFarlen, T.W. Cross infection and sterilization in dental practice. Br. Dent. J. 141(7):213–218, 1976.

28. Baier, R.E., et al. Degradative effects of conventional steam sterilization on biomaterial surfaces. Biomaterials 3(4):241–245, 1982.

29. Barrett, E.D. Sterilizer monitoring. J. Mich. Dent. Assoc. 64(6):243–244, 1982.

30. Bertolotti, R.L., et al. Minimizing corrosion of carbon steel dental instruments during autoclaving. Cert. Dent. Assist. J. 7(9):40–43, 1979.

31. Hegna, L.K., Kardel, K., and Kardel, M. Autoclaving of lubricated dental instruments. Scand. J. Dent. Res. 86(2):130–134, 1978.

32. Furuhashi, M., and Miyamae, T. Ethylene oxide sterilization of medical devices—with special references to the sporicidal activity and residual concentration of ethylene oxide and its secondary products. Bull. Tokyo Med. Dent. Univ. 29(2):23–35, 1982.

33. Rohner, M.D., and Bulard, R.A. Microwave sterilization. J. Am. Dent. Assoc. 110(1):194–198, 1985.

34. Christensen, R.P. Effectiveness of glutaraldehyde as a chemosterilizer used in a wrapping technique on simulated metal instruments. J. Dent. Res. 56(7):822–826, 1977.

35. Rowe, A.H., and Forrest, J.D. Dental impressions. The probability of contamination and a method of disinfection. Br. Dent. J. 145(6):184–186, 1979.

36. The Commission on Dental Practice. Recommendation for hygiene in dental practice. Int. Dent. J. 29(1):72–79, 1979.

37. ADA Council on Dental Therapeutics. Quaternary ammonium compounds not acceptable for disinfection of instruments and environmental surfaces in dentistry. J. Am. Dent. Assoc. 97(5):855–856, 1976.

38. Simpson, J.P., and Whittaker, D.K. Serum contamination of instruments in dental practice. Br. Dent. J. 146(3):76–78, 1979.

39. Ernst, R. Serum hepatitis: the hidden menace to the dental team. Dent. Assist. 47(3):22–24, 1978.

40. Ratcliff, R. Hepatitis and the dental hygienist. Dent. Hyg. 51(11):493–497, 1977.

41. Sanger, R.G. An inquiry into the sterilization of dental handpieces relative to the transmission of hepatitis B virus. J. Am. Dent. Assoc. 96(4):621–624, 1978.

42. The prevention of transmissible disease in dentistry: the example of serum hepatitis. Dent. Update 1(5):233–234, 1974.

43. Cooley, R.L., and Lubow, R.M. Hepatitis B vaccine: implications for dental personnel. J. Am. Dent. Assoc. 105(7):47–49, 1982.

44. Hepatitis in dentistry—a review. Quintessence Int. 13:1145, 1982.

45. Rothstein, S.S., and Goldman, H.S. Sterilizing and disinfecting for hepatitis B virus in the dental operatory. Clin. Prev. Dent. 2(6):9–11, 14, 1980.

46. Recognition and Prevention of Hepatitis. Health Studies Institute, Inc., 1983, pp. 1–55.

47. Chase, A. The Truth About STD. New York: William Morrow and Co., 1983.

48. Gross, M. Herpes: an overview of the diagnosis and treatment. J. K. Dent. Assoc. 33(3):26–29, 1981.

49. Herzberg, M. Herpes virus and the dental profession. Northwest Dent. 61(5):23–24, 1982.

50. How dentists cope with venereal herpes. Ill. Dent. J. 51(11):37, 1982.

51. Lee, M. Herpes. Miami: Premier Professional Seminars, 1984, pp. 1–85.

52. Lee, M. AIDS. Miami: Premier Professional Seminars, 1984, pp. 1–45.

53. Cahill, K. The AIDS Epidemic. New York: St. Martin's Press, 1983.

54. Masci, J.P., and Nichols, P. Precautions in treating patients with AIDS. N. Eng. J. Med. 308:156, 1983.

55. Truths about AIDS—dispelling eight common myths. Dent. Abstr. 364–368, 1985.

56. Silverman, S., et al. Oral findings in people with or at high risk for AIDS: a study of 375 homosexual males. J. Am. Dent. Assoc. 112:187–192, 1986.

57. Rothwell, P.S., Frame, J.W., and Shimmin, C.V. Mercury vapor hazards from hot air sterilizers in dental practice. Br. Dent. J. 142(11):359–365, 367, 1977.

58. Goldman, H.S., Hartman, K.S., and Messite, J. Occupational Hazards in Dentistry. Chicago: Year Book Medical Publ., 1984, pp. 1–193.

59. Shipp, I., and Shapiro, J. Mercury poisoning in dental practice. Compend. Cont. Ed. 4:107–110, 1983.

60. Recommendations in dental mercury hygiene. J. Am. Dent. Assoc. 107(10):617–619, 1984.

61. Johnson, K.F. Mercury hygiene. Dent. Clin. North Am. 22(3):447–488, 1978.

chapter 2

Health assessment and documentation

The dental hygienist begins the appointment by obtaining a thorough and complete health history of the patient (Fig. 2-1). Either a preexisting history is reviewed and updated or a new patient may be asked to fill out a medical history form (Figs. 2-2a and b). After the form is completed, the hygienist should discuss the history with a new patient for clarification and for the extrapolation of further information if indicated. A comprehensive health assessment is essential to planning the treatment of the patient. The current medical status, drugs that are currently part of the patient's regimen, and the presence of allergies and physical conditions that influence the approach to dental hygiene therapy must be identified. The result will be a profile unique to the particular patient for use in formulating a specific treatment plan for his or her dental health care.

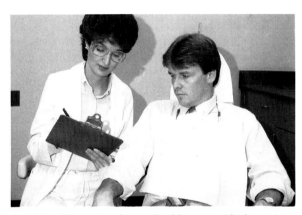

Fig. 2-1 Discussing the medical history with the patient.

Indications for antibiotic premedication

Some patients may require antibiotic premedication prior to the performance of instrumentation. Premedication may be indicated for patients with a previous history of rheumatic fever, congenital heart defects, calcified valvulitis, or heart disease; with valvular implants or pacemakers with implanted wires; who have undergone open heart surgery for correction of an intracardiac defect or closure of patent ductus arteriosus in the 6 months prior to dental treatment; or those patients with a prolapse of the mitral valve, kidney conditions such as glomerulonephritis, re-

duced capacity to resist infection (as a result of anticancer chemotherapy or corticosteroid treatment), or major prosthetic replacements such as hip replacements. Bacteria released during treatment might cause difficult-to-treat infections at sites of reduced resistance.[1,2]

Infective endocarditis is an infection of the endocardium that involves the heart valve, septal defect, or mitral endocardium. Acute endocarditis involves the normal heart, whereas subacute bacterial endocarditis is usually caused by streptococci of the viridans group attacking already damaged valves. The manipulation of the oral tissues or the rendering of any dental treatment that may result in the release of bacteria into the blood stream would be potentially dangerous to the patient who has a history of such

MEDICAL HISTORY (LONG FORM)

Date _____

Name _____ Address _____
    Last   First   Middle   Number & Street

City _____ State _____ Zip Code _____ Home Phone _____ Business Phone _____

Date of Birth_____ Sex_____ Height_____ Weight_____ Occupation _____

Social Security No._____ Single_____ Married_____ Name of Spouse _____

Closest Relative _____ Phone _____

If you are completing this form for another person, what is your relationship to that person? _____

Referred By: _____

In the following questions, circle yes or no, whichever applies. Your answers are for our records only and will be considered confidential.

1. Are you in good health? . . . . YES   NO
2. Has there been any change in your general health within the past year?. . . . . YES   NO
3. My last physical examination was on _____
4. Are you now under the care of a physician? . . . . YES   NO
   a. If so, what is the condition being treated? _____
5. The name and address of my physician is _____
   _____
   _____
6. Have you had any serious illness or operation? . . . . YES   NO
   a. If so, what was the illness or operation? _____
7. Have you been hospitalized or had a serious illness within the past five (5) years? . . . . YES   NO
   a. If so, what was the problem? _____
8. Do you have or have you had any of the following diseases or problems?
   a. Damaged heart valves or artificial heart valves . . . . YES   NO
   b. Congential heart lesions. . . . . YES   NO
   c. Cardiovascular disease (heart trouble, heart attack, coronary insufficiency, coronary occlusion,
      high blood pressure, arteriosclerosis, stroke) . . . . YES   NO
      1) Do you have pain in chest upon exertion? . . . . YES   NO
      2) Are you ever short of breath after mild exercise? . . . . YES   NO
      3) Do your ankles swell?. . . . . YES   NO
      4) Do you get short of breath when you lie down, or do you require extra pillows when you sleep?. . . . YES   NO
      5) Do you have a cardiac pacemaker? . . . . YES   NO
   d. Allergy. . . . . YES   NO
   e. Sinus trouble . . . . YES   NO
   f. Asthma or hay fever. . . . . YES   NO
   g. Hives or a skin rash . . . . YES   NO
   h. Fainting spells or seizures . . . . YES   NO
   i. Diabetes . . . . YES   NO
      1) Do you have to urinate (pass water) more than six times a day? . . . . YES   NO
      2) Are you thirsty much of the time? . . . . YES   NO
      3) Does your mouth frequently become dry? . . . . YES   NO
   j. Hepatitis, jaundice or liver disease . . . . YES   NO
   k. Arthritis. . . . . YES   NO
   l. Inflammatory rheumatism (painful swollen joints) . . . . YES   NO
   m. Stomach ulcers . . . . YES   NO
   n. Kidney trouble . . . . YES   NO
   o. Tuberculosis . . . . YES   NO
   p. Do you have a persistent cough or cough up blood? . . . . YES   NO
   q. Low blood pressure . . . . YES   NO
   r. Venereal disease . . . . YES   NO
   s. Other _____

B500   (over)

Fig. 2-2a   American Dental Association Medical History form (front).

9. Have you had abnormal bleeding associated with previous extractions, surgery, or trauma? . . . .   YES   NO
   a. Do you bruise easily . . . .   YES   NO
   b. Have you ever required a blood transfusion? . . . .   YES   NO
     If so, explain the circumstances _____

10. Do you have any blood disorder such as anemia? . . . .   YES   NO
11. Have you had surgery or x-ray treatment for a tumor, growth, or other condition of your head or neck? . .   YES   NO
12. Are you taking any drug or medicine? . . . .   YES   NO
    If so, what? _____

13. Are you taking any of the following:
   a. Antibiotics or sulfa drugs . . . .   YES   NO
   b. Anticoagulants (blood thinners). . . . .   YES   NO
   c. Medicine for high blood pressure . . . .   YES   NO
   d. Cortisone (steroids). . . . .   YES   NO
   e. Tranquilizers . . . .   YES   NO
   f. Antihistamines . . . .   YES   NO
   g. Aspirin . . . .   YÉS   NO
   h. Insulin, tolbutamide (Orinase) or similar drug . . . .   YES   NO
   i. Digitalis or drugs for heart trouble. . . . .   YES   NO
   j. Nitroglycerin . . . .   YES   NO
   k. Oral contraceptive or other hormonal therapy . . . .   YES   NO
   l. Other _____

14. Are you allergic or have you reacted adversely to:
   a. Local anesthetics . . . .   YES   NO
   b. Penicillin or other antibiotics . . . .   YES   NO
   c. Sulfa drugs . . . .   YES   NO
   d. Barbiturates, sedatives, or sleeping pills . . . .   YES   NO
   e. Aspirin . . . .   YES   NO
   f. Iodine . . . .   YES   NO
   g. Codeine or other narcotics . . . .   YES   NO
   h. Other _____
15. Have you had any serious trouble associated with any previous dental treatment?. . . . .   YES   NO
    If so, explain _____

16. Do you have any disease, condition, or problem not listed above that you think I should know about . . . .   YES   NO
    If so, explain _____

17. Are you employed in any situation which exposes you regularly to x-rays or other ionizing radiation? . . .   YES   NO
18. Are you wearing contact lenses? . . . .   YES   NO

WOMEN
19. Are you pregnant? . . . .   YES   NO
20. Do you have any problems associated with your menstrual period? . . . .   YES   NO
21. Are you nursing?. . . . .   YES   NO
CHIEF DENTAL COMPLAINT:

_____
SIGNATURE OF PATIENT

ADA American Dental Association

_____
SIGNATURE OF DENTIST

Fig. 2-2b American Dental Association Medical History form (back).

Table 2-1   Summary of recommended antibiotic regimens for dental/respiratory tract procedures

Standard regimen:

For dental procedures that cause gingival bleeding, and oral surgery	Penicillin V 2.0 gm orally 1 hour before, then 1.0 gm 6 hours later. For patients unable to take oral medications, 2 million units of aqueous penicillin G intravenously or intramuscularly 30 to 60 minutes before a procedure and 1 million units 6 hours later may be substituted.

Special regimens:

Parenteral regimen for use when maximal protection is desired (for example, for patients with prosthetic valves)	Ampicillin 1.0 to 2.0 gm intramuscularly or intravenously, plus gentamycin 1.5 mg/kg intramuscularly or intravenously, one-half hour before procedure, followed by 1.0 gm oral penicillin V 6 hours later. Alternatively, the parenteral regimen may be repeated once 8 hours later.
Oral regimen for penicillin allergic patients	Erythromycin 1.0 gm orally 1 hour before, then 500 mg 6 hours later.
Parenteral regimen for penicillin allergic patients	Vancomycin 1.0 gm intravenously slowly over 1 hour, starting 1 hour before. No repeat dose is necessary.
Pediatric doses	Ampicillin 50 mg/kg per dose; erythromycin 20 mg/kg for first dose, then 10 mg/kg; gentamycin 2.0 mg/kg per dose; penicillin V full adult dose if greater than 60 lb (27 kg), one-half adult dose if less than 60 pounds [27 kg]; aqueous penicillin G 50,000 units/kg (25,000 units/kg for follow-up); vancomycin 20 mg/kg per dose. The intervals between doses are the same as for adults. Total doses should not exceed adult doses.

Source: American Heart Association.

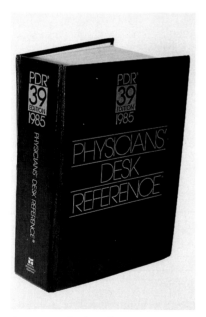

Fig. 2-3   Physicians' Desk Reference.

heart deformity.[2] Procedures for which endocarditis prophylaxis is indicated include all dental procedures likely to induce gingival bleeding (not simple adjustment of orthodontic appliances or shedding of primary teeth).

If antibiotic premedication is indicated, the American Heart Association recommended regimen for prophylactic antibiotic coverage should be followed[3] (Table 2-1).

Systemic and localized conditions may affect the treatment plan for the dental appointment. These will be discussed in Chapter 5.

Medications being taken

Medications that are being taken by the patient are notated in the patient's record. The reason for taking the drug, the routine of taking the drug, and the length of time it has been taken should be elicited from the patient. This should be done for both prescription and nonprescription medications. The dosage should be determined and indications and contraindications for use should be investigated. *The Physicians' Desk Reference* is useful when obtaining information about prescribed medications (Fig. 2-3).

The P.D.R. is the reference of choice for information relative to drug composition, dosages, indications, and contraindications. An updated version is published yearly. It provides indices of pharmaceutical products arranged alphabetically by manufacturers' names, brand (product) names, generic and chemical names, and drug categories. Information on each product is included and a picture section permits identification when the patient is unsure of the name but has a sample of the medication. Other sections deal with the increased use of diagnostic products in medicine and provide a guide to management of drug overdose.

As an example, suppose a patient advises you that he has been taking a tranquilizer twice a day for 2 years for tension. If he knows that the name of the drug is Valium, you would refer to the Product Name Index (pink section). If the patient knows the generic name of the drug, diazepam, you would refer to the Generic and Chemical Name Index (yellow section). If the patient does not know the name of the drug but can explain to you the condition for which he is using it, you would refer to the Product Category Index (blue section) for information.

Complete investigation and understanding of a patient's drug therapy is imperative in order to establish a profile of the patient. Medications may affect the patient's behavior or may be a major influence in the development of the treatment plan.

The vital signs

Taking the vital signs involves pulse rate, blood pressure, respiration, and temperature. These readings should be taken at the beginning of the dental appointment to establish a baseline for the patient against which future readings may be measured.

Pulse rate

The pulse should be evaluated with respect to rate, strength, and rhythm. The pulse rate is determined by placing the fingers (not the thumb) on the radial artery on the patient's wrist (Fig. 2-4). The artery is gently compressed and the pulse counted for one minute. The common practice of feeling the pulse for 15 seconds and multiplying the count by four provides too brief a period to detect cardiac abnormalities such as dropped beats, irregular beats, or irregular rhythms.

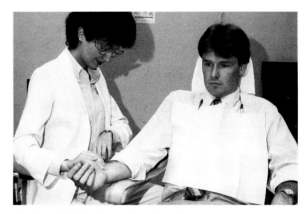

Fig. 2-4   Taking the patient's pulse.

The rate is indicated on the patient's record. An unusual pulse rate should be followed up with repetition of the measurement after a few minutes, and the findings should be called to the attention of the dentist. A rate of 60 to 90 beats per minute is considered normal for the adult patient. Pulse is slightly higher for women than for men. In children the pulse rate is usually faster and ranges between 90 to 140 beats per minute. The strength of a pulse may be referred to as weak (thready) or full. A weak pulse has a rippling quality and may indicate poor cardiac output. A full pulse has a bounding or explosive quality and usually occurs after exercise, in fevers, or in certain emotional states. The normal pulse has a regular rhythm.

Abnormalities of rhythm can be classified into two main categories: (1) regular irregularities and (2) irregular irregularities. A regular irregularity is a change in the pulse or heart beat at regular intervals. An example of a regular irregularity is when the heart speeds up during inspiration and slows down during expiration. An irregular irregularity is a change in the pulse or heart beat at irregular intervals. Atrial fibrillation is an example.

Blood pressure

The patient's blood pressure should be taken and recorded. This is of particular importance for the hypertensive patient who may be unaware of the condition.

Blood pressure is the pressure of the blood on the walls of the arteries. The first number, or Korotkoff's sounds, indicates the pressure in the blood vessel at the point of ventricular contraction of the heart—the systolic pressure. The sounds will continue to become louder from turbulent flow of the blood and then become muffled. The second number indicates the pressure in the artery during ventricular relaxation—the diastolic pressure, or static pressure.[4]

Normal blood pressure varies with age and from person to person. It is affected by a number of factors such as time of day; amount of recent exercise; and recent intake of caffeine, nicotine, and alcohol. The normal range is usually considered 100-140/55-90.[4] The patient who consistently presents systolic readings of 140 mm or higher and/or diastolic pressure of 90 mm or higher is likely to be hypertensive and should be referred to a physician for further testing.

Patients who exhibit high blood pressure are at a greater health risk than others when exposed to anxiety-producing situations. Because dental offices and treatment typically create anxiety in many people, the dental hygienist must identify hypertensive patients prior to dental therapy.

To measure the blood pressure, a stethoscope and sphygmomanometer are needed (Fig. 2-5). Stethoscopes may have a bell-shaped head, a diaphragm head, or a combination of both. The bell-shaped head lightly pressed against the skin is the best for conducting low-pitched sounds and murmurs. The diaphragm head closely applied is better for detecting high-pitched sounds or quiet murmurs. If frequent cardiac examinations are conducted, a combination stethoscope should be available. The two types of sphygmomanometers in current use are mercury and aneroid (Fig. 2-6). The mercury type is not as compact or as convenient to transport, but it has a highly sensitive calibration system and is dependable and durable. The mercury sphygmomanometer will remain accurate unless it loses mercury.

The components of a standard mercury sphygmomanometer are the mercury column, inflatable pressure cuff, pressure release screw, and inflation bulb. The mercury column shows the pressure in millimeters of mercury to which the cuff is inflated. Compression of the arm is achieved by inflating the cuff, which consists of a rubber bag (bladder) in an unyielding fabric covering. Inflation or deflation of the bladder is controlled by adjusting the pressure release screw. The hand bulb is used to fill the bladder with air.

The procedure for obtaining the systolic and diastolic readings with a sphygmomanometer and a stethoscope is as follows[5]:

1. Be sure patient is seated comfortably in the dental chair; legs should be uncrossed.
2. Wrap the cuff of the sphygmomanometer around the upper arm just above the elbow; if the patient is wearing a long-sleeved shirt or blouse, the sleeve should be rolled up loosely to expose the arm.
3. Locate the patient's radial pulse by placing the index and middle fingers on the thumb side of the patient's wrist (Fig. 2-7).
4. Once the pulse has been found, inflate the cuff until the pulse is lost; note the reading on the manometer and release the pressure, allowing the patient to rest for a moment.
5. Place the bell of the stethoscope over the antecubital space (inner aspect of patient's elbow).
6. Inflate the cuff 10 to 15 mm *above* the point where the pulse was lost; for example, if the pulse was lost at 115 mm, raise the pressure to 125 to 130 mm.
7. Open the release valve and deflate the cuff *slowly,* about 2 to 3 mm per second.
8. As the pressure is released, blood will begin to flow through the artery. Listen carefully for the first sound (systolic pressure) and note the reading on the manometer.
9. As the blood flow returns to normal, the pulsing sounds will disappear. The disappearance of sound indicates the lowest (diastolic) pressure; note the reading on the manometer as the sounds disappear.
10. Continue to slowly deflate the cuff for approximately 10 mm after the last sound is heard; at times, the pressure will seem to fade momentarily and return. This procedure will help to avoid false readings (Fig. 2-8).
11. Record the blood pressure reading in the patient's record as systolic/diastolic (e.g., 116/78 mm Hg). The blood pressure is always recorded in even numbers; if the reading seems to be between two numbers, always record the higher even number (for example, if the reading appears to be 113 mm, it is rounded up and recorded as 114 mm.) The complete date should also be indicated on the record.

Temperature

Temperature is the next vital sign that should be evaluated. Body temperature does not normally exceed

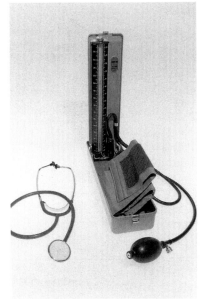
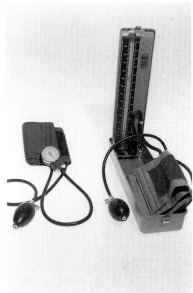

Fig. 2-5 (left) Stethoscope and sphyg-momanometer.

Fig. 2-6 (right) Aneroid and mercury manometers.

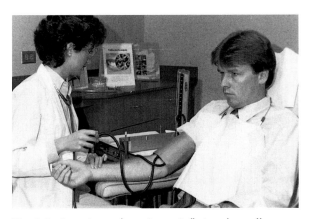

Fig. 2-7 Locating pulse prior to inflating the cuff.

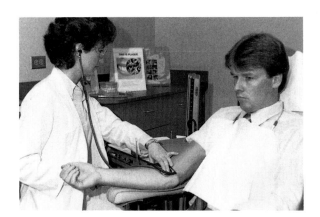

Fig. 2-8 Obtaining blood pressure reading.

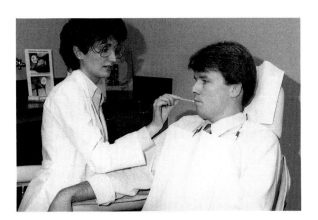

Fig. 2-9 Securing the patient's temperature with manual thermometer.

98.6°F (37° C) when taken orally. A variety of thermometers is available. Because they vary from manufacturer to manufacturer, the instruction sheet that accompanies the thermometer should be read carefully.

The procedure for taking a temperature is simply to shake down the thermometer to a point below the normal temperature reading and place it under the patient's tongue. The thermometer should remain in place for the recommended time period, which may be one-half minute, 1 minute, or 2 minutes (Fig. 2-9).

Respiration rate

The last vital sign that should be observed is the respiration rate. As respiration is normally an involuntary movement, the respiratory rate should be counted without the patient's knowledge. In the normal healthy adult, the frequency of respiration at rest is usually between 14 to 18 breaths per minute. The rate of respiration is easily determined by watching and counting the total breaths a patient takes in 60 seconds.

Medical consult form

The interpretation of abnormal vital signs is a medical decision that warrants the attention of a physician. As members of the dental health profession, dental hygienists have a responsibility to identify these abnormal signs. Also, if a significant finding such as a cardiovascular condition, infectious disease, or a bleeding disorder appears in the medical history, the patient should be given a medical consultation form to be filled out by his physician and returned at the next dental visit. The physician should indicate any precautions, premedications, or special needs of the patient or dental personnel during the dental appointment. Figure 2-10 is an example of a medical consultation form.

Past dental treatment

A summary of the patient's past dental treatment and experiences should be elicited. The treatment rendered, any adverse reactions, the anesthetic or conscious sedation utilized, the home care regimen employed, and general attitudes toward dentistry should be determined.

Fig. 2-10 (right) Medical consult release form.

MEDICAL CONSULT FORM

Patient's Name _____   Chart Number _____

REASON FOR CONSULT: General medical evaluation is sought prior to dental treatment. We are concerned specifically with the following:

HISTORICAL DATA:
☐ Heart Disease, MI, Rheumatic Fever, Murmur
☐ Hypertension   ☐ Diabetes Mellitus   ☐ Current Medications
☐ Thyroid Disease   ☐ Seizure Disorder
☐ Other: _____

IN ADDITION, THE FOLLOWING SYMPTOMS HAVE BEEN NOTED:
☐ None   ☐ Dyspnea
☐ Chest Pain   ☐ Other _____

ABNORMAL PHYSICAL FINDINGS:
☐ None   ☐ Elevated Blood Pressure   ☐ Edema
☐ Irregular Heart Murmur   ☐ Other _____
Blood Pressure _____ Rate _____ Rhythm   ☐ Regular   ☐ Irregular
_____ mmHg

Signed _____ D.D.S.   Date _____

REPLY (Disposition, medical status, medications, ability to undergo dental treatment, need for premedication, etc.):

Signed _____ , M.D.   Date _____

May be returned with the patient or mailed to:

_____ , D.D.S.

_____
(address)

_____
(telephone)

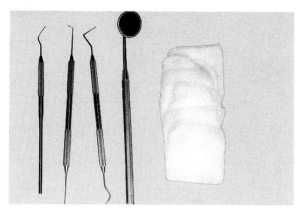

Fig. 2-11 Armamentarium for oral examination.

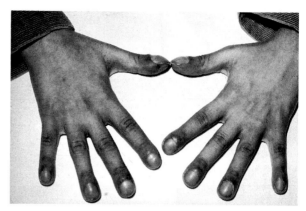

Fig. 2-12 Congenital heart disease patient with clubbed fingers.

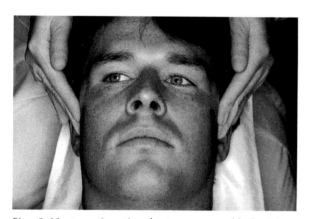

Figs. 2-13a to c Locating the temporomandibular joint.

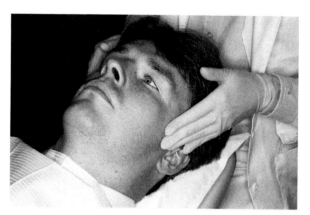

Figure 2-13b

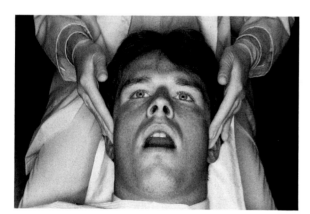

Figure 2-13c

Clinical examination: Extraoral and intraoral

The clinical examination of the head, neck, and mouth is the next phase in the formulation of all the necessary documentation for the patient. In the United States in recent years, dental hygienists have been involved in the detection of a high percentage of oral cancerous lesions. This requires a thorough knowledge of head and neck anatomy as well as normal and pathological conditions.

The dental hygienist detects the oral signs of disease, malfunction, and neglect through an oral examination that involves both visual and tactile components. The materials needed to perform the oral inspection are an intraoral mirror, explorers for calculus and caries detection, a periodontal probe, and

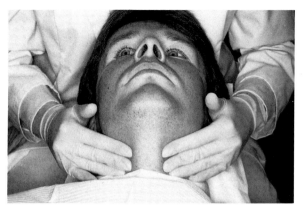

Fig. 2-14a Palpating of thyroid gland.

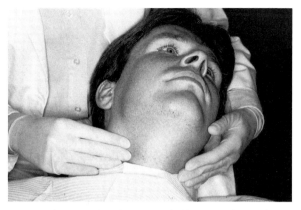

Fig. 2-14b Locating the sternocleidomastoid muscle.

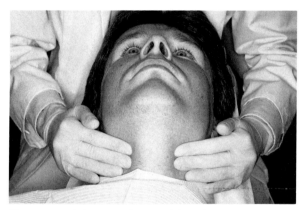

Fig. 2-14c Palpating of cervical lymph nodes.

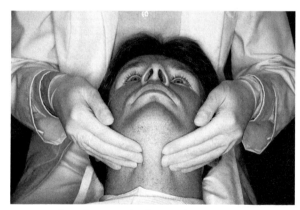

Fig. 2-14d Palpating of submental area.

2 × 2 gauze squares (Fig. 2-11). The procedures to be performed should be explained to the patient.

The examination itself consists of an extraoral and an intraoral component. The *extraoral examination* includes inspection of the head, skin, temporomandibular joint (TMJ), neck, thyroid gland, lymph nodes, and salivary glands. This phase is begun by assessing the patient's face and neck for symmetry, the presence of growths, and the color and appearance of the skin.

The patient's body should be observed for conditions that would alert the hygienist to medical problems; for example, clubbing of the fingers may be indicative of congenital heart disease or pulmonary disease (Fig. 2-12). Although dental treatment is performed on the mouth, the patient is the whole person.

The dental hygienist should observe the patient's profile for any enlargement of the temporomandibular

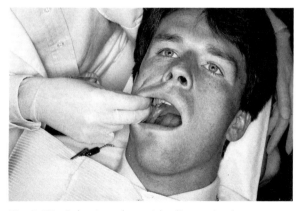

Fig. 2-15 Palpating of parotid salivary glands.

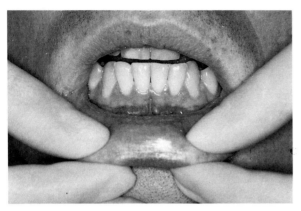

Figs. 2-16a and b   Examining the lips.

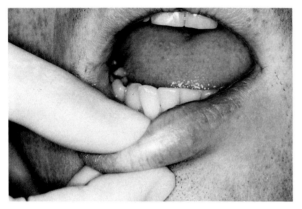

Figure 2-16b

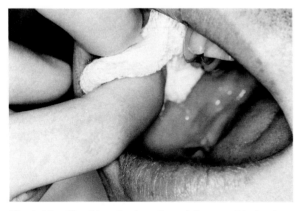

Fig. 2-17   Checking the function of the parotid gland.

joint (Figs. 2-13a to c). To examine the TMJ, the pads of the first and second fingers of each hand are placed just anterior and slightly inferior to the opening of the patient's ears and directly over the TMJ. The patient should be asked if there is any tenderness. Auscultation is employed at this point. As the patient opens and closes his or her mouth, the hygienist listens for any clicking sounds and feels for disjointed movement. As the patient opens his or her mouth halfway and moves the mandible from side to side, the hygienist listens and feels again. These techniques may identify the presence of temporomandibular joint dysfunction.[6]

Any deviation should be called to the attention of the dentist. Referral to a specialist or a university dental school may be necessary. The best way currently employed by many specialists to diagnose TMJ disorders involves injection of a contrast medium directly into the joint so that slices of radiographs can be made of the soft tissue.[7] Electronic stethoscopes, the kind used by cardiologists, are also being used as a diagnostic tool. The electronic stethoscope can detect sounds that cannot be heard by the human ear. It digitizes this information and produces a wave on a chart to characterize the sound.

The neck should be observed for asymmetry or the presence of lesions. As the patient swallows, the hygienist should observe the movement of the thyroid cartilage. The thyroid should be palpated at rest and during swallowing (Fig. 2-14a).

The hygienist should next locate the sternocleidomastoid muscle on each side of the neck (Fig. 2-14b) and palpate the area beneath, anterior, and posterior to it in order to examine the cervical lymph nodes (Fig. 2-14c). Tilting the patient's head forward may make the area more accessible.

The extraoral examination should be concluded with palpation of (1) the region just below the ear and the submandibular gland along and medial to the inferior borders of the mandible; (2) the lymph nodes and the tissues of the submental area upward toward the mandible (Fig. 2-14d); and (3) the parotid gland and the preauricular lymph nodes anterior to the ear (Fig. 2-15). This can all be accomplished relatively quickly.

The *intraoral examination* consists of inspection and evaluation of the lips, labial mucosa and anterior vestibule, buccal mucosa and posterior vestibule, hard palate and maxillary tuberosities, soft palate and pharyngeal area, tongue, sublingual area, gingiva, and teeth. For the examination, the patient should be properly positioned and the appropriate asepsis procedures followed.

Lips and vestibule

The lips should be observed while closed and the vermilion border examined. A quick overall check of the mouth for open lesions, which would indicate potential problems, should precede the detailed inspection. Any removable prosthetic appliances should be examined.

The dental hygienist should check the labial surface of the lower lip, the frenum attachment, mucobuccal fold, and alveolar mucosa (Fig. 2-16a). The same procedure should be followed for the upper lip. To locate any masses, the lips should be palpated with the thumb and index finger (Fig. 2-16b).

The mucobuccal folds and the alveolar mucosa should be palpated. The right buccal mucosa should be retracted and the entire surface inspected. The function of Stensen's duct should be checked by drying the area with a gauze square and noting the reappearance of saliva (Fig. 2-17). An intraoral mirror should be used to inspect the retromolar area. The sequence must be repeated for the left side. The examination of the vestibule should be concluded with palpation of the buccal mucosa with the thumb and index finger, the retromolar area and the pterygomandibular fold area with the index finger, and the mucobuccal fold and alveolar mucosa for the right and left side.

Palate

An intraoral mirror is used to view the hard palate. The dental hygienist should note the incisive papilla, the rugae, raphe, and the palatine suture (Fig. 2-18a); examine for the presence of torus palatinus (Fig. 2-18b); and view the junction between the hard and soft palates. The maxillary tuberosities and adjacent edentulous areas should be inspected. As the tongue is depressed and the patient says "ah," the soft palate, uvula, and oral pharynx area (Fig. 2-18c) can be inspected. The hard palate and the anterior segment of the soft palate should be palpated with the index finger. The right and left maxillary tuberosities should be palpated.

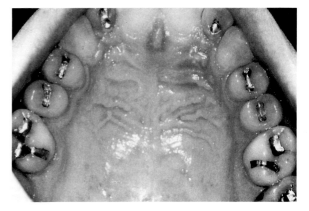

Fig. 2-18a Viewing the hard palate.

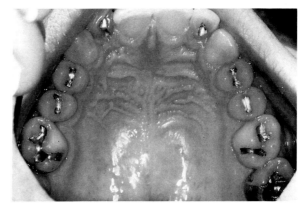

Fig. 2-18b Torus palatinus.

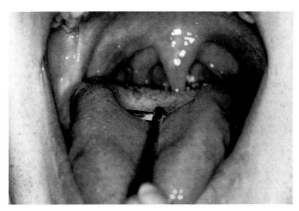

Fig. 2-18c Inspecting the soft palate and pharyngeal area.

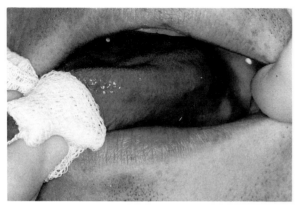

Fig. 2-19a   Examining the lateral borders of the tongue.

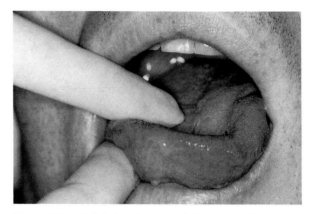

Fig. 2-19b   Bidigital palpation of the tongue for location of masses.

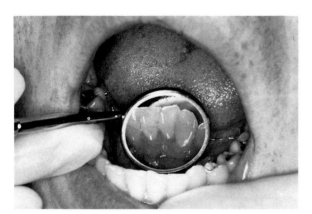

Fig. 2-20a   Viewing the lingual border of the mandible.

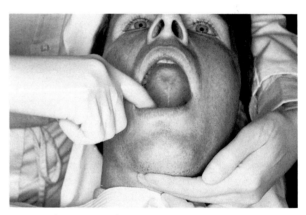

Fig. 2-20b   Bimanual palpation of the floor of the mouth.

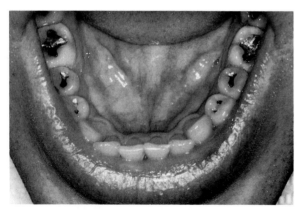

Fig. 2-20c   Mandibular tori.

Tongue and sublingual area

The patient should be asked to extend the tongue. After wrapping the tip of the tongue in a 2 × 2 gauze square to ensure a solid grasp, the dental hygienist should gently extend the tongue and have the patient move it to the right while the left lateral border is inspected (Fig. 2-19a). An intraoral mirror may be used to facilitate the inspection. The border and inferior surface of the tongue should be palpated and the procedure repeated for the other border of the tongue. The dental hygienist should inspect the dorsal surface of the tongue including the papillae while still holding the tongue. The tongue should be palpated (Fig. 2-19b). The patient should place the tip of the tongue on the hard palate, and the dental hygienist should note if there is any difficulty in lifting the tongue. The inferior surface of the tongue and the lingual frenum should be inspected. The hygienist should examine the floor of the mouth and request the patient to move the tongue from side to side so as to assess the symmetry of the movement.

An intraoral mirror should be used to assess the lingual border of the mandible (Fig. 2-20a). The floor of the mouth should be palpated using both index fingers, one intraorally and one extraorally (Fig. 2-20b). The entire surface of the mandible should be palpated. Mandibular tori would be discovered during this procedure (Fig. 2-20c). Finally, the hygienist should check the function of the sublingual salivary glands.

Detection of oral cancer

The dental hygienist's role in the detection of oral cancer cannot be overemphasized. Statistics from the American Cancer Society indicate 29,500 new reported cases of oral cancer in 1986 with 9,400 deaths attributed to oral cancer.[8] Five-year survival rates vary substantially depending on the site of the malignancy. Rates range from 31% for cancer of the pharynx to 92% for lip cancer. Overall, the 5-year survival rate for oral cancer patients is about 52%.[8] In oral cancer, early detection is of the utmost importance. Warning signs to which the dental professional should be alert include a lesion that bleeds easily or doesn't heal; a lump or thickening; a reddish area or ulceration; a whitish patch (leukoplakia); and difficulty in chewing, swallowing, or moving the tongue or mandible.[9]

Cytology smears and/or biopsy procedures may be indicated when the clinical examination or patient self-examination uncovers the presence of a suspicious lesion. Cytology smears and biopsy procedures are discussed in Chapter 4. In Chapter 5 dental hygiene involvement in the phases of oral cancer treatment are elaborated. Dental hygienists who practice in cancer therapy clinics in hospital settings are involved daily with clinical staging techniques for oral cancerous lesions. All dental hygienists should be familiar with the nomenclature, which may be part of the patient's chart.

The TNM classification system has been adopted by the American Joint Committee on Cancer as the system for clinical staging of cancerous lesions.[10] Proper staging of cancer is of major importance in the ultimate decisions that will be reached by the oral surgery team about therapy. The major classification categories that are used to stage a cancerous lesion are given in Tables 2-2 to 2-5. (T — tumor diameters;

Table 2-2 Definition of T categories of the oral cavity

T1	Greatest diameter of primary tumor 2 cm or less.
T2	Greatest diameter of primary tumor more than 2 cm but not more than 4 cm.
T3	Greatest diameter of primary tumor more than 4 cm.
T4	Massive tumor more than 4 cm in diameter, with deep invasion involving antrum, pterygoid muscles, base of tongue, or skin of neck.

Source: American Cancer Society.

Table 2-3 Definition of N categories*

N0	No clinically positive nodes.
N1	Single clinically positive homolateral node 3 cm or less in diameter.
N2	Single clinically positive homolateral node more than 3 cm, but not more than 6 cm in diameter, or multiple clinically positive homolateral nodes, none more than 6 cm in diameter.
N2a	Single clinically positive node more than 3 cm but not more than 6 cm in diameter.
N2b	Multiple clinically positive homolateral nodes, none more than 6 cm in diameter.
N3	Massive homolateral node(s), bilateral nodes, or contralateral node(s).
N3a	Clinically positive homolateral node(s), one of which is more than 6 cm in diameter.
N3b	Bilateral clinically positive nodes.
N3c	Contralateral clinically positive node(s) only.

Source: American Cancer Society.
*This regional lymph node classification is applicable to all cancers of the upper aerodigestive tract.

Table 2-4 Definition of M categories

M0	No (known) distant metastasis.
M1	Distant metastasis present—specify site(s).

Source: American Cancer Society.

Table 2-5 Stage grouping*

Stage I	T1 N0 M0
Stage II	T2 N0 M0
Stage III	T3 N0 M0
	T1, T2, or T3 N1 M0
Stage IV	T4 N0 or N1 M0
	Any T N2 or N3 M0
	Any T Any N M1

Source: American Cancer Society.
*These stage groupings apply to all squamous cell carcinomas of the upper aerodigestive tract. The prognosis for a given tumor is closely related to its clinical stage.

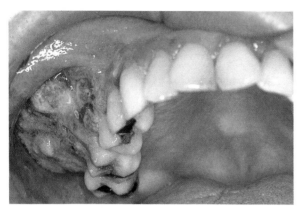

Fig. 2-21a   Squamous cell carcinoma of the alveolar ridge. (Courtesy of Dr. Peter Hurst, Northwestern Memorial Hospital, Chicago, Ill.)

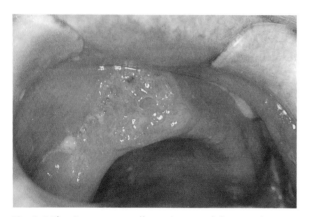

Fig. 2-21b   Squamous cell carcinoma of the anterior maxilla. (Courtesy of Dr. Peter Hurst.)

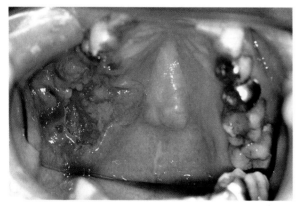

Fig. 2-21c   Squamous cell carcinoma of the alveolar ridge and tuberosity area. (Courtesy of Dr. Peter Hurst.)

Table 2-6   Anatomical distribution of 240 asymptomatic oral squamous cell carcinomas

Site	Number of lesions
Hard palate	1
Buccal mucosa	2
Alveolar ridge	3
Oral tongue	42
Soft palate complex:	
Lingual aspect of the retromolar tongue, 12	
Anterior tonsillar pillar, 29	
Soft palate proper, 35	76
Floor of mouth	116

Source: American Cancer Society.

N – lymph node categories; and M – categories for distant metastases). Table 2-6 gives the anatomical distribution of oral squamous cell carcinomas.

Squamous cell carcinomas   Squamous cell carcinomas comprise over 90% of malignant tumors in the oral cavity.[11] These tumors always arise in the surface epithelium, often in areas of leukoplakia or erythroplakia. Although tumors may arise in any site in the oral mucosa, the floor of the mouth, the sides of the mobile portion of the tongue, and the facial arches are the sites of predilection. Squamous cell carcinomas are almost always painless and may grow to a surprising size before causing symptoms. Figures 2-21a to c are examples of squamous cell carcinomas.

Adenocarcinomas   Adenocarcinomas are cancers of minor salivary glands that occur in scattered areas of epithelium of the oral cavity. These neoplasms of minor salivary glands are more likely to be malignant than those arising from the major salivary glands.[11,12] Adenocarcinomas generally appear as rounded, elevated masses covered by intact mucous membrane. The most common site of origin is the palate. Figure 2-22 shows an adenoid cystic carcinoma.

Lymphomas   The area encompassed by the nasopharynx, tonsils, and base of the tongue is the most common site of malignant lymphoma. Lymphomas have a rapid growth rate with early metastasis to regional lymph nodes.[11] Figure 2-23 shows a lymphoma of the palate.

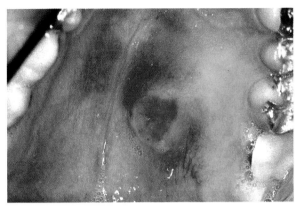

Fig. 2-22   Adenoid cystic carcinoma. (Courtesy of Dr. Peter Hurst.)

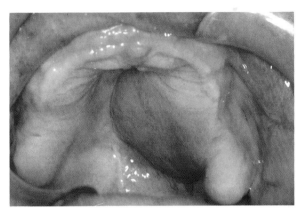

Fig. 2-23   Lymphoma of the palate. (Courtesy of Dr. Peter Hurst.)

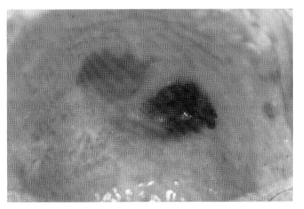

Figs. 2-24a to d   Malignant melanoma. (Courtesy of Dr. Peter Hurst.)

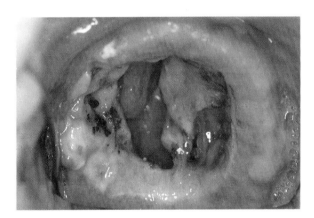

Figure 2-24b

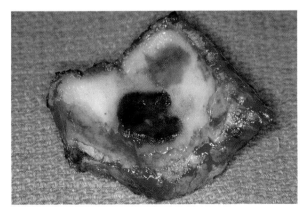

Figure 2-24c

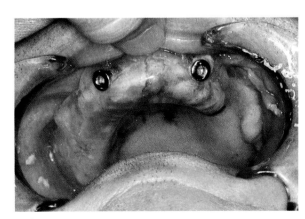

Figure 2-24d

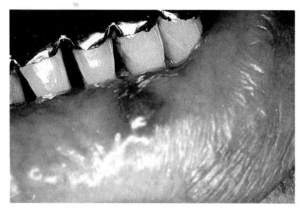

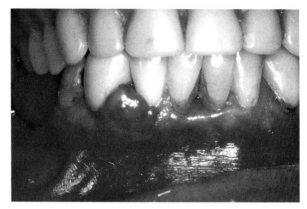

Figs. 2-25a to d   Benign oral conditions.

Figure 2-25b

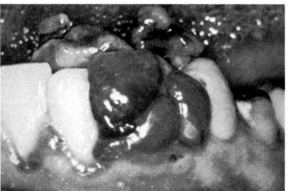

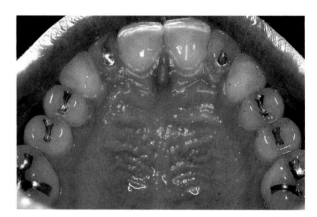

Figure 2-25c

Figure 2-25d

Melanomas   Pigmented lesions within the oral cavity require prompt attention. Malignant melanomas are uncommon in the oral cavity, but are particularly lethal.[9,11] Figure 2-24a shows a malignant melanoma of the palate; Fig. 2-24b, the site after surgical excision of the lesion; Fig. 2-24c, the specimen; and Fig. 2-24d, the area with the immediate surgical obturator in place.

Benign conditions   Many benign conditions may also be encountered in the oral examination.[11,13] They include:

- Papilloma—Epithelial neoplasm; most common site, the tongue.

- Pyogenic granuloma—Red, soft, easily bleeding mass; often follows trauma.
- Hemangioma—Benign proliferation of blood vessels (Fig. 2-25a).
- Epulis—Benign tumor from the periosteum (Fig. 2-25b).
- Pregnancy tumors—Associated with pregnancy gingivitis (Fig. 2-25c).
- Granular cell myoblastoma—Well circumscribed, firm, rounded mass within the muscle of the tongue.
- Giant cell reparative granuloma—Tumor-like lesion of the alveolar ridge usually found in children and adolescents.
- Torus—Benign exostosis most commonly found in the midline of the hard palate and the mandibular ridge (Fig. 2-25d).

- Mucocele—Retention cyst caused by occlusion of the ducts of the mucous glands, bluish in color, most commonly found on inner aspect of the lower lip.

The presence of these lesions should be called to the attention of the dentist; excision may be indicated. The hygienist should provide a complete description in the patient's record of the size, color, and location of the mass.[9] The periodontal probe is useful in gaining measurements of such lesions.

Gingiva

The examination continues with an evaluation of the periodontium, which involves inspection of the gingiva of the maxillary and mandibular arches.

The alveolar mucosa is the gingival tissue that lies between the lining of the floor of the mouth and the gingiva (Fig. 2-26). Blood vessels are visible through the tissue, which has a reddish color and shiny smooth surface in health. The scalloped line that separates the alveolar mucosa and the gingiva is the mucogingival junction (Fig. 2-27a). The alveolar mucosa is loosely attached to underlying bone, the attached gingiva (Fig. 2-27b) is firmly attached to underlying bone. In health, the color varies from pink to brown, depending on the skin pigmentation of the patient. The healthy gingiva has an appearance like an orange peel (Fig. 2-28). The presence of the stipples indicates the projection of the epithelial cells into the connective tissue; these projections are known as rete pegs. In the presence of inflammation, these stipples are not apparent because edema alters this pattern of connective tissue papillae and epithelial rete pegs (Figs. 2-29a and b).

The free gingival groove is a shallow depression running parallel to the gingival margin that marks the boundary between the attached gingiva and the marginal gingiva (Fig. 2-30a). The marginal gingiva is not attached to bone. It has a knife-edged margin, is smooth in texture, and is usually pink in color (Fig. 2-30b). The interproximal spaces are filled by the interdental papillae. Healthy papillae are firm and triangular in shape (Fig. 2-30c).

The col area is the interproximal depression of the gingiva in the buccolingual dimension. The sulcus area is the space between the marginal gingiva and the tooth enamel. In the healthy mouth, it is 1 to 2 mm deep (Fig. 2-31). This area is nonkeratinized tis-

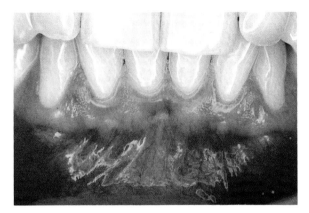

Figure 2-26

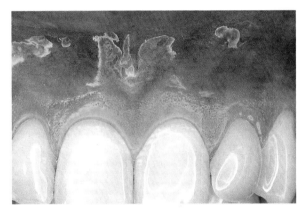

Figure 2-27a

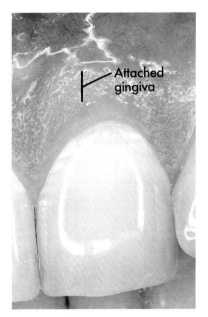

Figure 2-27b

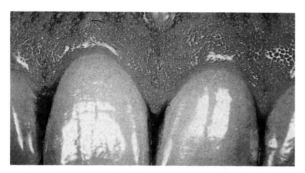

Fig. 2-28 From D. Lange: *Periodontology in Daily Practice,* Quintessence Publ. Co., 1981, in German.

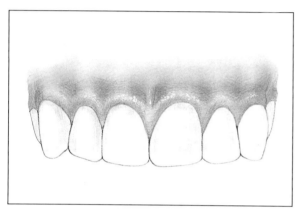

Fig. 2-29a Healthy gingiva. (From J. Berns: *What is Periodontal Disease?,* Quintessence Publ. Co., 1984.)

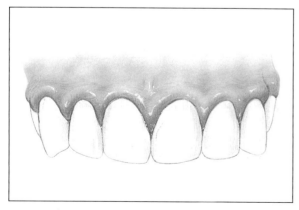

Fig. 2-29b Presence of inflammation. (From J. Berns: *What is Periodontal Disease?,* Quintessence Publ. Co., 1984.)

sue just superior to the epithelial attachment. The epithelium of the attached and marginal gingiva is either parakeratinized or keratinized. The sulcular epithelium and the epithelial attachment are nonkeratinized tissue.

Keratinization is the process by which cells that form as basal cells change characteristics as they migrate toward the surface of the tissue. Beginning as basal cells that are cuboidal in shape, the cells become spinous cells that are polygonal in shape. As the cells migrate, they flatten to become the stratum granulosum. Finally they migrate to a superficial layer, the stratum corneum, to become keratinized or parakeratinized (Fig. 2-32). The nonkeritanized sulcular area is extremely susceptible to pathological invasion, because the cells have not formed a cornified layer.

Periodontal probing A thorough periodontal assessment should include periodontal probing and recording of sulcus depth readings. A complete periodontal probing should be done the first time a patient is examined and followed up at least yearly at reexamination appointments. The probe is used for the gingival determinations of bleeding, consistency, and form and is therefore the most important tool in assessing periodontal health.

The probe is held in a modified pen grasp that is light enough to ensure tactile sensitivity, yet still maintains control of the instrument when performing the pocket survey (Fig. 2-33). Initially the working end is held as parallel as possible to the long axis of the tooth in both the buccolingual and mesiodistal dimensions (Fig. 2-34a). In order to reach the cementoenamel junction from the point of insertion, however, the tip must be rotated toward the center of the tooth (Fig. 2-34b).

The instrument is guided gently along the tooth surface until it reaches the soft spongy epithelial attachment (Fig. 2-35). From this point, the probe is moved in short, up and down strokes, maintaining the tip of the probe in the sulcus, around the entire circumference of the tooth (Fig. 2-36).

Probing is usually conducted after calculus removal. If there is calculus present, the probe might rest on the calculus instead of the epithelial attachment and thus mislead the dental hygienist as to the true reading. Performing the probing after calculus removal presents some difficulties, however. If extensive scaling has disrupted the epithelial attachment or caused an edematous reaction of the tissue, a false

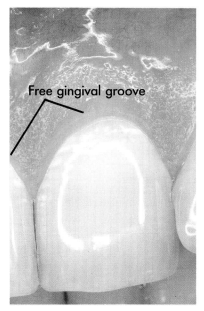

Fig. 2-30a Free gingival groove.

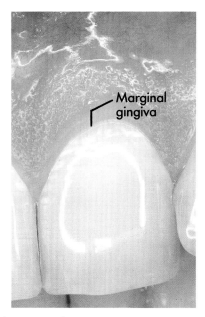

Fig. 2-30b Marginal gingiva.

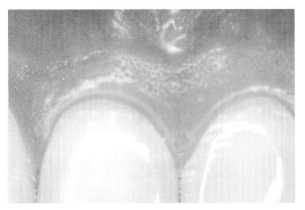

Fig. 2-30c Healthy interdental papillae.

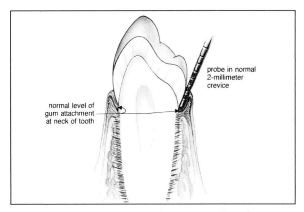

Fig. 2-31 From J. Berns: *What is Periodontal Disease?*, Quintessence Publ. Co., 1984.

reading may result. Routine probing at specific intervals after the initial readings are taken is the most prudent approach.

The reading recorded is the one that reflects the deepest point of each of six segments of the circumference determined by reading the millimeter marking at the margin of the free gingiva. If the reading is between markings, the higher number is used. Measurements are noted on the chart for the mesiofacial, facial, distofacial, mesiolingual, lingual, and distolingual aspects of the sulcus (Figs. 2-37a and b).

Proper performances of the pocket and sulcus sur-

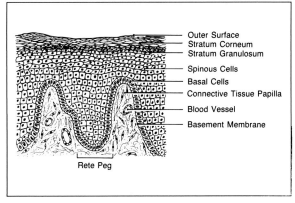

Figure 2-32

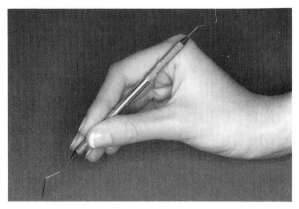

Figure 2-33

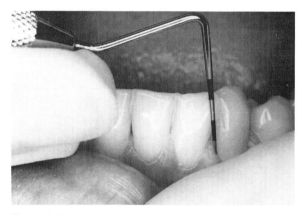

Figure 2-34a

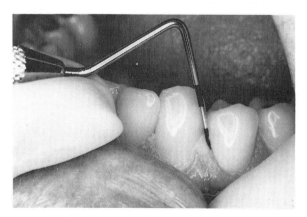

Figure 2-34b

vey locate variations in sulcus depths that exceed those normally associated with health (Fig. 2-38). Variations may be due to a decrease in the bony margin or to an increase in the gingival margin because of edema. In either case, this is an indication of an unhealthy condition. The disease process elicits a variety of topographic changes in the periodontium. Bony defects and the anatomic variations they uncover pose a problem to proper adaptation. In the case of multirooted teeth, furcations, developmental grooves, and root curvatures, instrumentation adaptions must be made. Roots tend to curve toward the distal aspect. Furcations begin about 4 to 6 mm apical to the cementoenamel junction.

Clinical observations Periodontal probing, radiographic findings, and clinical observations are all components of a thorough assessment of the periodontium. (Radiographic interpretations and charting will be covered in Volume 2.) Describing the condition of the periodontal tissues requires identification of the anatomical structures involved and evaluation of the characteristics of color, form, consistency, the presence of secretions, and mobility as well as the sulcular depth.

The color of healthy periodontal tissues varies from pink to brown or purple depending on the skin pigmentation of the person. Unhealthy tissues may appear red, usually indicating an acute condition or dark red to bluish color called cyanotic, which is due to the accumulation of unoxygenated blood that has not been circulating properly (Figs. 2-39a to c).

The form of the gingiva refers to the shape and contour of the tissue. Healthy gingiva has a knife-edged gingival margin. In the presence of disease, the marginal gingiva may become rolled or swollen. The interdental papillae in health fill the interdental space. In a diseased state, the papillae may be enlarged, blunted, or ulcerated as in the case of necrotizing ulcerative gingivitis (Figs. 2-40a and b).

The firmness and texture of the tissue is another determinant to gingival health. The tissue should be firm with stipples. In the presence of inflammation, loss of stipling results in smooth, glossy gingiva. Edema causes tissues to be spongy and depress easily when touched with a probe. Chronic conditions may result in tissue that is fibrotic.

Spontaneous bleeding upon use of compressed air or gentle manipulation of the tissue indicates an unhealthy condition. The presence of purulent exudate

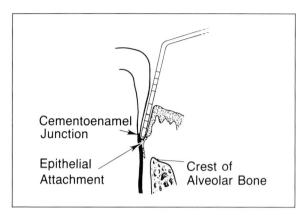

Figure 2-35

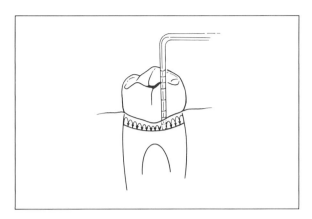

Figure 2-36

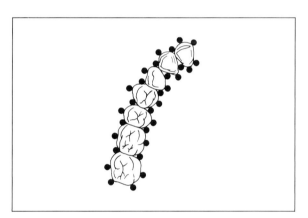

Fig. 2-37a Probing sites.

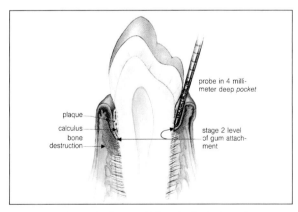

Fig. 2-38 From J. Berns: *What is Periodontal Disease?*, Quintessence Publ. Co., 1984.

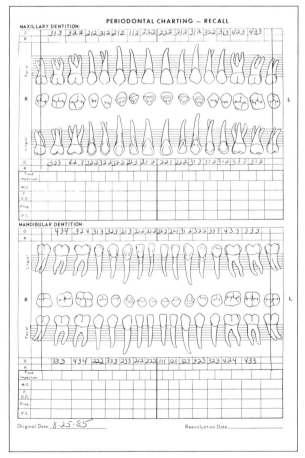

Fig. 2-37b Recording of completed probing.

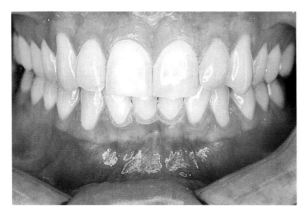

Fig. 2-39a Healthy gingiva.

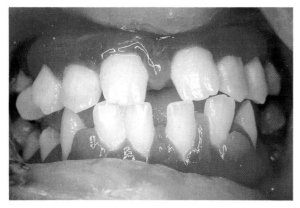

Fig. 2-39b Unhealthy (acute condition). (Courtesy of Dr. Anthony Gargiulo, Loyola University, Chicago, Ill.)

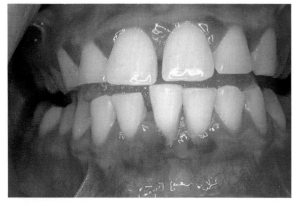

Fig. 2-39c Unhealthy (dark red tissue). (Courtesy of Dr. Anthony Gargiulo.)

indicates the presence of disease. Purulent exudate also is present at the site of a periodontal abscess. Incomplete removal of calculus by the dental hygienist may cause a periodontal abscess to occur. Gross scaling of heavy calculus deposits should never be attempted for the entire mouth at the initial appointment. Rather, complete debridement of a designated area would be the prudent treatment plan.

Tooth mobility evidenced by the ability to digitally or manually move the tooth or depress it in the socket is another indication of the presence of disease. Several methods exist for detecting mobility. The most desirable involves using two instrument handles to move the tooth facially and lingually (Fig. 2-41). A finger and an instrument handle or the blade of a curet may also be used in the fossa of a posterior tooth. Measurements are recorded as follows:

N = Essentially no movement, physiological only.
1° = Movement in a facial and lingual direction up to and including 1 mm.
2° = Movement in a facial and lingual direction greater than 1 mm.
3° = same as 2° *and* easily depressable in the socket.

The presence of any of the indicators is utilized to evaluate the periodontal status. The condition is then described as acute or chronic, applied to the anatomical structures involved. The extent of the involvement is described as generalized or localized, mild or severe.

The patient in Fig. 2-42 has mild, generalized, marginal gingivitis. The condition involves the entire mouth. There are changes in the indicators of color, form, and consistency. The marginal gingiva is the structure involved.

An acute gingival condition called acute necrotizing ulcerative gingivitis is indicated clinically by the ulceration of interdental papillae, a pseudomembrane, a foul breath, bleeding, and pain. The case in Fig. 2-40b is labeled as acute because it had a rapid onset and the tissue is bright red.

If bone loss through probing and radiographs, mobility, and/or secretions is detected (Fig. 2-43a), the description would be periodontitis because of the tissues involved (Fig. 2-43b).

Exploring to detect the presence of subgingival and supragingival calculus deposits should be completed. Some dental hygienists utilize forms to provide a chart of these deposits.

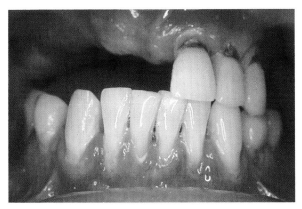

Fig. 2-40a   Blunted, cratered interdental papillae. (Courtesy of Dr. Anthony Gargiulo.)

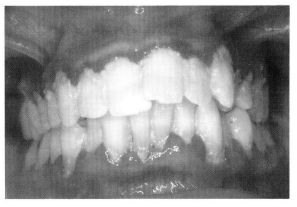

Fig. 2-40b   Diseased edematous papillae. (Courtesy of Dr. Anthony Gargiulo.)

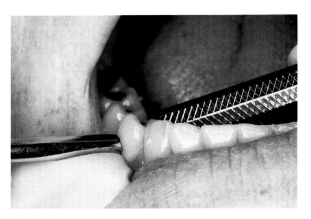

Figure 2-41

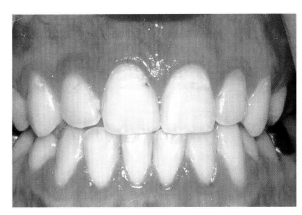

Figure 2-42

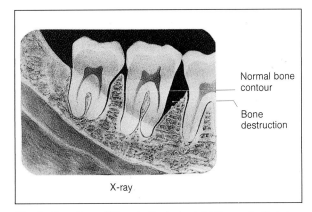

Fig. 2-43a   From *What is Periodontal Disease?*, Quintessence Publ. Co., 1984.

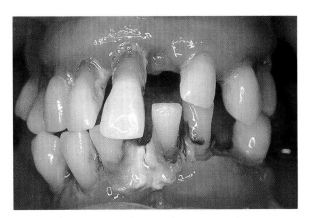

Fig. 2-43b   Courtesy of Dr. Anthony Gargiulo.

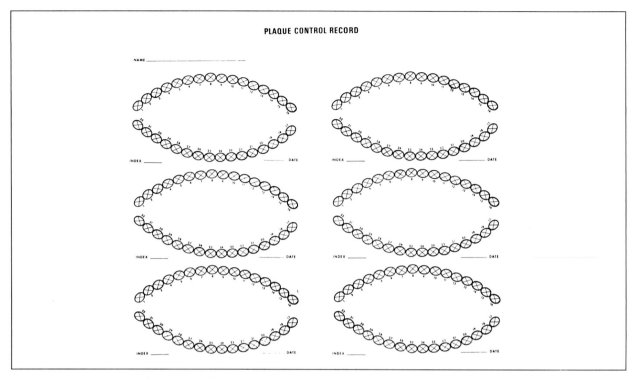

Fig. 2-44a O'Leary's local irritants index. (From T.J. O'Leary, R.B. Drake, and J.E. Naylor: The plaque control record. *Journal of Periodontology,* 43:38, 1972.)

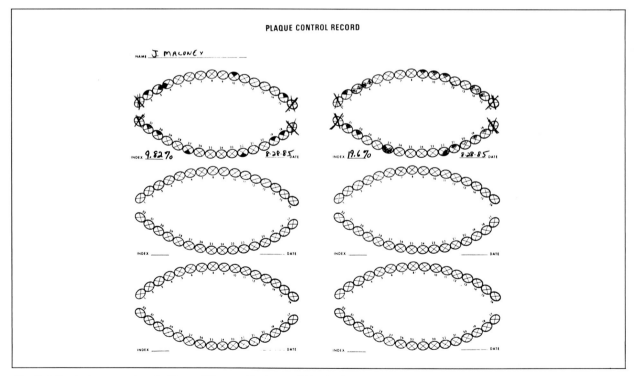

Fig. 2-44b Index completed. (From O'Leary, Drake, and Naylor.)

Gingival indices   Plaque and gingival indices may be part of the documentation. There are several types of indices. Some use selected teeth; some employ mathematic averaging; some use the presence of plaque and/or bleeding upon probing as the only criteria and do not involve qualitative assessment.

Hygienists employed in public health sectors where screenings are performed or hygienists involved in epidemiologic studies or research may use plaque indices that quantify the presence and amount of plaque. In private practice, however, where time constraints are a factor, the most typically used plaque indices are those that identify the presence or absence of plaque or those that provide a simplistic approach to its quantification.[14]

In the O'Leary Local Irritants Index, each diagram space represents a tooth and its four surfaces: mesial, distal, facial, and lingual (Fig. 2-44a). The presence of plaque in any quantity is recorded by coloring in the space representing that surface. All missing teeth are crossed out. The patient's plaque score is determined by multiplying the number of teeth present by 4 (surfaces) to obtain the total number of surfaces in the mouth; the number of surfaces where plaque is present is multiplied by 100 and divided by the total number of surfaces in the mouth (Fig. 2-44b).

The Simplified Oral Hygiene Index (OHI-S) uses six preselected tooth surfaces for measurement: the facial surfaces of the maxillary molars and the maxillary and mandibular central incisors and the lingual surfaces of the mandibular molars or the next tooth distal to each second premolar if the first molar is extracted. The presence of plaque is scored.[15]

0 = No debris or stain.
1 = Soft debris covering no more than one third of the tooth surface, or the presence of extrinsic stain.
2 = Soft debris covering more than one third but no more than two thirds of the tooth surface.
3 = Soft debris covering more than two thirds of the tooth surface.

The scores for the teeth are totaled and the sum is divided by the number of teeth examined.

The original Oral Hygiene Index (OHI) involved 12 instead of six surfaces, and teeth used for the scoring were those teeth with the most debris.

The Dental Plaque Index (PI) by Ramfjord involves scoring each tooth and dividing by the number of teeth.[16]

0 = No plaque.
1 = Plaque present on some but not all interproximal, facial, and lingual surfaces of the tooth.
2 = Plaque present on *all* interproximal facial and lingual surfaces, but covering less than one half of these surfaces.
3 = Plaque extending over all interproximal, facial, and lingual surfaces, and covering more than one half of these surfaces.

The Silness and Löe Plaque Index (PI-1) assesses the thickness of the plaque present on each tooth in the mouth. The presence of plaque at the cervical one third is scored.[17]

0 = No plaque.
1 = Plaque adhering to the free gingival margin and adjacent area of the tooth.
2 = Moderate accumulation of soft deposits within the gingival pocket or on the tooth and gingival margin.
3 = Abundance of soft matter within the gingival pocket and/or on the tooth and gingival margin.

Various types of disclosing solutions or agents are available to assist in the detection of plaque. Most contain some form of vegetable dye. Many of these are currently under scrutiny because of a possible carcinogenic hazard. Some disclosants contain sodium fluorescein, which must be used with a filtered light source.

Gingival indices are used to determine changes in several of the clinical characteristics of the gingival tissues that would indicate the presence of disease: changes in color, form, and consistency and the presence of bleeding spontaneously or upon probing.

The Gingivitis Index (GI) assesses the health of the gingiva in six locations: maxillary right first molar, left central incisor, left first premolar, mandibular left first molar, right central incisor, and right first premolar.[17]

0 = No signs of inflammation.
1 = Mild to moderate inflammatory gingival changes not extending around the tooth.
2 = Mild to moderately severe gingivitis extending *all* around the tooth.
3 = Severe gingivitis characterized by marked redness, swelling, tendency to bleed, and ulceration.

The Löe and Silness Gingival Index (GI) assesses the severity of gingivitis on the basis of color, consistency, and bleeding. The gingival area of each tooth is involved. The probe is used to evaluate the consistency of the gingiva and then used to identify bleeding points.

0 = Normal gingiva.
1 = Mild inflammation—slight changes in color, form (no bleeding upon probing).
2 = Moderate inflammation—redness, edema (bleeding upon probing).
3 = Severe inflammation—marked redness and edema, ulceration (spontaneous bleeding).

Scores are totaled and divided by the number of teeth.

The occlusion

The next aspect of the inspection relates to the classification of the occlusion and possible orthodontic needs of the patient. The relationship of the maxillary and mandibular arches and identification of related deviations is notated at this time.

Although a more comprehensive evaluation of the occlusion is made by orthodontists, Angle's classification is most often used by dental hygienists in general practices for record taking. This classification system is based on the relationship of the mesiobuccal cusp of the permanent maxillary first molar with the buccal groove of the permanent mandibular first molar. If the patient has primary teeth, the relationship is evaluated by the position of the mesiobuccal cusp of the maxillary second primary molar to the buccal groove of the mandibular second primary molar.

The term Class I is used to describe the normal sagittal relationship between the two dental arches (Figs. 2-45a and b). Malocclusion categories include Class I malocclusion, in which the molar relationship is normal but malposition of some teeth exists.

The Class II malocclusion category is subdivided into division 1 and division 2. In Class II malocclusion the position of the buccal groove of the mandibular first molar is distal to the mesiobuccal cusp of the maxillary first molar. This is called distocclusion (Figs. 2-46a to c). In Class II, division 1, all maxillary teeth are protruded. In Class II, division 2, in addition to the protrusion of most of the maxillary anterior teeth, one or more maxillary incisors are retruded (Figs. 2-47a and b).

In Class III malocclusion the buccal groove of the mandibular first molar is mesial to the mesiobuccal cusp of the maxillary first molar. This is called mesiocclusion (Figs. 2-48a to c). Malocclusion may be developmental in nature, may result from premature loss of the primary teeth, or may be caused by habits such as thumb sucking or tongue thrusting.

Other deviations that should be included in this aspect of the documentation are crossbite, overjet, overbite, edge-to-edge bite, and openbite. Crossbites involve abnormal relationships of opposing teeth. Anterior or posterior teeth may be involved (Figs. 2-49a and b), and the condition may be bilateral or unilateral. The maxillary teeth are in a lingual position to the mandibular teeth.

Overjet is the horizontal distance measured between the maxillary incisors "jetting" out over the mandibular incisors (Figs. 2-50a and b). The periodontal probe may be used to measure this horizontal space in millimeters. Overbite is the measurement of the vertical distance that the maxillary incisors overlap the mandibular incisors (Fig. 2-51). The periodontal probe may also be used to measure this deviation. Edge-to-edge bite relationships of the incisal surfaces of the maxillary and mandibular teeth should be noted.

An openbite exists when the maxillary and mandibular teeth cannot be occluded. There is an arching of the line of occlusion. This lack of normal vertical contact between opposing teeth is most often seen in the anterior region. These cases are usually the result of thumb- or finger-sucking habit or abnormal tongue position.

Surgical or clinical orthodontic treatment may be indicated for malocclusion or occlusal deviations. The patient shown in Figs. 2-52a to h had a Class II, division 1, deepbite. The surgical orthodontic procedure performed was a maxillary LeFort impaction (3-piece) with a sliding genioplasty to the mandible. The posttreatment cephalometric tracing illustrates the change in the palatal plane with the maxillary impaction procedure. Also illustrated is the autorotation upward and forward of the mandible.

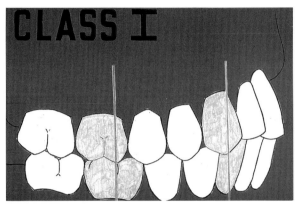

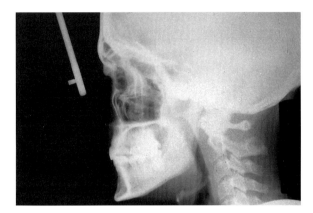

Figs. 2-45a and b   Courtesy of Dr. Harold T. Perry, North-western University, Chicago, Ill.

Figure 2-45b

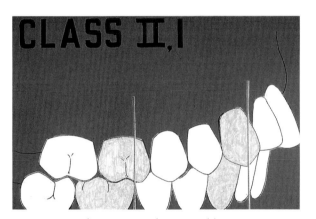

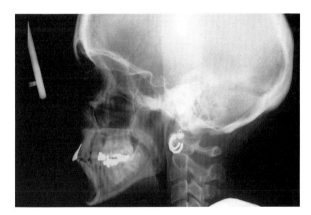

Figs. 2-46a to c   Courtesy of Dr. Harold T. Perry.

Figure 2-46b

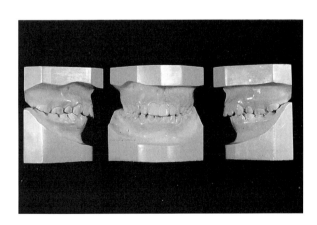

Figure 2-46c

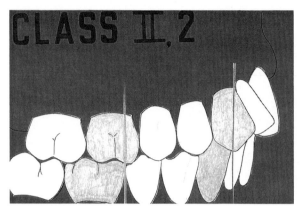

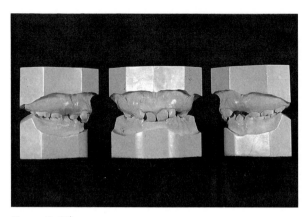

Figs. 2-47a and b   Courtesy of Dr. Harold T. Perry.

Figure 2-47b

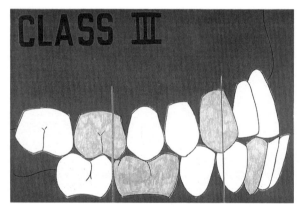

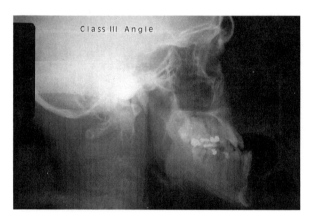

Figs. 2-48a to c   Courtesy of Dr. Harold T. Perry.

Figure 2-48b

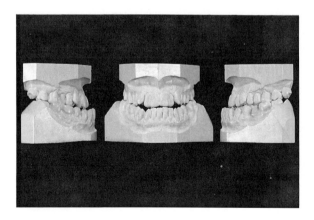

Figure 2-48c

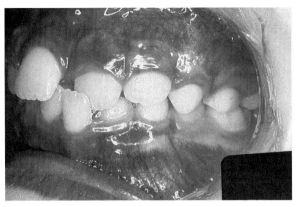

Fig. 2-49a Anterior crossbite. (Courtesy of Dr. Harold T. Perry.)

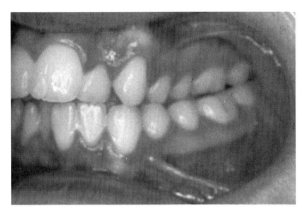

Fig. 2-49b Posterior crossbite.

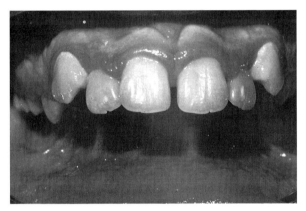

Fig. 2-50a Overjet. (Courtesy of Dr. Harold T. Perry.)

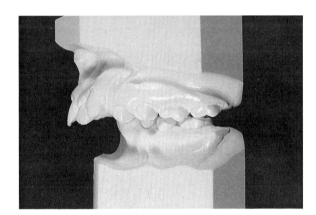

Fig. 2-50b Overjet.

Fig. 2-51 Overbite. (Courtesy of Dr. Harold T. Perry.)

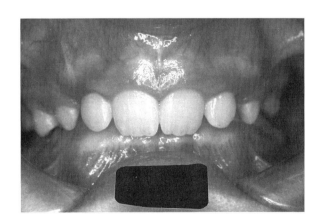

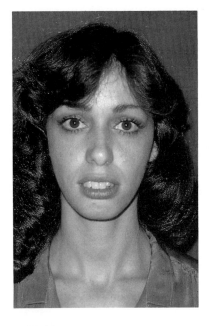 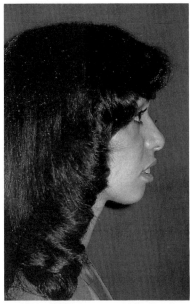

Fig. 2-52a   (left) Frontal view of patient before surgical procedure. (Courtesy of Dr. Roger Kallal, Northwestern University, Chicago, Ill.)

Fig. 2-52b   (right) Lateral view of patient before surgical procedure. (Courtesy of Dr. Roger Kallal.)

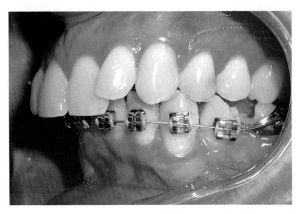 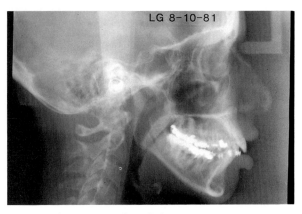

Fig. 2-52c Presurgical intraoral photograph of the maxillary-mandibular relationship. (Courtesy of Dr. Roger Kallal.)

Fig. 2-52d Presurgical cephalometric radiograph. (Courtesy of Dr. Roger Kallal.)

The dentition

The final aspect of health assessment documentation involves complete evaluation of the dentition. Identification and registration of pathological and nonpathological conditions and the presence of restorations and anomalies unique to each patient are important in treatment plan development. They also provide legal documentation related to the therapy and a source of identification in catastrophic occurrences.

Together the clinical findings and the radiographic findings present a pictorial diagnostic tool. Several types of graphic representation are used in dental charting. A geometric chart provides representations of the tooth surfaces with lines to indicate the marginal ridges and line angles (Fig. 2-53). The dental hygienist indicates the surfaces involved in disease or a restoration within the appropriate lines. Geometric charts do not provide for precise representation of the size of the lesion or particularities of the restoration.

An anatomic charting form involves the represen-

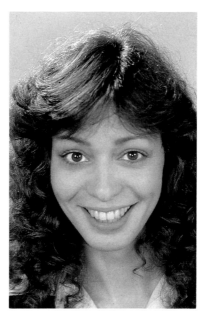

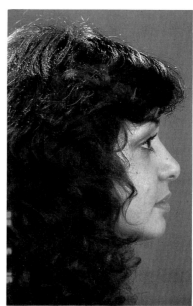

Fig. 2-52e (left) Frontal view of patient after surgical procedure. (Courtesy of Dr. Roger Kallal.)

Fig. 2-52f (right) Lateral view of patient after surgical procedure. (Courtesy of Dr. Roger Kallal.)

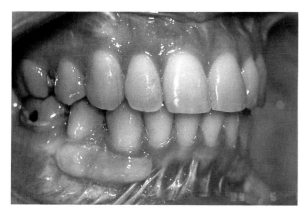

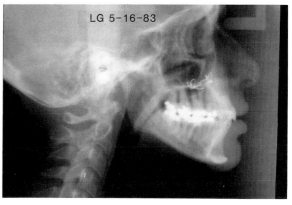

Fig. 2-52g Postsurgical intraoral photograph. (Courtesy of Dr. Roger Kallal.)

Fig. 2-52h Postsurgical cephalometric radiograph. (Courtesy of Dr. Roger Kallal.)

tation of each tooth. The crown and roots are depicted in several views so as to show the occlusal, facial, and lingual aspects (Fig. 2-54). When the presence of a lesion or restoration is indicated, precise descriptions may be drawn on the view of the teeth involved.

Tooth numbering systems The Universal System is the tooth numbering system most often used in dental charting. The numbering begins with the maxillary right third molar as number 1; the progression around the maxillary arch ends with the maxillary left third molar as number 16. The mandibular left third molar is then number 17; from left to right around the mandibular arch, the mandibular right third molar is number 32. In the primary dentition, small letters a through t are employed, starting with the maxillary right second primary molar (Fig. 2-55).

Less commonly used tooth numbering systems designate the quadrant in which a tooth is found. In the International System, numbers 1 through 4 indicate the quadrant, and numbers 1 through 8 indicate the tooth from incisor to third molar. In the Palmer Sys-

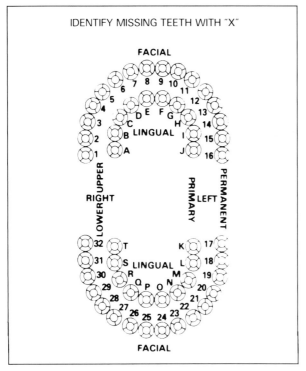

Figure 2-53

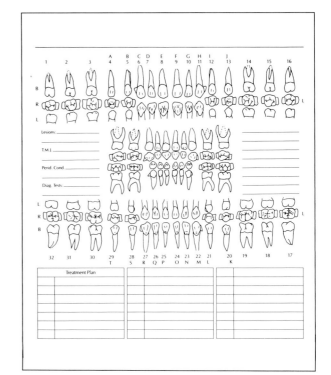

Figure 2-54

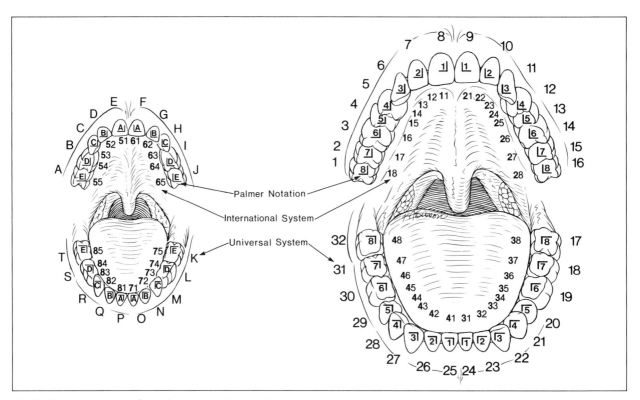

Fig. 2-55   Comparison of number systems for deciduous dentition (*left*) and adult dentition (*right*).

tem, the quadrants are designated by lines drawn alongside and above or below the tooth numbers.

To demonstrate a typical approach to the documentation of a dental chart, the Universal System of numbering and the anatomical form of chart will be employed because these are the most often used in dental practices.

A planned pattern of progression is suggested, beginning with tooth number 1 and proceeding sequentially to tooth number 32. The materials needed for the charting procedure are an intraoral mirror, an explorer, an air syringe, and black, blue, and red pencils. Pencils are used rather than pens to facilitate corrections.

Abnormalities In black pencil, the following abnormalities are noted: missing, tipped, or rotated teeth: submerged, unerupted, or impacted teeth; broken or fractured teeth; erosion, abrasion, attrition, and decalcification; open contacts, diastemata, dilacerated roots, and unusual contour of the gingival tissues (Fig. 2-56).

Missing teeth are indicated by a vertical line drawn through the tooth. The use of an X over the representation of the tooth is also a commonly utilized approach. Drifted or rotated teeth are represented by arrows indicating the direction in which the position is changed. An impacted tooth is indicated by a black curved line that indicates the presence of tissue over the tooth. A fractured tooth is indicated by drawing a black jagged line that represents the missing tooth structure. A tooth with abrasion or erosion is charted by drawing in black in the the location of the defect. Attrition—the gradual wearing away of tooth structure commonly found on mandibular anteriors of elderly patients—also is represented by drawing in black the tooth structure that has been worn away.

Hypoplastic defect or decalcification is notated by drawing black dots at the site of the involved area on the tooth. A diastema, frequently found between the maxillary central incisors, is depicted by two parallel lines indicating the space. If the measurement of the space is to be notated, a periodontal probe can be used as a millimeter ruler. A defective contact between two teeth is indicated by a zigzag black line. The presence of a dilacerated root is shown by drawing the deviation as it is seen on the radiographs. The presence of foreign bodies would also be indicated in black, usually by drawing some representation of the object.

Caries and other pathological conditions A red pencil is used to show carious lesions or other pathological conditions that require attention, such as retained root tips or abscesses (Fig. 2-57).

G.V. Black's classification is the standard method for classification of dental caries.[18]

Class I
Cavities in pits and fissures of the teeth: occlusal surfaces of premolars and molars.
Buccal and lingual surfaces of molars.
Lingual surfaces of maxillary incisors.
Class II
Cavities in the proximal surfaces of premolars and molars.
Class III
Cavities in proximal surfaces of incisors and canines not involving the incisal angle.
Class IV
Cavities in proximal surfaces of incisors or canines involving the incisal angle.
Class V
Cavities in the cervical one third of facial or lingual surfaces.

Carious lesions are represented by shading the area in red showing the approximate size of the lesion. Retained root tips are outlined in red to call attention to them, even though their presence may not be pathological in nature. Abscesses and periapical or nonperiapical rarefactions are indicated by charting a red circle above the roots of the tooth or in the area involved.

Existing restorations A blue pencil is used to show existing restorations that are in place and in good condition (Fig. 2-58). Amalgam restorations are outlined in blue and solidly filled in. The depiction should indicate the surfaces and approximate amount of tooth structure involved in the restoration. Esthetic filling materials such as composite resins are charted by outlining the restoration in blue and leaving it blank. Gold restorations, inlays, outlays, crowns, or foils are charted by outlining the restoration in blue and drawing diagonal parallel lines within the outline. Charting shows what is seen clinically: a full gold crown is charted to show entire coverage by the use of an outline and diagonal lines. A full crown with acrylic facing would have diagonal lines depicted on

1,5	Missing tooth		3&4,14&15	Defective contacts
16,17,32	Unerupted tooth		2	Etching
17	Impacted tooth		7	Abnormal tooth form
20,21	Rotated tooth		11,19	Dilacerated root
14,28	Extruded tooth		12,20,21	Abrasion
29	Submerged tooth		25,26,27,31	Attrition
Between 2&3,8&9,24&25	Open contacts		9,11	Erosion

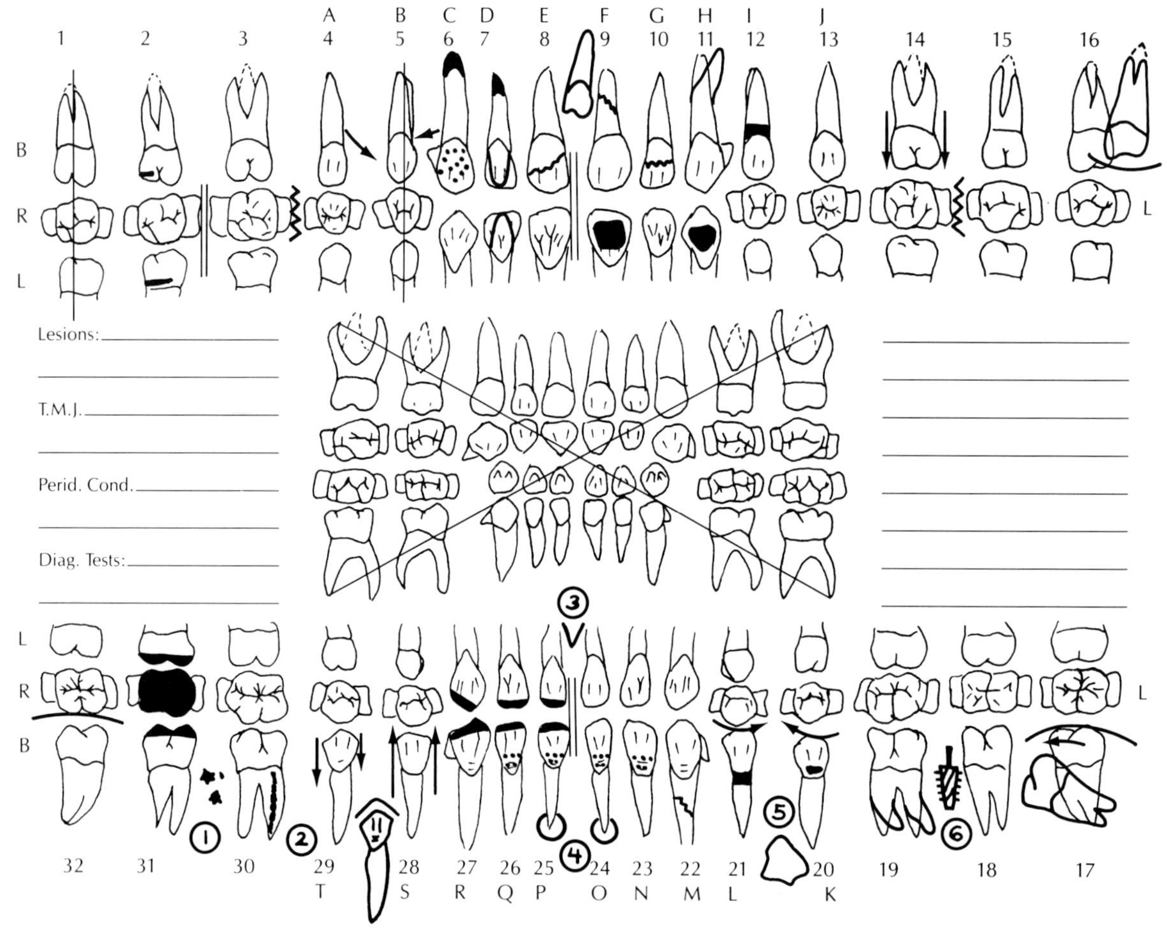

6,23,24,25,26	Hypoplastic defect		1.	Foreign body (amalgam)
6,7	Nonpathological root resorption		2.	Foreign body (broken endo file)
Between 8&9,28&29	Supernumerary tooth		3.	High lingual frenum
8,10	Fractured crown		4.	Cementoma
9,22	Fractured root		5.	Bone condensation
			6.	Foreign body (broken bur)

Fig. 2-56 Courtesy of Oral Diagnosis Department, Northwestern University, Chicago, Ill.

2,4,19	Class I caries	7,22	Cervical cementum caries
3,30	Buccal pit caries	16	Clinical crown destroyed by caries
2,7	Lingual pit caries	14	Retained root
3,4,19,20	Class II caries	3,4,7,19	Periapical rarefaction
6,7,8,9	Class III caries	Between 31&32	Nonperiapical rarefaction
8,10	Class IV caries	12,13	Root resorption due to
4,11	Class V caries		periapical rarefaction

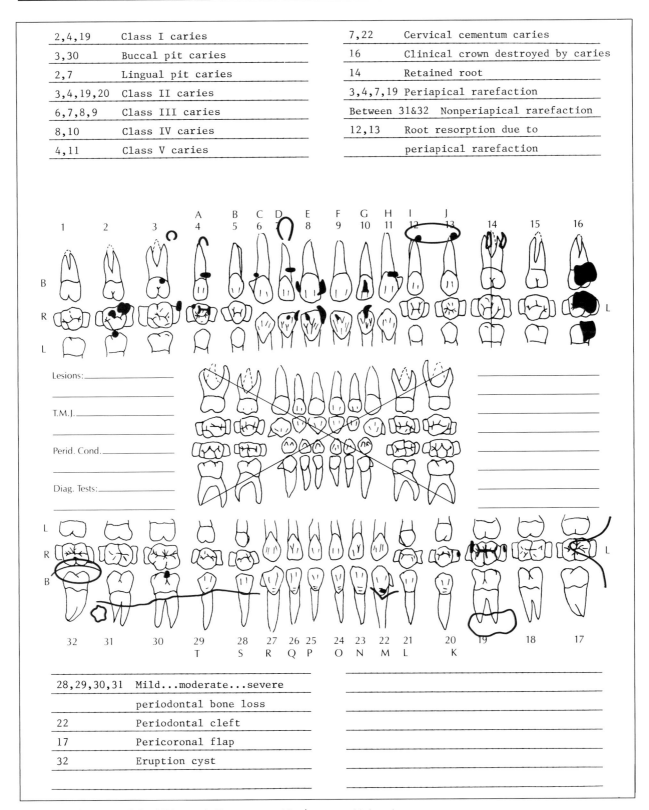

28,29,30,31	Mild...moderate...severe
	periodontal bone loss
22	Periodontal cleft
17	Pericoronal flap
32	Eruption cyst

Fig. 2-57 Courtesy of Oral Diagnosis Department, Northwestern University.

5,15	Class I restoration		4,9,11	Class V restoration
1,18	Buccal pit restoration		13,19,21,29	Full crown
3,8	Lingual pit restoration		19,21,29	Full crown with facing
2,3,14	Class II restoration		31	3/4 crown
2,3	Excess overhang		13	Post
7,8,9	Class III restoration		19 to 21	Fixed bridge
6,10	Class IV restoration		29 to 27	Cantilever bridge

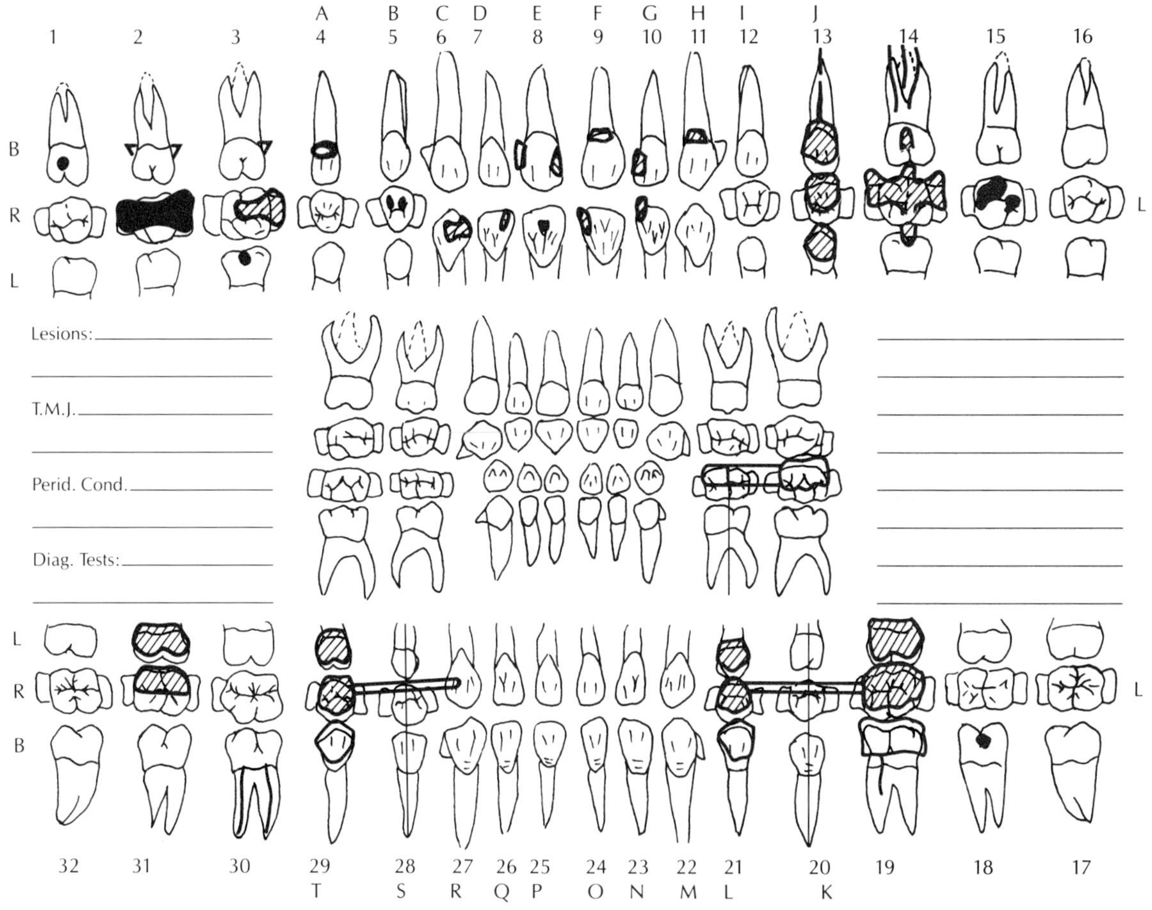

Lesions: _____
T.M.J. _____
Perid. Cond. _____
Diag. Tests: _____

13,14,30	Adequate root canal restoration
19	Inadequate root canal restoration
19	Defective crown
K to M	Space maintainer

Fig. 2-58   Courtesy of Oral Diagnosis Department, Northwestern University.

the occlusal and lingual views but blue outline on the facial surface, not filled in, indicating esthetic material used on the facial aspect. In this way, the reader of the chart has no difficulty determining the restorative materials present in this mouth.

Fixed partial dentures are indicated by drawing the restorations present on the abutment teeth and joining them by two horizontal lines in blue to indicate the presence of the partial denture. In Fig. 2-58, a black vertical line indicates that teeth 28 and 20 are missing, and the other notations indicate that the teeth have been replaced by fixed prostheses. Some fixed partial dentures have only one abutment. A cantilever prosthesis is indicated on teeth 29 to 27.

Also charted in blue are root canal fillings and space maintainers. Excess amounts of restorative material found in the interproximal area, designating overhangs, are labeled in blue on the appropriate interproximal space.

A complete approach to health assessment and documentation will provide the dental hygienist with a profile unique to each patient and is imperative to

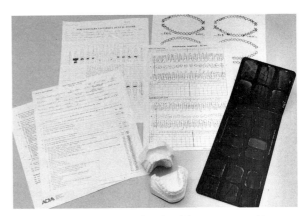

Fig. 2-59   Patient's complete health assessment file.

the formulation of the specific treatment plan for his or her dental health care delivery (Fig. 2-59). Supplementary components of the examination that may be employed for certain patients will be discussed in Chapter 4.

References

1. Ciancio, S.G. Prevention of bacterial endocarditis. Int. J. Periodont. Rest. Dent. 4(4):61–63, 1984.
2. Newman, M.G., and Goodman, A.D. (eds.) Guide to Antibiotic Use in Dental Practice. Chicago: Quintessence Publ. Co., 1984, pp. 144–150.
3. ADA Council on Dental Therapeutics. Bacterial endocarditis guidelines revised. ADA News, 99–100, 1985.
4. Burch, G.E., and Pasquale, N.P. Primer of Clinical Measurements of Blood Pressure. St. Louis: C.V. Mosby Co., 1962.
5. Maloney, K.L. The role of the auxiliary in hypertension screening. Quintessence J. 3(5):245–247, 1981.
6. Manzione, J.V., Katzberg, R.W., and Manzione, T.J. Internal derangements of the temporomandibular joint. I. Normal anatomy, physiology, and pathology. Int. J. Periodont. Rest. Dent. 4(4):9–16, 1984.
7. Manzione, J.V., Katzberg, R.W., and Manzione, T.J. Internal derangements of the temporomandibular joint. II. Diagnosis by arthography and computer tomography. Int. J. Periodont. Rest. Dent. 4(4):17–28, 1984.
8. American Cancer Society. Cancer Facts and Figures. New York: American Cancer Society, 1986.
9. Baker, H.W. Staging of cancer of the head and neck: oral cavity, pharynx, larynx, and paranasal sinuses. Ca-A Cancer J. Clin. 33(3):130–133, 1983.
10. Baker, G.W., et al. Cancer of the Head and Neck. Chicago: American Cancer Society, 1983, pp. 5–8.
11. Baker, G.W., et al. Oral Cancer. Chicago: American Cancer Society, 1973, pp. 6–10.
12. McKenna, R.J. Tumors of the Major and Minor Salivary Glands. Chicago: American Cancer Society, 1983, pp. 12–18.
13. Mashberg, A., and Garfinkel, L. Early Diagnosis of Oral Cancer: the Erythroplastic Lesion in High Risk Sites. Chicago: American Cancer Society, 1978, pp. 3–6.
14. O'Leary, T.J., Drake, R.B., and Naylor, J.E. The plaque control record. J. Periodontol. 43:38, 1972.
15. Greene, J.C., and Vermillion, J.R. The simplified oral hygiene index. J. Am. Dent. Assoc. 68(7):25–31, 1964.
16. Ramfjord, S.P. The periodontal disease index (PDI). J. Periodontol. 38:602–609, 1967.
17. Löe, H. The gingival index: the plaque index and the retention index systems. J. Periodontol. 38:610–614, 1967.
18. Blackwell, R.E. G.V. Black's Operative Dentistry. Volume 2, 9th ed. Milwaukee: Medico-Dental Publ. Co., 1955, pp. 1–4.

chapter 3

Preparation for emergencies

Treatment of dental patients requires knowledge about all aspects of dental treatment and management, whether routine or emergent in nature. Comprehensive dental therapy includes the application of current procedures for combating existing oral diseases or conditions. It also encompasses prevention and treatment of medical emergency situations should they occur in the dental office. A medical emergency is a sudden, urgent, usually unforeseen circumstance that requires immediate attention. This chapter provides an overview of the prevention and treatment processes for handling medical emergencies.

Stress and anxiety

The detection of a potential medical emergency requires dental personnel to be alert to signs of anxiety, stress, or fear exhibited by the patient prior to receiving dental treatment. These are usually the result of the patient's fear of the pain often associated with a dental appointment. Patients must be assured that pain incurred while undergoing dental treatment is controllable by a variety of techniques. The fear of pain, however, may be more difficult to address than the actual pain.[1] Therefore, the dental team must be skilled in anxiety management.

A dental auxiliary is usually the first person the patient encounters in the operatory. The auxiliary must be able to quickly assess the anxiety level of the patient. If the patient does not appear anxious, the auxiliary is free to continue with routine health assessment duties.

An anxious person is defined as someone apprehensive of perceived danger. This apprehension is accompanied by restlessness, tension, and a rapid heart rate, none of which can be attributed to a clearly identifiable stimulus. It disturbs the patient and keeps him or her in a state of uneasiness. The symptoms and signs of an anxious person include elevated blood pressure, sweaty palms, excessive talking, a flushed face, and the verbal expression of fear.

Several methods are available that may prove helpful in anxiety management. Scheduling appointments in the morning will help to decrease the time the patient has during the day to anticipate the pending appointment. Minimizing the time between the patient's arrival at the dental office and actual dental treatment is essential. If this time interval is controlled, the patient's mounting fears and anxiety brought on by antiseptic smells, or the sight and noise of dental equipment (such as syringes and high-speed handpieces), will not be as profound. Another technique to reduce anxiety involves the use of medication before the patient arrives at the dental office. Premedication with a mild tranquilizer, such as diazepam, can provide a light level of sedation that may be helpful in the control of anxiety.[2]

Adequate pain control during the appointment is extremely important in allaying the patient's fear and anxiety at subsequent dental appointments. Employment of nitrous oxide inhalation analgesia alone or in combination with anesthetic administration may make the anxious patient more comfortable during involved dental procedures. Selection of a particular anxiety reduction method is dependent upon the needs of the particular patient.

Emergencies

Despite the most careful screening efforts, the office staff may still be confronted with a life-threatening emergency. Therefore, all dental personnel should be able to recognize the signs associated with specific medical emergencies and should possess the skills needed to effectively and efficiently manage each emergency.

These skills include certification in basic life support, or CPR (cardiopulmonary resuscitation). The preparation of staff members in basic life support is the most significant prerequisite to be completed before an office emergency system can be established.[2] Many emergencies in the dental office can be managed solely through the use of basic life support and without the initiation of drug therapy.

Office personnel should also be trained in the securing of vital signs, namely, blood pressure, pulse, and respiration. The recording of vital signs can be utilized routinely as a screening tool or as a means to monitor the condition of a patient in an emergency.

In addition to the certification of all dental office personnel in basic life support skills, other steps in the preparation of a dental office for emergencies include:

1. The utilization of the team approach in handling emergencies.
2. The compilation of an office emergency manual.
3. The development of a specific plan of action or protocol to be initiated in the event of an emergency and the periodic rehearsal of this plan in simulated emergency situations.
4. The acquisition of emergency equipment, including an emergency kit.

Team approach

The team approach is considered the most effective method to treat emergencies that occur in the dental office. Should a crisis situation arise, each member of the team assumes specific duties. All employees should consider the extent of their professional educations and accept only the duties that they have the knowledge and the ability to perform. These duties must be decided upon at a meeting between the dentist and the staff and relayed in detail to each new employee. All emergency telephone numbers, including the nearest hospital and ambulance service,

should be obtained and posted in strategic areas around the office and beside each telephone.

With the entire team trained in basic life support, each individual member should be able to sustain life until trained medical personnel arrive. In most cases, the dentist accepts the major role in rendering emergency care and will direct the actions of the other team members. The dentist also assumes the primary responsibility of administering any necessary drugs to the patient.

All auxiliary personnel, if properly trained, can initiate and assist in performing CPR. One team member should be delegated the responsibility of retrieving the emergency kit and assisting in the preparation of drugs for administration, as instructed by the dentist. This member could also monitor the vital signs of the patient or notify medical authorities of the emergency. Another team member should be available to assist with emergency treatment as needed or to notify medical authorities. All other team members should be alert and available to aid those actively managing the emergency situation.

Office emergency manual

Emergency procedures should be recorded in the form of an office manual. The staff should meet to discuss exactly what information the manual will contain and how it will be organized. The manual should be designed to meet the needs of the individual office in a crisis situation. The manual should be placed in a central area where it is easily and quickly accessible for reference. While the specific manual will be unique to each individual office, certain items should be included in every emergency manual. These are listed in Fig. 3-1.

Emergency plan of action

The office emergency plan should be devised to accommodate any medical emergency. The staff should know the locations of all emergency exits and these exits should be well marked or lighted for easy recognition. The emergency protocol should be reexamined every few months to ensure its accuracy, and it should be revised when indicated.

A less-often utilized but critical step in the preparation of a dental office for an emergency is the rehearsal of the office emergency plan. Conducting regular drills will allow the members of the dental

TABLE OF CONTENTS

Emergency Telephone Numbers
   Ambulance Service
   Fire Department
   Hospital
   Physician
   Police

Emergency Equipment
   Emergency Kit
   Adjunctive Equipment
   Oxygen Delivery System

Emergency Protocol
   Notification of Medical Personnel
   Direction of Trained Medical Personnel Upon
     Arrival
   Transport of Emergency Kit to Scene of Emergency
   Periodic Check of Expiration Dates of
     Emergency Drugs
   Periodic Check of Oxygen Cylinders to Be Sure
     Tanks Are Full
   Update of Information in Emergency Manual
   Indications for Use of Emergency Drugs and
     Oxygen

Fig. 3-1   From *Office Emergency Procedures—Self-Study Course.* American Dental Hygienists' Association and Block Drug Company, 1979.

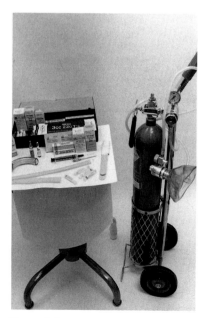

Figure 3-2

team to practice their duties in simulated office emergency situations. If the staff is familiar with the office protocol, they will more likely respond immediately in a well organized manner to manage any emergency. This will ensure a greater chance of patient survival in the event of an actual emergency.

Emergency equipment

Emergency equipment for the dental office consists of an oxygen delivering system and an emergency kit (Fig. 3-2). Standard first-aid supplies, such as gauze and bandages, should also be available for use.

Oxygen delivering systems   Oxygen is used routinely in dental office emergencies. Possible indications for oxygen use in emergency situations are to treat hypoxia and to establish or maintain respiration.[3] The methods for oxygen delivery include (1) exhaled air ventilation, (2) atmospheric air ventilation, (3) enriched oxygen ventilation, and (4) positive pressure oxygen ventilation.[4]

1. When an emergency situation occurs, the primary rescuer must determine the state of consciousness of the patient. If the patient is unresponsive and unconscious, the rescuer should secure an open airway and check for breathing. If apnea occurs—that is, the absence of spontaneous respiration—the rescuer would provide the patient with two full ventilations by pinching the nostrils and sealing his or her mouth over the mouth of the patient (Fig. 3-3). The rescuer would then check the carotid pulse of an adult or the brachial pulse of an infant (Fig. 3-4). If a palpable pulse is absent, the rescuer should begin chest compression. If a palpable pulse is present, the rescuer should administer artificial respiration.

Artificial ventilations provide the patient with air containing 16% oxygen. They are applied once every 5 seconds (12 times per minute), on an adult and one every 3 seconds (20 times per minute) on an infant. This procedure would be continued until the patient recovers or trained medical personnel arrive. This technique of artificial respiration is known as the mouth-to-mouth technique.

Mouth-to-nose ventilations can be effectively utilized when the mouth-to-mouth technique does not allow for proper ventilation. A patent airway must be maintained at all times. The rescuer places his or her mouth over the patient's nose and ventilates with the lips of the patient sealed. The same ventilation rates used in mouth-to-mouth ventilations are used in the mouth-to-nose technique.

2. Atmospheric air ventilation delivers air with 20% to 21% oxygen to the patient. This method is accomplished through the use of a device called the self-inflating bag-valve-mask unit. One such device commonly utilized in dental office emergencies is known as an Ambu bag. The rescuer, after securing a patent airway, would use one hand to stabilize and tightly seal the mask around the patient's mouth. The other hand would squeeze the bag to provide the ventilations. The ventilations would be applied at a rate of once every 5 seconds for an adult and once every 3 seconds for an infant.

If properly trained, all dental office personnel can safely and effectively use the self-inflating bag-valve-mask unit to administer oxygen. An advantage of this unit is that it can be easily transported to any part of the dental office, because emergencies can occur in places other than in the operatory.

3. The enriched oxygen ventilation method uses oxygen from tanks or cylinders colored green to differentiate them from tanks containing other gases. The cylinders have a regulator that controls the pressure of the oxygen being delivered to the patient. The regulator has a pin index safety system designed to control the pins that fit into the cylinder outlet valve. The configuration of the pins is such that they will fit only into the outlet valve designated for the particular gas being utilized. This system prevents the inadvertant exchange of various gases.

Cylinders are available in various sizes from 2¼ by 11 inches (AA cylinder) to 9 by 55 inches (H cylinder). The size most commonly utilized by dental personnel is the E cylinder, which is 4¼ by 29¾ inches and contains 22 cubic feet of oxygen.[3] This cylinder fits into a mobile stand that allows it to be easily transported to all areas of the office (Fig. 3-5).

4. Positive pressure oxygen is administered by depressing a button on the face mask. Oxygen from the E cylinder can also be delivered on demand to assist patients who are not capable of maintaining respiration. The rate of respiration is once every 5 seconds (12 times per minute) for an adult and once every 3 seconds (20 times per minute) for an infant.

When oxygen is delivered from compressed cylinders, the amount of oxygen in the tank must be carefully monitored. The tank will be useless in an

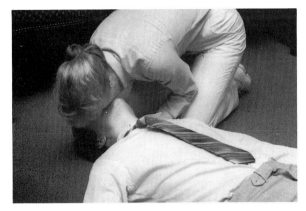

Figure 3-3

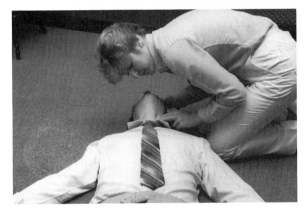

Figure 3-4

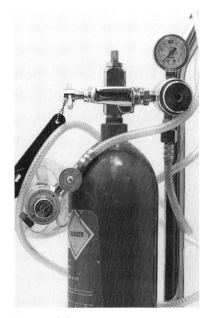

Fig. 3-5 Oxygen delivery system.

Table 3-1 Sample emergency drug list for oral or intramuscular administration

Drug	Indication(s) for use	Dosage	Suggested supply for emergency kit
Epinephrine	Anaphylaxis	0.01 mg/kg subcutaneously or intramuscularly	
Diphenhydramine (Benadryl)	Anaphylaxis	25 to 50 mg intramuscularly	2 doses of 50 mg/ml
Methylprednisolone	Anaphylaxis Aspiration Shock	125 mg or more intramuscularly	2 doses of 125 mg/vial
Nitroglycerin	Angina pectoris	0.3 mg (1/200 grain) to 0.6 mg (1/100 grain) sublingually (0.4 mg, 1/150 most common)	100 tablets 0.4 mg
Metaproterenol	Mild bronchial asthma	One inhalation 0.65 mg repeated every 3 minutes up to three inhalations	Two inhalers
Hard candy, juice	Insulin reaction		1 or 2 rolls of candy 2 to 3 cans

Source: Adapted from W.H. Davis. Emergency drugs and allergy, pp. 266–268. *In* F.M. McCarthy (ed.) Medical Emergencies in Dentistry: Emergencies in Dental Practice, abr. ed. Philadelphia: W.B. Saunders Co., 1982.

Table 3-2 Adjunctive equipment

Equipment	Description	Suggested quantity
Oxygen delivery system	Self-inflating bag-valve mask E Cylinder of oxygen Clear face masks	1 to 2 cylinders 1 small (child) size 1 large (adult) size
	Valve for positive pressure oxygen	
Suction and suction tips	Large-diameter, round-ended suction tips or tonsil suction tips (high volume suction)	Two
Syringes for drug	Disposable syringes	3 to 4 syringes, 5 ml, with 18- or 21-gauge needle
Needles	Disposable needles for intramuscular injections Intravenous needles	
Intravenous infusion sets		
Tourniquets	Rubber tourniquet or latex tubing	
Sphygmomanometer		
Stethoscope		
Artificial airways	Oral Nasal	
Alcohol sponges		

Sources: Adapted from F.M. McCarthy. Medical Emergencies in Dentistry: Emergencies in Dental Practice, abr. ed. Philadelphia: W.B. Saunders Co., 1982; S.F. Malamed. Handbook of Medical Emergencies in the Dental Office, 2nd ed. St. Louis: C.V. Mosby Co., 1982, p. 49.

Table 3-3 Sample emergency drug list for intravenous administration (I.V. sedation used)

Drug	Indication(s) for use	Dosage	Suggested supply for emergency kit
Metaproterenol	Mild bronchial asthma	One inhalation 0.65 mg repeated every 3 minutes up to three inhalations	Two inhalers
Nitroglycerin (Nitrostat)	Angina pectoris	0.4 mg sublingually (1/150 grains)	100 tablets 0.4 mg
Diazepam (Valium)	Status epilepticus or severe recurrent convulsions	5 mg/min intravenously (if possible) until seizures are controlled	10 doses of 5 mg/ml
Naloxone (Narcan)	Reversing narcotic excess	Titrate 0.1 mg intravenously every 2 minutes until desired effect	5 doses of 0.4 mg/ml
Dextrose 50%	Hypoglycemic coma Initial use in any seizure disorder	50 mg intravenously	3 doses of 2.5 mg/50 ml
Dextrose 5% in Water	Diluting drugs for slow intravenous dosage, for correction of hypovolemia, for maintaining a patent intravenous route		2 units of 500 ml
Epinephrine	Severe bronchospasm Anaphylaxis	0.01 mg/kg 0.01 mg/kg	
Diphenhydramine (Benadryl)	Anaphylaxis (not for asthma)	25 to 50 mg intramuscularly or slowly intravenously	2 doses of 50 mg/ml
Methylprednisolone (Solu/Medrol)	Anaphylaxis Asthma Aspiration Shock	125 mg or more intramuscularly or intravenously	3 doses of 125 mg/vial
Atropine	Marked bradycardia accompanied by hypotension that is symptomatic	0.5 mg as an intravenous bolus repeated as necessary	4 doses of 0.4 or 0.5 mg/ml
Morphine	Myocardial infarction or acute pulmonary edema	10 to 15 mg intramuscularly or 5 to 10 mg intravenously	3 doses of 10 mg/ml

Source: Adapted from W.H. Davis. Emergency drugs and allergy, pp. 266–268. *In* F.M. McCarthy (ed.) Medical Emergencies in Dentistry: Emergencies in Dental Practice, abr. ed. Philadelphia: W.B. Saunders Co., 1982.

emergency situation if it is empty. For maximum safety, cylinders should be changed when the controls read below 500 psi.[3]

The amount of oxygen a cylinder can deliver during an emergency should be noted. Use of an E cylinder provides sufficient oxygen to administer approximately 30 minutes of positive pressure breathing.[4] Once the oxygen supply has been depleted, other means of oxygen delivery must be employed until a full tank is available or until the patient's breathing is restored.

Emergency kit A number of drugs that may be utilized in the management of emergencies should be kept in the office emergency kit, along with other adjunctive equipment. The emergency kit should be designed to include medications that the dentist is capable of administering comfortably to a patient. He or she should be knowledgeable about the indications for use of each drug, its route of administration, and its dosage. Tables 3-1 and 3-3 summarize the emergency drugs to be administered orally, intramuscularly, and intravenously. Table 3-2 lists adjunctive equipment suggested for inclusion in a dental office emergency kit.

Medical-legal considerations

A complete written record of all treatment rendered in an emergency situation should be kept for legal purposes. This record should include:

1. Time of onset of emergency.
2. Symptoms observed.
3. Vital signs of patient.
4. Basic life support rendered.
5. Drugs administered by the dentist, time given, dosage, and route of administration.
6. Comments regarding reaction of patient to the drug or overall patient condition.[5]

A thorough treatment record will ensure that the dentist and his office staff are protected in the event of possible litigation.

Basic life support

Members of the dental health care team should practice basic life support techniques only after they have been certified through an accepted course given by the American Heart Association or the American Red Cross. Basic life support is the phase of emergency cardiac care that either (1) prevents respiratory or circulatory arrest through prompt recognition and intervention or (2) externally supports the respiration or circulation of a victim through artificial ventilations or cardiopulmonary resuscitation (CPR).[6] Basic life support also emphasizes early entry into the emergency medical services system (EMS).

The steps of CPR

As illustrated in Fig. 3-6, the steps of CPR include:

1. Establishing unresponsiveness.
2. Calling for help (entry into the EMS system).
3. Positioning the victim.

These should be followed by the ABCs of CPR:

4. **A**irway
   a. Open the airway.
   b. Determine status of respiration (present, impaired, or absent).

5. **B**reathing
   a. Restore breathing through artificial respiration.
   b. Check for foreign body airway obstruction.
6. **C**irculation
   a. Establish presence or absence of a pulse.
   b. If pulse is absent, restore circulation by beginning chest compressions.[6]

These steps should be started immediately and continued until one of the following occurs:

1. The patient recovers.
2. The resuscitation effort is transferred to another person who continues CPR.
3. A physician assumes responsibility.
4. The resuscitation effort is transferred to trained medical personnel.
5. The rescuer becomes totally exhausted and is unable to continue.[6]

The steps of CPR should be performed only after it has been determined that the patient is unconscious. This is accomplished by tapping or lightly shaking the patient's shoulder and shouting near the ear to arouse him or her. If the patient does not respond, the rescuer should activate the EMS system by designating another member of the office staff to telephone for help.

The rescuer should then position the patient on his or her back on a firm, horizontal surface. If the patient is face down, the rescuer must be careful to roll the patient as a unit so as not to cause any neck or spinal injury. The time allowed to recognize unconsciousness is 4 to 10 seconds.

Airway   The airway should be opened using the head tilt–chin lift method. The rescuer places one hand on the patient's forehead to maintain the head tilt. The fingers of the other hand are placed under the bony part of the mandible on the side closest to the rescuer (Fig. 3-6, 1). The rescuer lifts upward and forward until the teeth are nearly closed, taking care to lift the jaw so as not to obstruct the airway. The rescuer's thumb may be used to open the lips to allow free air passage. This replaces the previous technique of head tilt (Fig. 3-7).

If the head tilt–chin lift maneuver is not effective in opening the airway, alternative methods may be employed, such as the jaw thrust. This is the preferred choice when a mask is used.

This is accomplished by the rescuer's placing both

Cardiopulmonary Resuscitation (CPR)

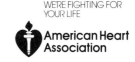
Place victim flat on his/her back on a hard surface.

1 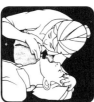 ### If unconscious, open airway.

Head-tilt/chin-lift.

2 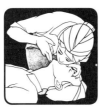 ### If not breathing, begin rescue breathing.

Give 2 full breaths. If airway is blocked,
reposition head and try again to give breaths.
If still blocked,
perform abdominal thrusts (Heimlich maneuver).

3 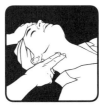 ### Check carotid pulse.

4 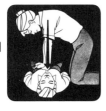 ### If there is no pulse, begin chest compressions.

Depress sternum 1½ to 2 inches.
Perform 15 compressions (rate: 80–100 per minute)
to every 2 full breaths.

Continue uninterrupted until advanced life support is available.

Fig. 3-6   The steps of CPR. (Reprinted with permission. © The American Heart Association.)

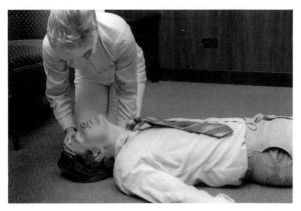

Fig. 3-7   Head tilt.

hands under the angles of the patient's lower jaw (mandible) and lifting upward while tilting the head backward. The rescuer can then use his or her thumbs to open the patient's mouth. In cases of suspected neck injury, a modified jaw thrust maneuver should be performed. The technique is the same as the jaw thrust maneuver except that the neck is not extended backward.

Breathing   Once a patent airway is secured, the rescuer should establish the presence or absence of breathing in 3 to 5 seconds. The rescuer should *look* toward the victim's chest to see if it is rising and falling, *listen* for air escaping during exhalation, and *feel* for the flow of air on the side of his or her cheek. Many times an open airway is all that is needed for a patient to begin breathing. If this is the case, the rescuer should maintain the open airway and monitor the patient until trained medical personnel arrive. If the rescuer determines that the patient is not breathing, then he or she should begin artificial respiration.

Initially the rescuer should administer two slow full breaths, allowing for full deflation of the lungs between breaths. The rescuer does this by pinching the nostrils of the patient and sealing his or her mouth completely over the patient's mouth. Following the two full breaths, the rescuer should check the carotid pulse of an adult or child patient and the brachial pulse of an infant for 5 to 10 seconds. If a palpable pulse is present, the rescuer should continue with artificial ventilations, providing one breath every 5 seconds for an adult (12 times per minute), one breath every 4 seconds for a child (15 times per minute), and

one breath every 3 seconds for an infant (20 times per minute).

Circulation   Artificial circulation can be created through the use of external cardiac compressions. External cardiac compression consists of rhythmic pressure over the lower portion of the sternum to compress the heart between the sternum and the spine. External cardiac compression should always be utilized in conjunction with artificial respiration. When cardiac arrest occurs, circulation stops, the pulse disappears, and breathing stops at the same time or shortly thereafter. Both artificial respiration and artificial circulation are required to oxygenate the blood and circulate it to the tissues throughout the body. These emergency techniques are required immediately in the case of cardiac arrest to prevent irreversible brain damage. This condition may occur if the brain is deprived of oxygen for a period of 4 to 6 minutes.

If a palpable pulse cannot be obtained, the rescuer should position himself or herself next to the chest of the victim with his or her knees shoulder-width apart. The hand closest to the patient's feet is used to trace the margin of the rib cage. The rescuer follows along the rib margin to the substernal notch, where the ribs meet the sternum (Figs. 3-8a and b). The middle finger is placed into it. The heel of the other hand is placed next to the index finger on the lower half of the sternum. The fingers of the two hands may be interlocked to keep the fingers off the chest wall (Fig. 3-9). Hand position must be checked each time the rescuer returns to the patient's chest to perform compressions. Great care must be taken to avoid compressing over the xiphoid process, as this may cause laceration of the internal organs, such as the liver.

Once the correct hand placement is determined, the rescuer should straighten both elbows by locking them and position his or her shoulders directly over the hands. This will ensure that the force of the compressions is directed straight down. Pressure is then exerted to depress the sternum of the adult 1½ to 2 inches. Relaxation should follow compression without changing hand positions. This will permit adequate cardiac refill. The compressions should be smooth, even, and uninterrupted. Bouncing or jerking compressions must be avoided because they are less effective and more likely to cause injury.

A single rescuer should perform artificial respiration and artificial circulation at a 15:2 ratio. This consists of two lung inflations after each set of 15 chest compressions. To achieve optimal effectiveness, the rescuer should perform four cycles of the 15:2 ratio in approximately 1 minute. This is accomplished at a rate of 80 to 100 compressions per minute.

The rescuer should palpate the pulse of the patient periodically to check the effectiveness of the compressions while performing CPR and should determine whether or not the patient resumes spontaneous breathing and circulation. The pulse should be checked after the first minute of CPR and every few minutes thereafter.

Two-rescuer CPR is taught primarily to health care and emergency medical professionals. When two such individuals arrive together at an emergency situation and CPR is not in progress, one rescuer activates the EMS system to summon medical assistance. The other rescuer assumes responsibility for assessing unresponsiveness, positioning the victim, opening the airway, and evaluating breathing.

If the victim is breathless, the rescuer ventilates twice slowly, observing the rise of the chest and allowing for exhalation between breaths. If the rescuer observes adequate chest rise and does not detect air resistance, she/he will check the carotid pulse. In the interim, the other rescuer locates the correct anatomic landmarks on the victim's chest, in preparation for administering chest compressions. If the first rescuer states that no pulse is present, the second rescuer begins chest compressions at a rate of 80 to 100 per minute. After five compressions, the second rescuer pauses in order to allow the first rescuer to give one slow breath. The ratio of compressions to breaths is 5:1. A count of "one and two and three and four and five and breathe" is established to help the second rescuer maintain a smooth, even rhythm and allow a pause for the breath. Ten cycles of five compressions to one ventilation should take 40 to 53 seconds (Fig. 3-10).

When the second rescuer becomes tired, she/he may call for a switch by saying "change and one and two and three and four and five and breathe." The switch occurs at the completion of the cycle, when the second rescuer completes the fifth compression. She/he quickly moves to the position at the victim's head. The first rescuer completes the cycle by giving a breath, and then moves to the position at the victim's chest. The second rescuer opens the airway and assesses breathing and pulse for five seconds. During the pulse check, the first rescuer locates the proper landmarks on the victim's chest and waits for direc-

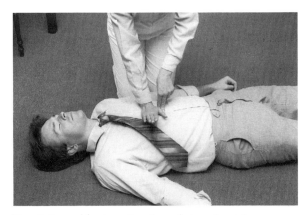

Figs. 3-8a and b   Locating the substernal notch.

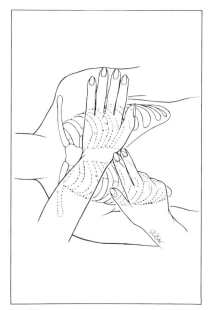

Figure 3-8b

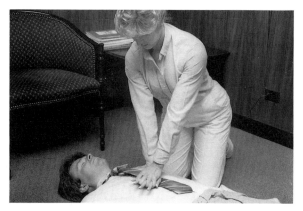

Figure 3-9

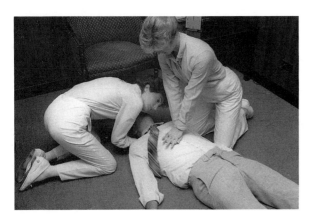

Figure 3-10

tions. If the second rescuer determines that the victim is still pulseless, she/he says "no pulse," gives one ventilation, and says "continue compressions" or "continue CPR."

Two-rescuer CPR may be performed with both rescuers on the same side of the victim, but it is most effective when rescuers are on opposite sides of the victim, to facilitate switching positions.

The rescuers should check for spontaneous pulse and respiration after every few minutes of CPR. The rescuer at the patient's head also has the responsibility to check the effectiveness of the compressions of the second rescuer. If an artificial pulse is not detected, the rescuer at the chest should be instructed to check his or her technique.

CPR for children

CPR for children includes the same basic procedures as CPR for adults with a few slight modifications. In general, CPR technique is determined by the size of the child. The technique for children is performed from the ages of 1 to 8 years. After 8 years of age, adult procedures apply. When providing rescue breathing to a child, the rescuer should deliver one breath every 4 seconds, instead of one breath every 5 seconds. When providing chest compressions, the same anatomic landmarks utilized for adults are employed for children. However, using both hands to provide chest compressions is not necessary. For children, the heel of one hand provides adequate compression. The sternum should be depressed 1 to 1½ inches. The compression rate is 80 to 100

compressions per minute and the ratio is 5 : 1 (five compressions to one breath).

Airway obstruction

When respiratory difficulties are caused by a foreign body obstruction, the following procedures should be utilized to properly manage conscious and unconscious victims (Fig. 3-11). If the victim is conscious and can speak, cough, or breathe, interference is not required. If the victim is conscious and displays the universal choking sign (hand to the throat), then the correct sequence to follow is to deliver six to ten abdominal thrusts, known as the Heimlich Maneuver. If the victim is conscious but obese or pregnant, chest thrusts should be delivered.

An unconscious choking victim is managed by first opening the airway and attempting to ventilate. If this attempt to ventilate is unsuccessful, the rescuer will feel resistance. The rescuer should then reposition the head in order to secure an open airway and then attempt to ventilate again. If ventilation attempts fail, the rescuer should administer six to ten abdominal thrusts, perform a finger sweep in the mouth, and attempt to reventilate. A finger sweep is performed on a child only if the foreign object is visible. This sequence should be continued until the foreign body is expelled or advanced life support is available.

Specific emergency situations

Basic life support skills provide a foundation for the management of a number of specific emergency situations that may occur in the dental office. Some of those most often encountered are listed and described below and on the following pages.

Altered states of consciousness

CEREBRAL VASCULAR ACCIDENT (STROKE)
A neurological disorder resulting from the destruction of brain substance due to intracerebral hemorrhage, embolism, cerebral vascular thrombosis, or cerebral vascular insufficiency.

Symptoms and Signs—Neurologic Abnormalities
– altered mental status (confusion to coma)
– visual change (blurred to blindness)

FIRST AID FOR CHOKING

CALL-FOR-HELP NUMBER:
_____

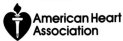

WE'RE FIGHTING FOR YOUR LIFE

American Heart Association

CONSCIOUS VICTIM

1 Ask the victim: "Are you choking?"
If the victim can speak, cough, or breathe, do not interfere.

2 If the victim cannot speak, cough, or breathe,
apply subdiaphragmatic abdominal thrusts (the Heimlich maneuver)
until the foreign body is expelled or the victim becomes unconscious.

IF VICTIM BECOMES UNCONSCIOUS

1  Open mouth and perform finger sweep.

2 Open airway and try to ventilate.

3 If unsuccessful, apply 6-10 subdiaphragmatic abdominal thrusts.

BE PERSISTENT

Activate the EMS system as soon as possible.

Repeat sequence: thrusts, finger sweep, attempt to ventilate.

Continue uninterrupted until advanced life support is available.

Fig. 3-11   Managing patients with airway obstruction. (Reprinted with permission. © The American Heart Association.)

– weakness (facial and/or extremity, usually unilateral)
– numbness (unilateral)
– speech change (slurred, difficulty with word choice or language syntax)
– incoordination
– dizziness

Symptoms and Signs—Systemic Abnormalities
– tachycardia
– hypertension
– hyperventilation

Management
– Terminate dental procedures.
– Support vital signs (ABCs).
– Administer oxygen.
– Keep patient upright and comfortable.
– Notify and transport to hospital (paramedics).

DIABETIC KETOACIDOSIS

Clinical hyperglycemic syndrome that occurs when there is a relative lack of insulin. This insulin deficiency (in untreated diabetics and/or in treated diabetics with increased insulin requirements secondary to emotional stress, infection, trauma, or heart attack) causes hyperglycemia with a resulting urinary osmotic diuresis (increased urinary output), hypovolemia leading to shock, and increased fatty acid metabolism resulting in ketone production and acidosis.

Symptoms and Signs
– dizziness (hypovolemia)
– thirst (dehydration)
– polyuria (increased urinary output)
– stomach pain with nausea and vomiting (acidosis)
– chest pain (stress-induced myocardial infarction)
– mental status changes (shock, ketoacidosis)
– fruity, sweet breath (ketosis)
– tachycardia, dry cool skin, hypotension (hypovolemic shock)

Management
– Support vital signs (ABCs).
– Administer oxygen.
– Treat for shock (supine position, warmth).
– Administer intravenous fluids (normal saline).
– Notify and transport to hospital (paramedics).

HYPERGLYCEMIC HYPEROSMOLAR NONKETOTIC COMA (HHNK)

Clinical hyperglycemic syndrome typically occurring in the elderly with mild diabetes and multiple medical problems and an insulin deficiency that induces hyperglycemia without ketosis. As blood glucose rises, urinary osmotic diuresis (increased urinary output) induces dehydration and very high serum glucose levels, which in turn induce a hyperosmolar state. The combination of whole body dehydration and hyperosmolar serum (increased concentration) leads to cellular dehydration and dysfunction (especially brain cells) that results in progressive lethargy and coma.

Symptoms and Signs
– mental status changes, may mimic stroke (confusion, lethargy, coma)
– thirst (dehydration)
– polyuria
– tachycardia, dry cool skin, hypotension (hypovolemic shock)

Management
– Support vital signs (ABCs).
– Administer oxygen.
– Treat for shock.
– Notify and transport to hospital (paramedics).
– Administer intravenous fluids.

HYPOGLYCEMIA (INSULIN SHOCK)

A metabolic disorder caused by an insulin overdose, inducing hypoglycemia (low blood sugar) with resulting insufficient energy course for cerebral function.

Symptoms and Signs
– weakness, fatigue, shakiness, hunger
– nausea and vomiting
– tachycardia, cool moist skin, hypotension (hypovolemic shock)
– diaphoresis
– pallor
– mental status changes
– possible seizures

Management—Conscious Patient
1. Administer oral carbohydrates (i.e., orange juice, sugar cubes, etc.).
2. Contact physician and/or notify and transport to hospital (paramedics).

Management—Unconscious Patient
1. Support vital signs (ABCs).
2. Administer oxygen.
3. Place a sugar cube under tongue.
4. Contact physician and/or notify and transport to hospital (paramedics).

Drug Management (qualified personnel only)
— Administer dextrose I.V. (50 m of 50% glucose solution).

ORTHOSTATIC HYPOTENSION

A clinical syndrome secondary to avascular regulatory dysfunction that inhibits the body's control of heart rate and blood pressure. This dysfunction allows positional changes without decreased cerebral perfusion.

Symptoms and Signs
— syncope or dizziness when suddenly placed in an upright position
— positional changes in blood pressure (drops when upright)
— baseline or slightly higher heart rate

Management
— Position patient in supine position.
— Maintain airway.
— Positional changes from supine to upright should be made in stages.
— Dismiss patient after retaking blood pressure and comparing reading to original reading.

CARDIOGENIC SHOCK

Shock that occurs when the injured or diseased heart muscle is incapable of a forceful contraction, and there is diminished output with each contraction.

Symptoms and Signs
— confusion
— cool, damp, mottled skin
— tachycardia; may have normal blood pressure reading
— respiratory distress (shortness of breath to frank pulmonary edema)
— edema of extremities (ascites)
— chest pain with acute myocardial ischemia
— decreased urination

Management
— Establish an airway, ventilation, oxygenation.
— Position patient with head and trunk upright.
— Control sources of bleeding, if any exist.
— Relieve pain.
— Prevent loss of body heat.
— Give nothing by mouth.
— Monitor blood pressure.
— Notify and transport to hospital (paramedics).

HYPOVOLEMIC SHOCK

A syndrome of inadequate tissue organ perfusion resulting from loss of blood or blood volume from external or internal bleeding, or dehydration from any cause (vomiting, diarrhea, heatstroke, or polyuria).

Symptoms and Signs
— mental status changes (confusion, lethargy)
— pulse change (tachycardia to weak, thready pulse)
— cool, pale, clammy skin
— decreased urinary output
— blood pressure drop
— complaints of thirst and lightheadedness

Management
— Establish an airway, ventilation, oxygenation.
— Position patient with head and trunk at the same level.
— Control sources of bleeding, if any exist.
— Elevate lower extremities to assist return of blood to the heart.
— Prevent loss of body heat.
— Give nothing by mouth.
— Monitor blood pressure.
— Notify and transport to hospital (paramedics).

Drug Management
— Start I.V. if possible (normal saline).

VASODEPRESSOR SYNCOPE

A transient loss of consciousness resulting from decreased cerebral blood flow following a drop in blood pressure and/or pulse caused by anxiety, pain, fatigue, or fear (especially fear of local anesthetics).

Symptoms and Signs
(presyncope symptoms typically last longer than 5 seconds)
— weakness or nausea
— perspiration on forehead
— skin and mucosa noticeably blanched
— dilated pupils
— initial tachycardia followed by bradycardia
— marked hypotension
— mental status changes
— unconsciousness
Management
— Position patient in the supine position.
— Support vital signs (ABCs).
— Administer oxygen.
— Spirits of ammonia placed under patient's nose may be helpful.

– Loosen tight clothing.
– A cool, moist towel may be applied to the forehead.
– After recovery, slowly resume upright position.

Cardiovascular emergencies

ACUTE CONGESTIVE HEART FAILURE

A clinical syndrome with occasional acute exacerbations in which the heart does not maintain an adequate output, resulting in diminished blood flow to tissues and congestion in the pulmonary and/or systemic circulation.

Symptoms and Signs
– fatigue and weakness
– dyspnea upon exertion (even short of breath with speech)
– orthopnea (short of breath when supine)
– periods of hyperventilation
– chronically ill in appearance

Management
– Prior to dental treatment (1) consult with patient's physician, (2) schedule early morning dental appointments, and (3) place patient in upright position in dental chair for treatment.
– Support vital signs (ABCs).
– Administer oxygen.
– Notify and transport to hospital (paramedics).

ACUTE MYOCARDIAL INFARCTION

Syndrome resulting from occlusion (blockage) of a coronary artery due to the formation of a blood clot with resulting ischemia, dysfunction, and death of a variable portion of myocardial tissue.

Symptoms and Signs
– chest pain (often with extension to neck, arm, or jaw)
– nausea
– dyspnea
– weakness
– dizziness
– palpitations
– cold perspiration
– sense of doom
– cool, pale, moist skin
– restlessness
– cardiac arrest

Management
– Terminate appointment if symptoms and/or signs occur.
– Support vital signs (ABCs).
– Administer oxygen.
– Place patient in 45° sitting position.
– Treat for shock.
– Notify and transport to hospital (paramedics).
Drug Management
– Reduce stress with diazepam, 5 to 10 mg.
– Start I.V. (D^5W or Ringer's lactate).

ANGINA PECTORIS

Syndrome typified by chest pain resulting from an insufficient blood supply to a portion of heart muscle with possible resulting cardiac dysfunction.

Symptoms and Signs
– chest pain induced by exertion or stress
– radiation of pain to left shoulder or arm
– history of previous attacks
– pallor
– cold perspiration
– possible shallow respiration

Management
– Support vital signs (ABCs).
– Administer oxygen.
– Place patient in 45° sitting position.
– If patient takes nitroglycerin, encourage its use.
– Notify and transport to hospital (paramedics).

Drug Management
– Premedicate with diazepam, 5 to 10 mg.
– Administer sublingual nitroglycerin if blood pressure is adequate.

CARDIAC ARREST

Clinical syndrome characterized by loss of consciousness, arterial pulse, pulse pressure, and respiration; arrest may be due to cardiac standstill, ventricular fibrillation, tachycardias, or bradycardias.

Symptoms and Signs
– loss of consciousness with complete unresponsiveness
– loss of respiration, heartbeat, and pulse

Management
– Support vital signs (ABCs).
– Administer oxygen.

– Administer CPR, making sure to check for adequate pulse with chest compressions.
– Notify and transport to hospital (paramedics).

Drug Management
– Start I.V. (D⁵W or Ringer's lactate) if possible.
– Administer no medications without cardiac monitor.

HYPERTENSION

Abnormally elevated blood pressure: mild diastolic pressure, 90 to 100; moderate diastolic pressure, 100 to 120; severe diastolic pressure, greater than 120 mm Hg.

Symptoms and Signs
– usually asymptomatic
– severe, pounding headache
– nausea
– vomiting
– irritability
– confusion and disorientation
– possible cerebral dysfunction and/or cardiac dysfunction

Management
– Make patient comfortable.
– Check vital signs.
– Seek medical attention.
– Control stress and pain.

Local anesthetic related emergencies

ALLERGIC REACTIONS
(typically due to local
anesthetics or antibiotics)

The result of an antigen antibody response to a specific drug or chemical agent that triggers an abnormal immune reaction releasing histamine and other vasoactive chemicals; these chemicals induce reactions varying from hives to anaphylaxis.

Symptoms and Signs
– skin rashes
– hives
– pruritis (itching)
– angioedema
– bronchospasm (asthma attack)
– anaphylaxis (may indicate cardiac arrest)

Management
– Support vital signs (ABCs).

– Administer oxygen.
– Place patient in supine position.
– Loosen clothing.
– Notify and transport to hospital (paramedics).

Drug Management
– If necessary, administer 0.5 ml epinephrine 1:1000 either I.V. or subcutaneously.
– Administer antihistaminic agents (Benadryl, 20 to 50 mg PO, I.M., I.V.).
– Administer isoproterenol or epinephrine inhalants.
– Start aminophylline 0.5 gm I.V.

TOXIC OVERDOSE TO LOCAL ANESTHETICS

Toxicity occurring when the rate of systemic absorption exceeds the rate of metabolism and the local anesthetic exceeds toxic serum levels, inducing systemic side effects.

Symptoms and Signs
– cerebral cortical stimulation: talkativeness, restlessness, apprehension, excitement, convulsions
– cerebral cortical depression: lethargy, sleepiness, unconsciousness
– medullary stimulation: increased blood pressure, increased pulse rate, increased respirations, possible nausea and vomiting
– medullary depression: blood pressure normal in mild cases to zero in severe cases, pulse from normal to weak, thready, or absent, and respiratory changes slight to apneic

Management
– Support vital signs (ABCs).
– Administer oxygen.
– Place patient in supine position.
– Loosen tight clothing.
– Notify and transport to hospital (paramedics).

Drug Management
– If convulsions occur, give patient oxygen between seizures; if unable to do this, give patient diazepam I.V.

Other hazards

FOREIGN OBJECT IN EYE

An injury caused by a foreign object blown or rubbed into the eye.

Symptoms and Signs
– pain

- tearing
- injection into the conjunctiva (causing redness of the eye)
- blurry vision

Management
- Pull down the lower lid to determine whether or not the object lies on the inner surface.
- If the object lies on the inner surface, lift it gently with the corner of a clean handkerchief, paper tissue, or cotton tipped applicator.
- If the object has not been located, it may be lodged beneath the upper lid.
- While the patient looks down, grasp the lashes of the upper lid gently.
- Pull the upper lid forward and down over the lower lid.
- Tears may dislodge object.
- If cannot locate object, patch over eye and seek further medical assistance.

OPEN WOUND

Occurring when there is a break in the skin or mucous membrane.

Symptoms and Signs
- abrasions: outer layers of skin scraped and damaged, bleeding limited
- incisions: skin cut on sharp objects, bleeding possibly rapid and heavy
- lacerations: jagged, irregular appearance of skin, bleeding possibly rapid and extensive
- punctures: skin pierced, creating a hole in tissues, external bleeding limited

Management
- Stop bleeding immediately with local compression.
- Protect wound from contamination and infection.
- Provide care for possible shock.
- Obtain medical attention.

Respiratory emergencies

AIRWAY OBSTRUCTION

One of the most common life-threatening emergencies; may be caused by foreign objects blocking air passages or by anaphylaxis.

Symptoms and Signs
- completely blocked airway: patient unable to speak, cough, or breathe
- partially blocked airway resulting in (1) weak, in-

effective cough; (2) high-pitched sounds upon inhalation; (3) increased respiratory difficulty; (4) ashen-grey color of skin; and (5) possible cyanosis of nails and lips

Management—Conscious Choking Patient
- Give four abdominal or chest thrusts.
- Repeat sequence as long as necessary.

Management—Unconscious Choking Patient
- Check to see if airway is open.
- Give two breaths.
- Give four abdominal or chest thrusts.
- Fingersweep airway.
- Repeat sequence as long as necessary.

ASTHMA

The result of stimuli (an allergen or stress) to hyperactive airways (bronchi) and mucous-secreting glands, inducing bronchospasm and reduced air passage with respirations.

Symptoms and Signs
- possible noisy breathing and chronic cough
- wheezing
- dyspnea (shortness of breath)
- high blood pressure
- increased anxiety
- increased heart rate
- orthopnea
- cyanosis of lips and nails
- perspiration
- flushing of face
- mental status changes

Management
- Terminate dental procedures.
- Position patient comfortably.
- Allow patient to use bronchodilator if available.
- Administer oxygen.
- Notify physician and/or hospital.

Drug Management
- If mild attack, allow patient to use bronchodilator—one or two deep inhalations. Repeat as needed in 3 to 5 minutes.
- If acute attack (adults less than 50 years old and without heart disease), administer epinephrine, 0.3 to 0.5 cc of 1:1000 subcutaneously. Repeat as needed in 10 to 15 minutes.

HYPERVENTILATION

A clinical syndrome induced by rapid or deep breathing that causes a lowering of carbon dioxide levels resulting in alkalosis; typically brought on by anxiety, stress, pain, or fear.

Symptoms and Signs
— lightheadedness and anxiety
— feeling of lump in throat
— chest pain
— tingling and numbness of fingers and toes
— increased rate of respiration
— increased depth of breathing
— increased pulse

Management
— Terminate dental procedures.
— Remove cause of anxiety (syringe, for example) from patient's line of vision.
— Position patient upright to facilitate breathing.
— Remove any foreign materials from patient's mouth (rubber dam, for example).
— Calm patient and try to regulate rate of breathing: four to six breaths per minute.
— If this does not work, allow patient to breathe into a brown paper bag at the rate of six to ten breaths per minute.

Seizure disorders

EPILEPSY

A chronic seizure disorder usually of unknown origin.

Symptoms and Signs—Grand Mal Seizure
— possible premonition or aura immediately before the onset of the seizure
— biting or chewing of tongue
— involuntary urination or defecation
— unresponsive during seizure
— excessive muscular activity
— loss of consciousness
— muscular rigidity

Symptoms and Signs—Petit Mal Seizure
— lip smacking or staring into space
— interrupted speech
— minor convulsive movements of an extremity or eyes

Management
— Protect the patient from causing himself injury during seizure.
— Bite block should *not* be placed between teeth.
— Support vital signs.
— Administer oxygen.
— Notify and transport to hospital (paramedics) when seizure terminates.
— A written or verbal history given to medical team is quite beneficial to patient care.

References

1. Stahl, S.S. What Dentists Do: A Patient's Guide to Modern Dentistry. East Norwalk, Conn.: Appleton-Century-Crofts, 1982, p. 29.
2. Malamed, S.F. Handbook of Medical Emergencies in the Dental Office, 2nd ed. St. Louis: C.V. Mosby Co., 1982, pp. 28–31.
3. Brown, D.T. Oxygen therapy in the dental practice. Ohio Dent. J. 57(3):29–32, 1983.
4. McCarthy, F.M. Medical Emergencies in Dentistry, 3rd ed. Philadelphia: W.B. Saunders Co., 1982, p. 227.
5. Rose, L.F., and Hendler, B.H. Medical Emergencies in Dental Practice. Chicago: Quintessence Publ. Co., 1981, pp. 224, 229–241.
6. American Heart Association. Cardiopulmonary Resuscitation, 2nd ed. Tulsa: C.P.R. Publ., 1980, p. 10.
7. Parcel, G.S. Basic Emergency Care of the Sick and Injured, 2nd ed. St. Louis: C.V. Mosby Co., 1982, p. 165.

4

Supplemental components of the examination

When the initial phase of health assessment and documentation has been completed, several other components of the pretherapy examination may be employed. Some of them are performed routinely, for example, study models. Others are utilized as needed for special cases. This chapter will discuss the rationale for and techniques involved in the performance of these tasks.

Study models

Diagnostic study models serve a number of purposes in overall patient treatment. As accurate reproductions of the teeth and adjacent surrounding structures, study models are an excellent means of recording the patient's current dental status. They can aid the dental hygienist in charting procedures, particularly in the documentation of gingival position, shape, and size, and in assessment of frenum attachment. Study casts are often utilized as patient education devices to explain necessary restorative, surgical, or periodontal therapy as well as specific oral hygiene recommendations. A series of study models can serve as a visual component of the patient's record and document therapy from initial treatment to the conclusion of all procedures, as is the case during orthodontic correction.

Study models are obtained by preparing impressions of the maxillary and mandibular arches, usually utilizing an irreversible hydrocolloid material known as alginate. Alginate is commercially available as a powder either in large-volume metal containers or premeasured individual pouches. Because contami-

nation of the powder via exposure to high levels of humidity and temperature can cause deterioration, storage in tightly closed containers in a cool, dry environment is necessary.

Impression trays are available in metal and plastic and may be perforated or nonperforated. Metal trays may be sterilized by conventional methods; plastic ones are usually disposable, because the heat associated with sterilizing would melt the plastic. The perforations in the trays aid in holding the alginate securely in the tray, which is especially helpful when removing trays from the patient's mouth. However, adhesive agents are available with which to coat nonperforated and plastic trays to avoid accidental separation of the alginate from the tray.

Preparation

Prior to taking the impressions, the required armamentarium should be assembled:

1. Alginate powder.
2. Rubber mixing bowl.
3. Wide-blade mixing spatula.
4. Beading wax strips.
5. Alginate impression trays.
6. Intraoral mirror.
7. Saliva ejector.
8. Water measuring vial.
9. Baseplate wax.
10. Plastic drape for patient.
11. Mouthwash.

The patient should be seated in an upright position

to allow the dental hygienist optimum access and to decrease the possibility of stimulating the patient's gag reflex. The procedures to be performed should be explained to the patient. The patient should be draped with a plastic cover, because impression taking is often a messy procedure. The dental hygienist should inspect the mouth for general anatomy, malposed teeth, mandibular tori, and any other conditions that may affect the size or fit of the trays to be selected for the impressions.

If gross debris is present in the patient's mouth, the patient should be requested to brush the teeth. Otherwise, a cup of commercial mouthwash is given so that the patient can rinse prior to taking the impressions. This rinsing helps to free the mouth of excess saliva, to decrease surface microorganisms, and to lower surface tension in order to prevent the occurrence of bubbles in the impression material.

A large selection of tray sizes is available to fit almost every patient's mouth. With experience, estimating the approximate size of trays needed is not difficult. Nevertheless, the dental hygienist should try in the trays to assure proper fit prior to taking an impression.

The empty trays should be inserted into the patient's mouth, one at a time, to determine if the fit is adequate. The trays should be long enough to cover the tuberosities and retromolar areas, thereby assuring inclusion of all teeth in the final casts. At least a quarter inch of clearance space is needed between the anterior portion of the tray and the incisors. The trays should be wide enough to allow enough impression material on both facial and lingual surfaces to provide the necessary rigidity and strength. If a tray is slightly narrow, the flanges may be spread gently.

Once the trays have been selected, a strip of soft utility wax is applied to the borders of the trays. Additional wax strips are added from canine to canine areas on both trays; the wax should be indented midline to allow for the presence of the labial frena. The wax is placed on the trays for several reasons:

1. To obtain a deeper, more complete impression of the mucobuccal areas.
2. To prevent the teeth from penetrating through the impression material to the tray, resulting in defects in the final models.
3. To aid in retention of the alginate material in the trays.
4. To increase the comfort of the patient.

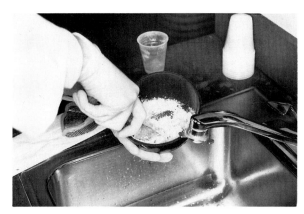

Figure 4-1

Once the trays have been prepared, the next step is to measure and mix the alginate powder with water. Directions are always provided by the manufacturer for measuring and mixing and should be read and followed carefully. When using regular set alginate, the hygienist has approximately 2 minutes for mixing, loading the tray, and inserting it into the patient's mouth. The temperature of the water can affect the setting time of the impression material. The cooler the water, the longer the setting time; the warmer the water, the faster the material will set. Water at room temperature (20° C to 21° C, or 68° F to 70° F) is considered to be ideal for preparing alginate.

The specified amount of water is measured and dispensed into a clean, dry rubber mixing bowl. The specified amount of alginate is sprinkled into the water. The mixture is quickly stirred with a wide-blade spatula and then spatulated against the sides of the bowl for about 1 minute, until a creamy smooth consistency is achieved (Fig. 4-1).

The mandibular tray is filled from one side to the other (Fig. 4-2). The alginate is pressed gently down into the tray. The hygienist tries to avoid trapping air bubbles as the tray is loaded. The tray is filled to just below the edge of the beading wax on the tray rims. The surface of the alginate is smoothed with the index finger, which is moistened with cold water. A slight depression is made in the middle of the material where the teeth will insert.

Excess alginate remaining in the bowl is gathered on the spatula and applied with the index finger to coat areas in the mouth where bubbles are more likely to occur: the impression's occlusal surfaces, the ves-

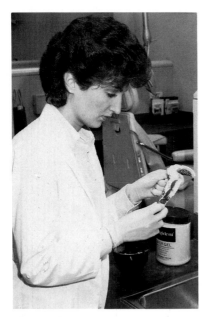

Figure 4-2

tibule (especially at frenum attachments), and cervically abraded or eroded tooth surfaces.

Taking the impression

Standing in front and to the side of the patient, the dental hygienist retracts the lip and cheek with one hand; with the other hand holding the tray, the opposite lip and cheek are retracted gently, using the side of the tray itself (Fig. 4-3). The mandibular tray is inserted with a rotary or side-to-side motion. The tray is centered and then pulled forward about a quarter inch. The hygienist asks the patient to lift his or her tongue and gently presses the tray down into place, seating the anterior portion first, then the posterior segment. The hygienist presses gently over the premolar–molar area with equal pressure on both sides. The patient is asked to extend his or her tongue outward to free the sublingual area. The hygienist gently frees the lip and cheeks by running the index fingers of both hands around the area and lightly pulling out on the soft tissues. The saliva ejector is placed in the patient's mouth and the tray stabilized by holding it in place with the fingers of one or both hands until the alginate has set. If perforated trays are used,

the material protruding from the perforations can be used to test the set. Otherwise, excess alginate in the bowl can be used. The material is set when it has lost its surface stickiness.

The tray is removed by releasing the edges near the buccal mucosa and pulling up with a quick snap. The tray should *not* be rocked back and forth with the handle, because this can cause distortion of the impression.

The tray is rinsed under cool running water and inspected for accuracy. The impression should show clear imprints of all teeth present and should have an adequate representation of the vestibular area. There should be no bubbles or holes. If the impression is not adequate, it should be redone. If it is judged satisfactory, it is wrapped in a wet towel while the maxillary impression is taken.

The primary reason for taking the mandibular impression first is that it usually does not induce the patient's gag reflex whereas gagging is more common with the maxillary impression. By taking the mandibular impression first, the patient is more confident and less likely to fear gagging as a sequela to the subsequent impression.

Before the maxillary impression is taken, the patient is asked to rinse to remove remaining bits of impression material and excess saliva. The alginate is prepared as before and the maxillary tray is loaded. In order to minimize potential gagging, excess alginate should not be placed in the posterior region of the tray; rather, the tray is filled slightly more in the anterior area.

Standing to the back and side of the patient, the hygienist inserts the tray by retracting the soft tissues with the hand and tray (Fig. 4-4a). The tray is positioned with a rotary motion, centered, and then pulled forward about a quarter inch. The tray is seated in a posterior–anterior manner by pushing it gently in the molar area first, then seating the anterior portion (Fig. 4-4b). This will prevent excess alginate from flowing down the patient's throat, decreasing the likelihood of stimulating the gag response. The patient is asked to breathe through the nose. The hygienist frees the soft tissues by lifting the lip and cheek out; requests the patient to form an O with the lips to mold the buccal area; and stabilizes the tray with one or both hands until the alginate sets.

If the patient tends to gag, rinsing with very cold water or holding an ice cube in the mouth or swabbing the posterior section of the hard palate with a topical

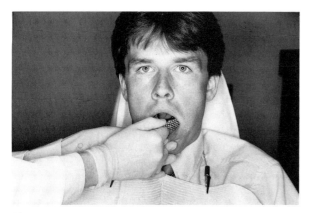

Figure 4-3

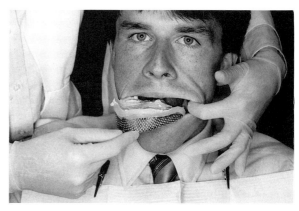

Figure 4-4a

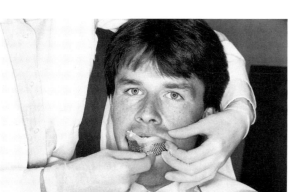

Figure 4-4b

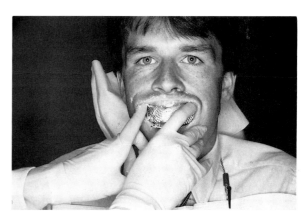

Figure 4-5

anesthetic agent will often lessen the gag reflex. Another technique, once the maxillary tray has been inserted, is to tilt the patient's head forward and provide a paper towel in case of drooling. The patient should be reminded to breathe through the nose.

Once the alginate has set, the tray is removed by breaking the palatal seal: the index fingers of both hands are used to loosen the tray at the buccal rims (Fig. 4-5). The impression tray is snapped down and out by using the handle. The impression is rinsed, inspected to assure the inclusions of all pertinent structures, and wrapped in a wet towel. Both mandibular and maxillary wrapped impressions are placed in a plastic bag until they can be poured. Impressions should not be stored in water or left exposed to air. Both situations would cause distortion of the final models.

The interocclusal record (wax bite)

In order to accurately align and interrelate the maxillary and mandibular models, an interocclusal record is obtained. Also known as a wax bite, this record is further used during the trimming phase of study model preparation and while models are stored, to protect the casts and avoid accidental breakage of the teeth. Although usually most study models will easily occlude in only one position, certain conditions such as openbites, crossbites, edge-to-edge bites, end-to-end bites, and edentulous areas may cause interferences with normal occlusion. The wax bite will aid in assuring the proper occlusal relationship in such instances.

To obtain the interocclusal record, the patient is asked to bite together to check the customary occlusal

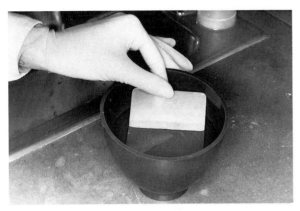

Figure 4-6a

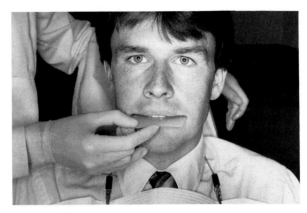

Figure 4-6b

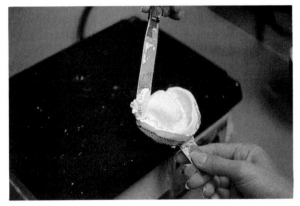

Figure 4-7

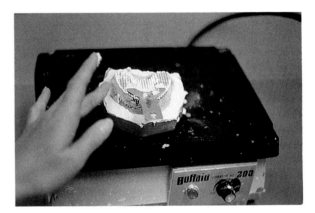

Figure 4-8

relationship between the arches. In a bowl of warm water the dental hygienist softens a piece of baseplate wax that has been cut to fit the curve of the arch (Fig. 4-6a). The wax is placed in the patient's mouth, centered, and checked to make sure it covers all posterior teeth. The patient is asked to gently close together. The hygienist shapes the wax upward over the maxillary teeth (Fig. 4-6b), carefully removes it, and places it immediately in cold water.

Pouring the impression

Alginate impressions should be poured as soon as possible. If the impressions are exposed to air for even relatively short periods of time, or are stored under water, distortion of the alginate occurs and the final model will not be an accurate representation of the dental arches.

Prior to pouring the models, the necessary armamentarium should be assembled. This includes:

1. Mixing bowl.
2. Wide-blade spatula.
3. Dental stone or plaster.
4. Plaster knife.
5. Vibrator.
6. Model base formers or nonabsorbent slab or paper (such as ceramic slab, glass slab, or waxed paper).

The impressions should be rinsed quickly under cool running water and dried gently with compressed air. The hygienist creates an artificial floor of the mouth for the mandibular impression by mixing a small amount of alginate and filling the space between the flanges of the tray. The surface of the alginate is smoothed with a wet finger and the material is allowed to set up. The stone or plaster is mixed with water according to the manufacturer's directions. The hygienist turns the vibrator on to low speed and places one of the impressions on the table of the vibrator at an angle, holding it by the handle. Using the spatula, she or he lifts a small dab of stone and gently touches the spatula against the side of the impression tray (Fig. 4-7). The vibrating motion will cause the stone to flow from the spatula into the impression and should be continued until the imprints of all the teeth have been filled. Care must be taken not to press the tray with undue force against the vibrator. Excess force will cause bubbles to form that may then be incorporated into the final cast. The purpose of the vibration is to remove air bubbles during the pouring stage. Care should be taken to avoid creating additional bubbles.

Additional stone is added slowly until the impression is filled to the rim. It is then set aside temporarily to make the base. In terms of time and effort the easiest way to pour the base of the impression is to use preformed base formers. These are rubber molds shaped to the correct height and contour for the bases of the final models. The base former is filled with additional stone or plaster and vibrated for several seconds to remove bubbles (Fig. 4-8). It is then placed on a flat surface and the poured impression is inverted on top of it. The tray is centered and aligned so that it is positioned evenly on the base former, with the tray handle parallel to the table or surface on which it rests. The process is repeated for the second impression. The poured impression must remain undisturbed until the stone or plaster has set (approximately 1 hour). During the reaction phase, heat is eliminated as the stone or plaster sets. Once the model feels cool to the touch, the material has set, and the casts may be separated from the impressions.

If base formers are not available, two other ways to formulate the base are (1) with boxing wax or (2) free forming the base on a nonabsorbent surface. In the wax technique, a strip of utility wax is formed around the rim of the tray, to which boxing or base-plate wax is then attached to a height of about a half inch. The impression is poured to the top edge of the wax. This technique does not require the impression to be inverted onto additional stone.

The second way to make the base is to pour the impression, place a mound of stone on a nonabsorbent surface, and invert the impression on it, settling it gently into the stone. The tray must be centered on the mound and the tray handle must be parallel to

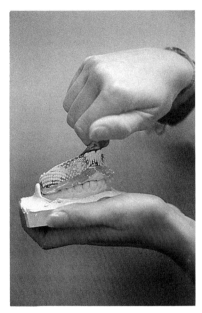

Figure 4-9

the surface. The basic outline of the final base shape may be roughed out before the stone sets by using the spatula to achieve the desired shape. This will make trimming easier once the models have set. When this technique is used, the stone or plaster mix must not be too thin or the tray will sink into the material, giving too thin a base.

Separating the cast from the impression

Once the casts have fully set, the casts are separated from the impressions. Care must be taken to avoid accidental breakage of the teeth, especially with the mandibular cast, during the separation process. If base formers were used, they are removed first. If the wax technique was used, the wax is removed from around the cast. A sharp plaster knife is used to remove any stone or plaster that may be impinging on the rims of the trays (Fig. 4-9). The tray is loosened by moving the handle up and down gently. The tray is lifted off the cast by pulling straight up.

Trimming

Trimming of study casts is the next step in the preparation of final models. In the contemporary practice of dental hygiene, the reproduction of the arches is of prime importance, not the exact angulations of the bases. For the dental hygienist employed in an orth-

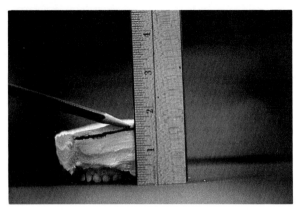

Figure 4-10

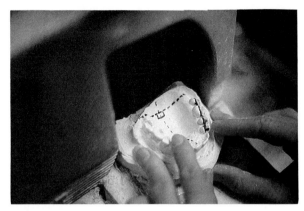

Figure 4-11

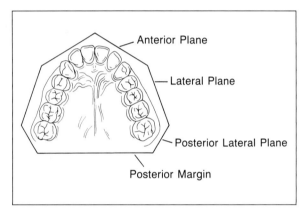

Anterior Plane

Lateral Plane

Posterior Lateral Plane

Posterior Margin

Figure 4-12

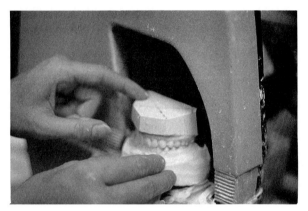

Figure 4-13

odontic practice, exact dimensions become more critical. The beginning student, however, should concentrate on obtaining a usable cast.

The first step is to trim the base of the maxillary cast so that it is parallel to the occlusal plane, with a height of about 1½ inches from the occlusal plane to the top of the base (Fig. 4-10). Next, the posterior border is trimmed so that it is flat and even (Fig. 4-11). They should not be trimmed excessively because final trimming of both casts in occlusion will be performed later so that they are exactly even. The heels, sides, and anterior portions of the maxillary cast are trimmed to approximate the dimensions shown in Fig. 4-12. Symmetry between sides is important.

The two casts are placed in occlusion and the posterior border of the mandibular cast is trimmed so that it is exactly even with the maxillary (Fig. 4-13). The base of the mandibular cast is trimmed to approximately 1½ inches thick. The heels, sides, and anterior

portions of the mandibular cast (Fig. 4-14) are trimmed to approximate the dimensions shown in Fig. 4-15. Again, both sides should be symmetrical. While the anterior portion of the maxillary cast comes to a point between the maxillary central incisors, the mandibular anterior segment is rounded.

Once basic trimming has been completed, the casts are finished by filling all voids or bubble areas with stone or plaster and using a plaster knife to smooth rough edges and remove excess (Figs. 4-16a and b). Each cast is marked with the patient's name and date and stored in a safe place.

Pulp vitality testing

Patients will occasionally have dental conditions that require the use of pulp vitality testers to determine the extent of vitality in a given tooth or teeth. Teeth may

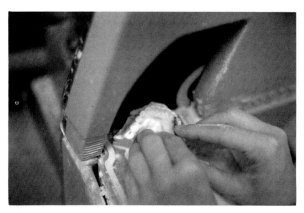

Figure 4-14

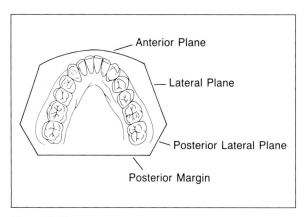

Anterior Plane

Lateral Plane

Posterior Lateral Plane

Posterior Margin

Figure 4-15

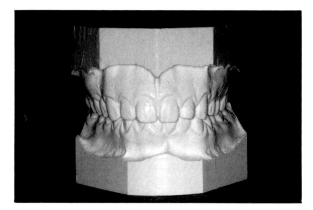

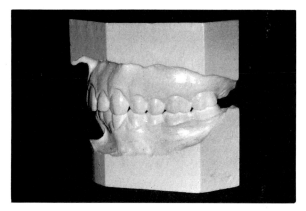

Figs. 4-16a and b   Finished study models.

Figure 4-16b

lose vitality from a wide variety of causes, such as pulpal invasion from either periodontal disease or caries, traumatic injuries, extreme thermal conditions, or iatrogenic dentistry.

Certain clinical and radiographic findings may prompt the dental hygienist to suspect potential loss of pulpal vitality:

1. Obvious large carious lesion.
2. Very large restoration.
3. Fractured tooth.
4. Intrinsic discoloration of the tooth.
5. Presence of fistula near the apex of a tooth.
6. Radiolucency near the tooth apex.
7. Fracture of the root of the tooth.
8. Large carious lesion or restoration very close to the pulp of tooth.
9. Thickening of periodontal ligament space to the apex of the tooth, accompanied by bone loss.

Both thermal and electrical testing systems have been used to determine tooth vitality, but the electric testers are generally preferred because of greater reliability and consistency of results. The electric testing device functions by generating a stimulus that the patient perceives as pain. The vitality of the pulp is determined by its blood supply and not the innervation itself. Because of this, the readings obtained during pulp testing may not reflect an accurate assessment of the health of the pulp.

Electric pulp testers may be either plug-in or battery-operated types. The basic technique for use is the same, regardless of type. Each tester is accompanied by instructions from the manufacturer, which should be read thoroughly prior to use. Consistency in the performance of pulp testing procedures is essential in order to obtain consistent results.

Before the actual test is run, all equipment should be assembled and tested to assure optimum working

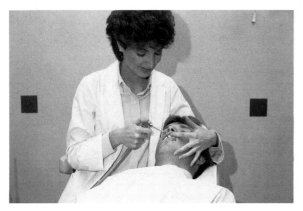

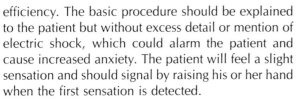

Figure 4-17

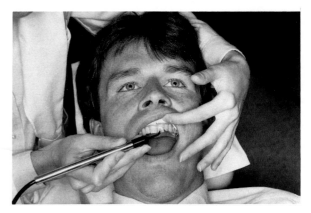

Figure 4-18

efficiency. The basic procedure should be explained to the patient but without excess detail or mention of electric shock, which could alarm the patient and cause increased anxiety. The patient will feel a slight sensation and should signal by raising his or her hand when the first sensation is detected.

The test area is isolated with cotton rolls and the specific teeth are air dried (Fig. 4-17). A small amount of toothpaste is placed on the tip portion of the tester, and the tester is applied to a tooth adjacent to the one in question. The tip is placed on the middle third of the crown on a single-rooted tooth, or the middle third of each cusp of a multirooted tooth. That tooth is tested, then the same tooth on the contralateral side, and finally the tooth in question (Fig. 4-18). This pretesting allows the hygienist to observe and determine the patient's normal response pattern.

The tester tip must not be allowed to contact the gingiva or other mucosal tissues. Metallic restorations should also be avoided, because metal conducts the current more rapidly. If there are restorations that extend to the proximal surfaces, and the tip is placed on the metal, the current may be transmitted to the adjacent tooth, giving a reading for the wrong tooth.

The rheostat is placed at zero and advanced slowly, with very brief stops at each number. The first discernible sensation felt by the patient is recorded. Each tooth should be tested twice, with the readings then averaged and recorded in the patient's chart. All readings taken must be recorded, not just the readings for the tooth or teeth in question.

Cytology smears

When performing the intraoral examination, the dental hygienist will, on some occasions, note lesions or suspicious areas that may be indicative of potential oral cancer. Suspicious areas require further investigation, either through referral to a specialist or cytological smear at the time the suspected area is first identified.

The exfoliative cytology smear is a diagnostic procedure in which surface cells of a potential lesion are removed and studied under a microscope. Because it is a surface test, heavily keratinized and deeper lesions do not lend themselves to this technique. Treatment for the lesions is not determined by results of the smear alone. If the smear results are positive, a biopsy is required for further information and definitive diagnosis. The cytology smear is a screening test only and cannot be considered reliable from a diagnostic point of view. (False negative cytologic reports can yield positive results with a biopsy.)

With these limitations in mind, the smear may still be utilized when indicated by the dentist. In order to secure a smear, the appropriate armamentarium should be gathered:

1. Glass microscope slides with frosted end.
2. Flexible metal or plastic spatula.
3. Fixative (70% alcohol).
4. 2 × 2 gauze sponges.
5. Plastic slide holder.

The patient's name and the date are written on the frosted segment of the glass slides (two slides for each

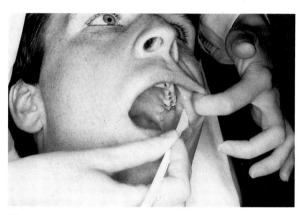

Figure 4-19

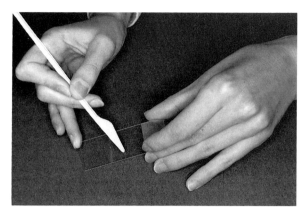

Figure 4-20

lesion to be smeared). The area to be scraped is gently irrigated to remove any surface debris present. If any debris or blood remains, the area is gently wiped with a wet gauze sponge. It should not be dried.

The plastic spatula is used to scrape the entire area firmly several times, with all strokes in the same direction (Fig. 4-19). The collected cells are smeared across the glass slide, starting at the center of the clear area and spreading evenly across the slide (Fig. 4-20). The slide is immediately flooded with the 70% alcohol fixative. The procedure is repeated to obtain the smear for the second slide.

The slides are allowed to fix for 30 minutes; excess alcohol is drained after 20 minutes by tipping the slides slightly. The slides must air dry away from contamination by dust, dirt, and other foreign matter. When completely dry, they are packed in a plastic slide container for mailing to the laboratory. A form is enclosed containing pertinent information for the pathologist: patient's name and address, dentist's name and address, detailed description of the lesion (including location, size, color, consistency, and shape), and any other clinical observations or patient-related information that may be of importance.

The pathologist will examine the slides and report his findings in one of the following categories:

Unsatisfactory:
The slide is not utilizable as presented; either the smear was inadequate or the cells dried prior to fixation. Another smear is necessary.
Class I:
Normal.

Class II:
Atypical, but not suggestive of malignancy.
Class III:
Uncertain (possibly may be cancer).
Class IV:
Probable for cancer.
Class V:
Positive for cancer.

A biopsy is definitely indicated in the event of a Class IV or V report; it is usually performed with a Class III result. For a Class I or II evaluation, careful monitoring of the lesion by the dental hygienist and dentist is necessary. If the lesion has not healed or disappeared after 2 weeks, the smear should be repeated or a biopsy performed.

A biopsy is not within the purview of the dental hygienist to perform, but she or he should be familiar with the basic technique and rationale for the procedure. Biopsies may be incisional, with only a portion or segment of the lesion removed, or excisional, with the entire lesion removed for microscopic examination of the tissues or other material. In inaccessible areas such as the larynx or posterior section of the hard palate, a punch biopsy technique is incorporated. A special instrument that punches out a small segment of tissue is used. Curettage may occasionally be used to obtain biopsy material, although it has limited accuracy. It may be used to extract material from tooth sockets, sinuses, and other bony areas.

The type of biopsy to be performed is dependent upon the type and size of the lesion. Any unusual unidentifiable oral lesion, any lesion that has not healed in 2 weeks, any persistent, white hyperkeratinized lesion, and any mass that does not break through the surface epithelium are usually referred for biopsy.

Throat culture

In some pedodontic offices, throat culturing may be an additional component of the examination procedure. This is a health screening tool designed to identify the presence of streptococcal infections that may lead to more serious medically compromising situations for the child patient. The technique of obtaining a throat culture is very simple; special long culture swabs are utilized, the pharynx area is swabbed, and the applicator is placed in its accompanying vial and sent to the laboratory for analysis.

Dental images

Photographs and videos are extremely valuable communicative tools, providing easily made and accurate records. For this reason, dentistry has incorporated the use of imaging into both general and specialty practices.

Many orthodontists take full-face and profile portraits of each patient prior to and following treatment. Prosthodontists may send the patient's photographs to the laboratory technician for guidance in preparing veneers and crowns. Pedodontists report that instant photos are effective in reducing anxiety in the child dental patient. Pictures serve as a nonthreatening introduction to the first dental visit as well as to unfamiliar procedures throughout treatment.

Photographs taken before treatment are especially valuable for documenting the extent of facial injuries prior to emergency treatment. Insurance companies consider accident reports to be more complete and handle them more expediently if photographs are included. Patient education can be made more personalized and meaningful through the use of orientation videos and instant photos. As an example, many patients are unable to see dental plaque, gingival inflammation, and other conditions in their own mouths. Photographs can assist them in evaluating their oral health and thus lead to more effective learning of preventive concepts. Photographs of incipient lesions can also be added to a patient's permanent record to allow more precise and consistent follow-up.

Some dental practices keep up-to-date manuals that include photographs of tray setups and drawer or room arrangements; some record office techniques on videos. New staff members are more easily oriented to office policies when photographs and videos are used in their training. Most important, photographs complete a patient's personal dental record. Intraoral photographs not only record conditions before and after treatment but can be used as an accurate reminder of past oral conditions at recall time.

In a comprehensive dental practice, dental imaging is thus an integral part of the learning process, an essential part of the patient record, and a primary means of professional communication. From photographs for use in longitudinal studies of clinical cases to documentary videos for peer presentations, there are applications for imaging that improve procedures and patient care. Moreover, even amateur photographers can operate imaging systems for dental subjects, provided some general principles are understood and applied.

Characteristics of equipment

The main objectives in rendering dental subjects are: achieving adequate depth of field and resolution, reproducing color and tone, and viewing hard-to-see areas in the mouth. These become easier and less expensive to attain on a routine basis as materials and equipment are improved. In recent years there have been exciting advances in both the quality of materials and in the automatic facilities of imaging equipment, which are now affordable for the student and practitioner alike.

The four main ranges of magnification in imaging are general (infinity to 1:10), close-up (1:10 to 1:1), photomacrographic (1:1 to 20:1), and photomicrographic (20:1 to 1000:1). Dental imaging is primarily concerned with close-up and photomacro magnification ranges. These two ranges cover a full-face portrait or a single detail of a tooth.

In the past, many of the components necessary for these ranges were unavailable or cobbled together by specialists in the field. Now, in still photographic systems, a wide range of optics span the range of 1:10 to 12:1 with auto diaphragm control and a selection of specialized flash sources such as ring lights, point lights, and diffuse lights, all with automatic exposure control. Combining them with autofocus, auto-winders, and sophisticated program exposure control, the student and practitioner alike can produce quality images easily and at low cost.

A similar situation has occurred in video. Although ½-inch video has been plagued with incompatible formats (VHS and Beta), the 8mm format is an international standard. This format holds great promise for low-cost, high-quality video in an easy-to-operate camera/recorder.

Each imaging medium has characteristics that make it appropriate for communication, both in production ease and distribution efficiency. The basic characteristics of the still photography medium are high resolution, color realism, inexpensive materials, versatility (print and projection uses), and a high degree of automation available at low cost. The basic characteristics of the video medium are sound/motion simultaneity, instant access to recording image, inexpensive materials, and a high degree of automation available at low cost. Matching assets to the specific situation will improve the usefulness of each medium.

A photographic imaging system

A still photographic system should be a 35mm single lens reflex camera from a reputable manufacturer (such as Olympus, Canon, Nikon, Minolta, or Pentax) or a specialized-systems vendor (such as Lester Dine or Peter Gray) (Fig. 4-21). For projection and processing services, 35mm is the standard medium. Depending on the results of a needs survey, the following components will be required: macro optics, generally 50mm or 100mm lenses to start, followed by extension tubes, teleconverters, bellows, and specialized photomacro objectives. A longer focal length permits greater working distance, which is usually preferred.

The lighting system should be electronic flash, which has the benefits of good color, repeatable output, brief durations (motion stopping), and low-cost operation. The quality of light greatly affects the rendering of the subject. Ring lights (surrounding the lens) help eliminate shadows and bring out the subtle colors of the subject, but often make the subject look two dimensional, especially with cross-polarization. Point lights (small in relation to the subject) are more effective in making the subject look three dimensional, but often cause extreme contrast and specular reflections that detract from a realistic portrayal. Dif-

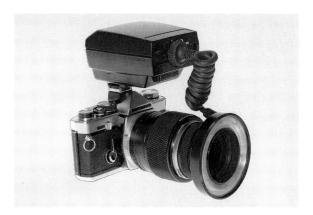

Figure 4-21

fuse lights (source size much larger than the object) are effective in three-dimensional rendering but are difficult to employ in macro ranges where working distance is restricted.

Many variations of these three main classifications are available from different manufacturers. An effective strategy for selection is to negotiate a trial period with a supplier. The choice of a camera body preselects a proprietary lens mount for the system. It also determines what automated accessories will be available to integrate with the system.

The main criteria for selection should relate to the optics and lighting components needed, because these contribute the most to the final image. Most camera bodies offer automated exposure control and film handling. In special circumstances, certain features such as autofocus, programmed exposure, or special metering facilities will dominate the selection process, but this should be infrequent. Currently a wide variety of equipment is available at low cost.

A video imaging system

The assembling of a video imaging system involves choosing a format (½-inch VHS or Beta; 8mm) and an equipment style (unitized or component). Most systems are made by one of two manufacturers (even though many have private labels), and so the quality is generally equivalent. The principle features that differ are miniaturization, optics, autofocus, titling facilities, and camera tube. Those that most affect image quality are type of tube (Newvicon, Saticon, and Vidicon are considered best) and optics. Having macro optic facilities, without the need to resort to accessories, is a definite advantage in dental imaging.

There are advantages and disadvantages to both the unitized (Camcorder) and component-equipment styles. The choice is usually related to tripod usage, because unitized equipment is too heavy to hand hold in extended periods of close-up use. An additional consideration, the importance of program interchange, applies to ½-inch VHS and Beta formats but not to 8mm.

Calibration of an imaging system

After mastering the specific operations of the equipment from the manufacturer's manuals, the user should calibrate any new system for the types of situations most often encountered. Whether an automated or a manual system is calibrated, it is important to set up a test that changes one variable at a time. A test series should be planned and written down in advance of performing the exposures. Accurate notes on every setting should be kept. This will greatly aid the interpretation of the results. Record keeping is greatly simplified by exposing a record of the exposures on the film or tape that remains with the images for reference. The small cost of materials is easily repaid by time saved in clerical tasks.

In calibrating a photographic system, the first step is to choose one film with an ASA/ISO rating from 25 to 100 and daylight color balance. A slide film is preferable because it requires the most accurate exposures. Second, the outfit is assembled with lens and flash, and a magnification and subject are chosen that are typical for the user. If the system is manually controlled for exposure, a series of exposures is taken at every f-stop on the lens. If the system is automatically controlled, the lens is set at the recommended stop (using the largest number or smallest f-stop), and the ASA/ISO setting is varied from ¼ to 2 times the film's rating.

The exposed film should be processed and returned unmounted. The film is then examined to identify the best exposure among those that properly include both dark tones and light tones in one frame. The test is repeated for each significant situation, for example, a different light source. Discipline at this stage will produce a consistent technique.

Calibrating a video system begins with the selection of a tape. (Use house brands for copying tapes, name-brand consumer grades for documentation, and a name-brand professional grade when editing or post-production is planned). When reading manuals provided with the system, special attention should be paid to the section on white balance. Because each light source is different, proper setup of the camera for accurate color reproduction is important. It is also important to review the manual on the use of the color bars to properly set up the monitor or receiver for accurate reproduction. Finally, the user should be aware that any color camera needs a certain level of light intensity for good color; even the so-called low-light cameras perform better with higher than ambient levels (with the side benefit of more depth of field).

When using a white card for the balance setup, the f-stop should be checked for good levels. Thirty seconds of color bars should be recorded at the beginning of each tape. This allows the monitor to be checked before each showing and makes the high-wear section of the tape expendable.

Operation of an imaging system

Once the system has been successfully calibrated, the recurring task is to follow the procedure carefully (possibly with a checklist) and apply the procedure to appropriate situations. After the basic uses are mastered, variations can be introduced to cope with subject characteristics or esthetic considerations. Experimenting with different rendering techniques, in a disciplined way, can become a stimulating adjunct to routine documentation.

The specific issues in rendering dental subjects are: depth of field and resolution, tone and color reproduction, the quality of light, and the manipulation of the patient for viewing hard-to-see areas in the mouth.

Achieving adequate depth of field and resolution requires the proper lens and f-stop setting. Fortunately, there is a good selection of close-up lenses (commonly called macrofocusing) that are designed for use between 1:10 and 1:1. These lenses will produce high resolution images and commonly have small f-stops (f/22, f/32) for situations needing the most depth of field. Depth of field is not a panacea. As a lens is stopped down (beyond f/8 or f/11), resolution suffers. A compromise is always best made by using the f-stop that just covers the area needed.

Tone and color reproduction accuracy begin with matching the film type to the light source used (e.g., daylight films with electronic flash). Slide films have inherently high contrast, requiring very accurate ex-

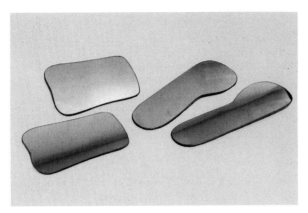

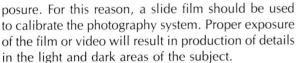

Figure 4-22

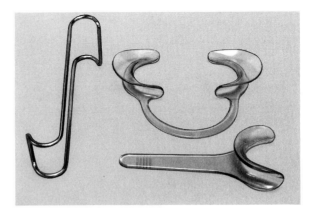

Figure 4-23

posure. For this reason, a slide film should be used to calibrate the photography system. Proper exposure of the film or video will result in production of details in the light and dark areas of the subject.

The quality of the light source determines the way the subject is illuminated. Because the image produced will always be two dimensional, some mechanism will be needed to portray those features of the subject, in whatever priority of rendering decisions are to be made. Generally, the size of the light source or sources in relation to the subject influences the type of shadows created. Shadows are a key factor in the perception of three dimensionality. Because most flash units are larger than structures in the oral cavity, they are usually easy to use in providing an evenly lit image.

Ring lights (surrounding the lens) produce the fewest shadows. Diffuse lighting (bounce flash) produces more. Point lights cause even more shadows and are best used when surface texture is very important to show. Specular highlights (no detail reflections of the light source) can be controlled by keeping the subject dry with cotton daubing or, in extreme situations (i.e., metallic subjects), by using cross-polarization. This is accomplished by putting a vertical polarizer over the light source and a horizontal polarizer over the lens.

Because of the current interest in cosmetic dentistry and the use of resin bonding and ceramics, it is also important to filter ultraviolet wavelengths from the light source. This is easily done by taping over the light source an ultraviolet filter obtained from a photo or lighting supply vendor. The choice of light source will become easier if identical images are made with different sources for reference.

Manipulation of the patient

Working with a patient to obtain the best view is a key factor in producing the needed images. The patient will experience minor discomfort while cheek retractors and mirrors are in use, similar to that experienced when bite-wing radiographs are taken. An unscratched set of tools should always be kept for making photographs, because the rhodium-plated mirrors that are recommended are easily damaged (Fig. 4-22). A selection of full arch, adult and child size retractors of clear plastic construction should be available (Fig. 4-23). The major courtesy to the patient is to work quickly, making all settings and adjustments to the equipment before patients assume their positions.

Guidelines for photography

This section on producing dental images is intended as an aid to the beginner. The troubleshooting chart in Table 4-1 may help diagnose the most common problems in photography and provide solutions. Practice, patience, and perseverance in the operation of all imaging systems will result in increased professional confidence and ability.

The following ten-step checklist provides guidelines for intraoral photographs:

1. Use these camera settings: light meter and flash, ASA/ISO 64, shutter speed at 1/60 second, and aperture between $f/8$ and $f/22$.
2. Get close. Exclude all extraneous structures surrounding the area of interest. This includes retractors and mirror edges. If a mirror image is

Table 4-1 Troubleshooting guide for dental photography

Appearance	Causes	Corrections
All black	Nothing exposed	Check loading technique.
		Have shutter and aperture checked professionally.
Dark, off-color, with highlights from flash visible	Not enough light entering camera	Increase aperture opening.
		Check flash batteries.
		Increase flash intensity.
		See test roll.
Dark, off-color, with no flash highlights visible	No flash activation	Check flash synchronization cable and/or batteries.
Half black	Flash and shutter not synchronized	Set shutter speed at 1/60 second.
Clear	– Film exposed to light or radiation	Keep away from radiation.
	– Camera back opened	Rewind film into cassette before opening camera back.
Blurred	Patient/photographer movement	Instruct patient to sit very still.
		Keep camera steady, squeeze shutter.
		Set shutter speed at 1/60 second.
Tissue color not desirable	Personal preference	Use filters on camera lens and/or flash.
	Incorrect lighting (color temperature)	Refer to test roll.
Light red, yellow smears	Picture made on exposed portion of film	"Click off" three frames prior to taking first photograph.

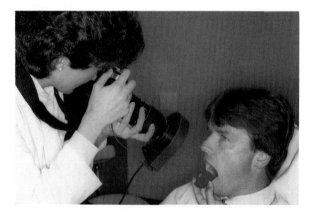

Figure 4-24

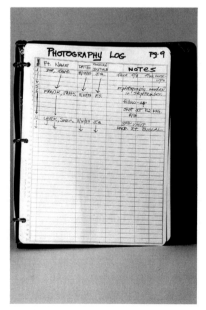

Figure 4-25

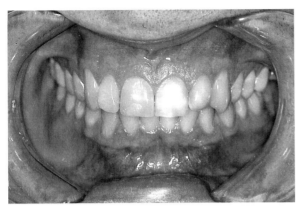

Fig. 4-26a Frontal view photograph in intraoral series.

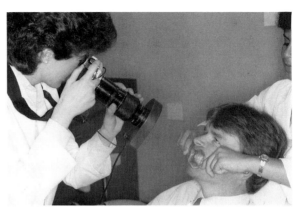

Fig. 4-26b Photographer–patient position for frontal view photograph.

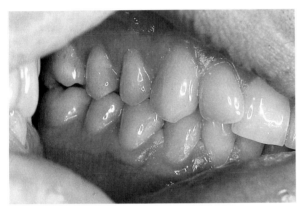

Fig. 4-27 Buccal view (*right*).

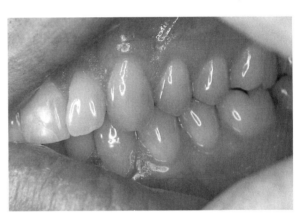

Fig. 4-28 Buccal view (*left*).

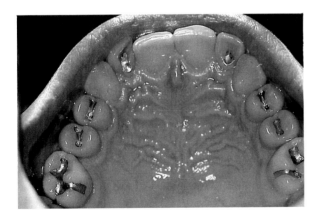

Fig. 4-29a Maxillary occlusal view.

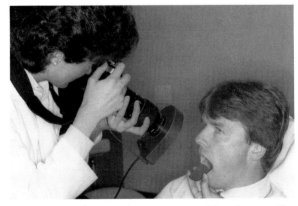

Fig. 4-29b Photographer–patient position for maxillary occlusal view.

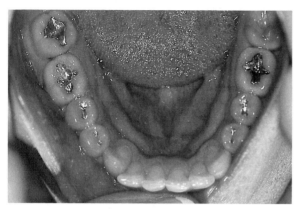

Fig. 4-30a   Mandibular occlusal view.

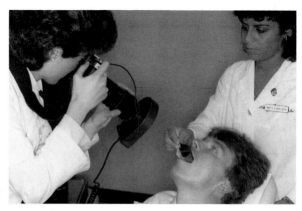

Fig. 4-30b   Photographer–patient position for mandibular occlusal view.

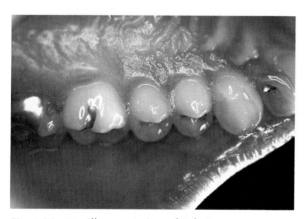

Fig. 4-31   Maxillary posterior palatal view.

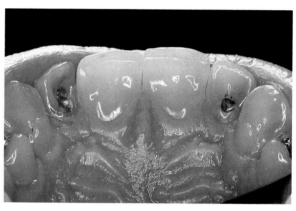

Fig. 4-32   Maxillary anterior palatal view.

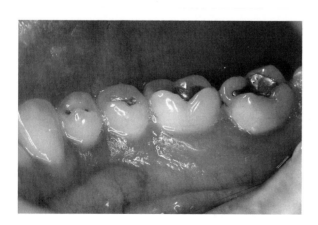

Fig. 4-33   Mandibular posterior lingual view.

being photographed, eliminate the actual oral structure from the viewfinder. If the subject and the mirror image are both visible, the audience will become confused. Fingers should be excluded from the view whenever possible.

3. Perform adequate tissue retraction. Use the appropriate size of retractor, moisten before inserting, place the retractor onto the edge of the lower lip, and then rotate parallel to the corner of the mouth.

4. Support the patient's head. This will reduce subject movement.

5. Adjust the patient and dental chair. Different views require different photographic angles, and so adjustment of the patient's head and the entire dental chair may be necessitated.

6. Keep the field of view dry. Use gentle, compressed air to eliminate glare on teeth and to reduce mirror fogging. Blood interferes with the area of interest and distracts the viewer's attention.

7. Use a lens-to-mirror angle of 45°. Align the length of the lens so that it forms a 45° angle with the mirror. An angle greater than 45° may cause the flash to bounce back through the shutter. This would be similar to taking your own picture in a mirror (Fig. 4-24).

8. Support the camera and lens. Keep elbows close to the body for added support. Make final focusing adjustments by rocking yourself back and forth until the image is in sharp focus. "Squeeze" the shutter release button. Do not "punch" it down, because this causes camera movement.

9. Be consistent in before and after views. Use the same camera, settings, lighting conditions, camera–subject distance, and camera–subject angle for before and after views.

10. Calibrate the imaging system for consistent results.

A ledger in which to record the date, patient name, and corresponding frame number is a vital record-keeping tool. This information can be transferred onto slide mounts or prints when they are returned by the processing laboratory. The ledger is also helpful when calibrating and testing new equipment or techniques and for noting camera settings, camera–subject position, and other detail (Fig. 4-25). The most convenient method of storing slides is to file them in clear vinyl sheets that hold 20 slides each.

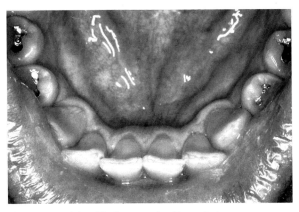

Fig. 4-34a Mandibular anterior lingual view.

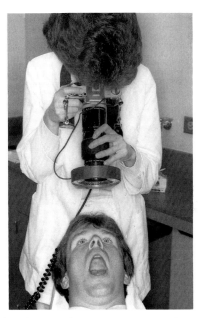

Fig. 4-34b Photographer–patient position for mandibular anterior lingual view.

Although an intraoral series requires no specific number of photographs, a full mouth survey will require the five separate views in Figs. 4-26 to 4-30. Additional photographic angles may be indicated in certain cases. Supplementary views may include full face and profile or any of these intraoral views: maxillary posterior palatal view, maxillary anterior palatal view, mandibular posterior lingual view, or mandibular anterior lingual view (Figs. 4-31 to 4-34).

part 2

The treatment plan: Formulation and implementation

chapter 5

Individualization of treatment

Previous chapters have discussed techniques for the prevention of communicable disease transmission. Many systemic diseases, although they do not pose the problem of contagion for the dental hygienist, result in oral or physiological manifestations that require alterations in the hygiene treatment plan. Different therapies, appointment scheduling, and postoperative procedures may be necessitated by the presence of these conditions.

Hematological disorders

Hematological disorders such as leukemia, anemia, hemophilia, and a thrombocytopenic purpura may cause changes in the oral cavity.

Leukemia manifests itself in the oral cavity by rounding and tenseness of the gingival margin due to packing of leukemic cells in the submucosa (Fig. 5-1). Blunting of the interdental papillae and varying degrees of gingival inflammation with ulceration, necrosis, and pseudomembrane formation occur. Infection is a major concern when delivering dental treatment to a leukemia patient. The symptoms are often present prior to a medical diagnosis. The dental hygienist must be alert to the oral signs and symptoms of leukemia, because dental treatment of an undiagnosed case may be very dangerous.

Consultation with the medical professionals responsible for treatment of the diagnosed leukemia patient is mandatory. Dental treatment allowed is very limited because of the danger of infection. If any dental care is to be delivered, preparatory techniques may be established by the physician, including prophylactic antibiotic coverage.

In anemic patients changes occur in the gingiva, the oral mucosa, lips, and most often the tongue (Fig. 5-2). The tongue appears red, smooth, and shiny because of the uniform atrophy of the fungiform and filliform papillae. The tongue may be painful and burning, and numbness may occur. The tongue is sensitive to hot or spicy food and swallowing is difficult. The mucosa and the lips may have a pallor. The gingiva appears hemorrhagic with petechiae on the mucous membrane.

The American black population has a one in ten incidence of sickle cell anemia. It is an hereditary form of hemolytic anemia that manifests itself in the oral cavity by the pallor often seen in other anemias (Fig. 5-3). In addition, some of the tissues may have a jaundiced color indicative of destruction of liver tissues. Bone loss and osteoporosis are also often seen in these patients.

Hemophilia is an hereditary abnormality of the blood characterized by prolonged hemorrhaging following lacerations. The coagulation time of the blood is prolonged. The disease is due to a deficiency of a coagulation factor. Classic hemophilia is caused by a deficiency in Factor VIII (hemophilia A). Christmas disease is caused by a deficiency in Factor IX (hemophilia B). Von Willebrand's disease is due to a deficiency in Factor VIII as well as a deficiency in the synthesis of the plasma factor necessary for platelet function.[1]

Prior to dental treatment of the hemophiliac patient (Fig. 5-4), information concerning the severity of the condition and possible need of factor replacement should be obtained from the physician. Anesthetic administration should be limited, and block anesthesia should never be given. Aspirin or aspirin-contain-

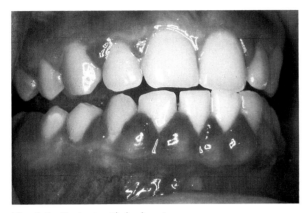

Fig. 5-1   Patient with leukemia.

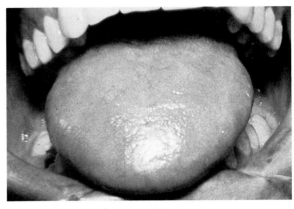

Fig. 5-2   Tongue of patient with anemia.

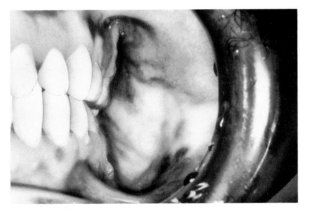

Fig. 5-3   Buccal mucosa of patient with sickle cell anemia.

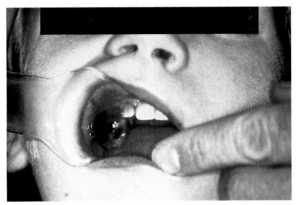

Fig. 5-4   Child hemophiliac patient.

ing compounds must never be prescribed. The soft tissues must always be protected. The most difficulty occurs from high speed evacuation or saliva ejector devices with the potential for causing a hematoma on the floor of the mouth.[1] Care must be taken so that corners of radiographic film and impression trays do not lacerate the patient's oral tissues. Because hemophiliac patients are commonly exposed to blood transfusions, health care personnel should wear gloves, mask, and glasses and maintain the sterilization techniques recommended for possible hepatitis and AIDS patients.

Thrombocytopenia results in inadequate platelet numbers and is clinically manifested by prolonged bleeding. Thrombocytopenia rarely results from genetic factors. It is acquired by drug inducement and alcohol. The bleeding is usually from small superficial blood vessels. Oral manifestations include petechiae in the mucosa.[1]

Diabetes

The diabetic patient has an altered response of the tissues to local irritants and occlusal forces. Although diabetes does not cause periodontal disease, it may expedite the condition. The healing process tends to be retarded in the diabetic patient so that anticipated clinical results may not occur.

The diabetic patient (Fig. 5-5) has a dry mouth, usually redness in the gingiva, and can have an acetone breath. The dental hygienist must be alert to the symptoms of the diabetic emergencies of hypoglycemia, or insulin shock, and hyperglycemia, or dia-

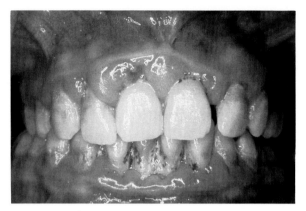

Fig. 5-5 Diabetic patient.

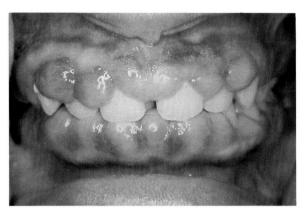

Fig. 5-6 Hyperplasia of patient taking Dilantin. (Courtesy of Dr. Anthony Gargiulo, Loyola University, Chicago, Ill.)

betic coma. Alteration in the treatment plan can help to prevent these emergencies. Appointments for the controlled diabetic patient should be scheduled 1½ hours after the morning meal and the patient's medication. The patient should not be kept waiting in the reception area, because anxiety may cause a glucose imbalance.[2] If extensive instrumentation is performed, the treatment plan should be adjusted so that scaling and related therapies are performed on half of the mouth and the other half is scheduled for a subsequent office visit.[2] The diabetic must eat regularly and must therefore be comfortable on at least one side of his mouth.

Epilepsy

An epileptic patient has oral manifestations, not of the disease, but of the drug taken for treatment of the disease, diphenylhydantoin (Dilantin). Use of the drug may cause excessive bleeding and overgrowth of the gingival tissues, called Dilantin hyperplasia (Fig. 5-6). The hygienist must always be alert to signs of epileptic seizure and take precautions not to contribute to the potentiality of a seizure. The dental operatory light should be used with care to avoid shining it in the patient's eyes. When taking radiographs or impressions, cold water rinses or topical anesthetic agents must be used to avoid triggering an unnecessary gag reflex or anxiety on the part of the patient.

Congenital defective diseases such as Down's Syndrome or Papillon-Lefèvre syndrome can result in oral manifestations that may affect the dental hygiene treatment plan. These include macroglossia, malformed dentition, and gross alveolar bone loss.

The presence of herpetic lesions should result in delay of scheduled dental treatment if at all possible. Exposing the host to possible further outbreaks—and exposing the operator as well—is contraindicated. If dental care must be administered, the operator should wear gloves, mask, and glasses and follow strict sterilization procedures.

Cancer

The dental hygienist plays a significant role in the team management of the patient with cancer. The greatest contribution made by any health care professional is early diagnosis. The routine performance of a thorough head and neck exam for all patients facilitates early identification of head and neck cancers and ultimately promotes a more positive prognosis and increases survival rate. Symptoms such as delayed healing, unusual or prolonged bleeding, and severe tenderness following routine dental procedures, should be investigated. These are often indicative of undiagnosed cancers such as leukemia or Hodgkin's disease.

Once the diagnosis of cancer has been ascertained, treatment modalities are determined by the medical and dental team. Treatment may be limited to surgery, radiation, or chemotherapy. Often, treatment will include a combination of these therapies. All patients receiving cancer therapy become highly susceptible to dental diseases, particularly the patient receiving

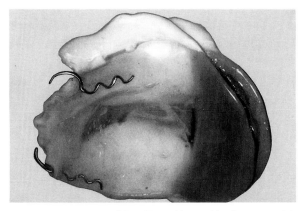

Fig. 5-7 Courtesy of Dr. Peter Hurst, Northwestern Memorial Hospital, Chicago, Ill.

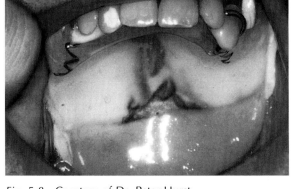

Fig. 5-8 Courtesy of Dr. Peter Hurst.

radiation therapy. Prevention and patient education are essential components of dental management. The hygienist provides valuable therapy for this patient population.

Hygiene care is divided into three management phases according to the stage of cancer therapy.

Pretreatment phase

An initial dental visit prepares the patient for upcoming treatment and expected oral changes. This visit should include a complete dental evaluation and a thorough prophylaxis. Ideally, this appointment should be scheduled at least 10 days prior to surgery, radiation, or chemotherapy. This time period gives the dental team the opportunity to eliminate or control caries and periodontal diseases. It also permits complete postoperative healing, if necessary. Patients are also better able to tolerate and to cooperate with the dental treatment plan.

A plaque control program should be incorporated at this visit. Maintaining optimal oral health will minimize the severity of oral complications. Home care instructions should include a general description of expected oral changes, but care should be taken not to alarm the patient.

Oral changes with surgery For the patient managed by surgery, instructions are limited to cleansing the surgical site. This is accomplished with a bulb syringe, an oral irrigation device, or by rinsing with a 0.9% sodium chloride solution four to six times a day.

If the surgical site leaves a significant defect, a prosthesis will be designed to help restore form and function. This prosthesis is referred to as an obturator (Fig. 5-7). Study models are taken prior to surgery to aid the oral surgeon and the dentist in its design to replace the hard and soft tissues sacrificed in the surgery. The obturator is placed immediately after surgery (Fig. 5-8). This allows the patient to eat, drink, and speak immediately following surgery, which encourages a faster recovery time postoperatively. Without an obturator, patients are fed intravenously and must use a note pad to communicate; hospital stays are extended.

Specific home care instructions for the obturator and final prosthesis are reserved until actual placement.

Oral changes with radiation Significant oral changes occur during the course of radiation therapy. Within 5 to 7 days of treatment, patients will experience mucositis, stomatitis, and xerostomia.[3]

Mucositis and stomatitis are transient changes that occur only during radiation.[3] The severity of symptoms is proportional to the dose of radiation. Doses vary from 5,000 to 7,500 rads. To ease the painful burning sensations, mouth rinses are utilized four to six times daily. Rinses commonly recommended include peroxide and baking soda or salt diluted in warm water. Diluted milk of magnesia is also helpful.

Xerostomia may be either a transient or a permanent change.[3] Dramatic reduction in salivary flow occurs in 5 to 7 days when the major salivary glands are included in the field of radiation. Salivary flow for some patients will return to normal within 6 months of completion of therapy. For others, salivary flow will never return to normal function. The remaining saliva becomes thick, ropy, and viscous. This inhibits the patient's ability to eat and to speak. It also compromises the patient's ability to maintain oral hygiene. Patients should be cautioned to avoid relieving xerostomia with candies and liquids containing sucrose because these foods cause the patient to be particularly susceptible to caries.

Saliva substitutes may be utilized to ease dryness. Several commercial products are available: Orex,* Xero-Lube,† Moi-Stir,‡ Salivart synthetic saliva.§ Most consist of a humectant and the predominant electrolytes balanced in natural saliva. Some have added fluoride to promote tooth remineralization. Many patients, however, prefer to sip water throughout the day rather than utilize a saliva substitute. Home rinses of glycerol and water, mineral oil and water, or saline rinses are also useful.

Alternatives to artificial saliva substitutes are being investigated. The drug philocarpine has been used to stimulate normal saliva production. Given orally, it induces saliva flow by stimulating receptors on the surface of the salivary glands without harmful side effects.[3] In addition, a method of inducing reflex salivation within the tongue and oral mucosa has been utilized. A battery-powered hand-held probe is inserted into the mouth for approximately 3 minutes. This method is painless and results in no tissue trauma. Patients reported increased salivary flow following three stimulations.[4]

With the onset of xerostomia, radiated patients also experience a marked change in the oral flora. The number of *Streptococcus mutans* and lactobacilli increases dramatically. The change in the oral flora and the xerostomia render the patient highly susceptible to radiation caries.[5] Radiation caries occurs at the cervical thirds of the teeth. It may also involve the incisal thirds of canines and premolars and molars. Its course is rapid and destructive. Without preventive dental care, the entire dentition can be lost.

In addition to effective sulcular tooth brushing and flossing, adjunctive therapy is needed to control

*Young Dental Manufacturing Co., Maryland Heights, Mo.
†Schever Laboratories, Dallas, Tex.
‡Kingswood Laboratories, Inc., Carmel, Ind.
§Westport Pharmaceuticals, Inc., Westport, Conn.

radiation caries. A fluoride supplement program is essential. A 1.23% acidulated fluoride gel is most commonly recommended. However, with recent innovations in research, many viable fluoride alternatives are available.[6] Patients should administer fluoride treatments at home, once a day, for 5 minutes. Custom trays, designed from study models, are recommended to aid in patient comfort and to ease delivery.

Another adjunct under current investigation is the use of the chemical plaque inhibitor chlorhexidine. Used in a 0.1% concentration, it significantly reduces the number of *Streptococcus mutans* in the oral flora. Chlorhexidine binds to the tooth surface and salivary proteins. It is retained in the oral cavity and released slowly over a 24 hour period.

Chlorhexidine is now available for oral use in the United States. It has been under investigation by the Federal Drug Administration, although it has been used in Europe for 30 years. Chlorhexidine causes superficial staining of the teeth. This stain is extrinsic and is easily removed by professional prophylaxis. Mucosal irritation has also been reported, but usually with a 0.2% concentration. Chlorhexidine has also been combined with fluoride as an adjunctive form of therapy. It has been used for the successful maintenance of a group of patients undergoing radiation therapy who utilized this combined mode of therapy as a mouth rinse.[6] Now that chlorhexidine is approved by the FHA for oral use, it will be available by prescription only.

Nutritional counseling Most patients receiving radiation for head and neck tumors will receive 5,000 to 7,500 rads. The treatments are often fractioned into 30 sessions, with 5 per week. Patients are usually seen on an outpatient basis. Before each treatment, patients are weighed. If weight loss exceeds 10 pounds, the patient is referred for nutritional counseling. By this time, the patient is nutritionally depleted and counseling is a great challenge.

The hygienist can provide supportive nutritional counseling from the onset of therapy before a major weight loss has occurred. Patients should increase protein intake and minimize sucrose intake. Liquids should be taken with all meals to facilitate chewing and swallowing. Citrus fruits and juices should be taken with caution because of mucositis. Diluting them with water will minimize irritation. Commercial mouthwashes also irritate mucosa and should be

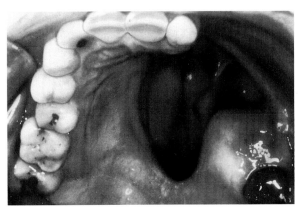

Fig. 5-9a Stoma. (Courtesy of Dr. Peter Hurst.)

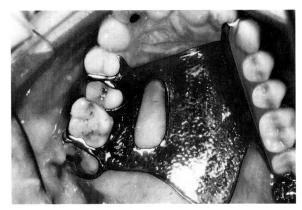

Fig. 5-9b Stoma with obturator in place. (Courtesy of Dr. Peter Hurst.)

avoided. Smoking and drinking alcohol should also be avoided.

To combat anorexia and ageusia patients should eat small but frequent meals. Daily caloric goals should be set. Food diaries help the patient attain a set goal each day. A text, *Eating Hints,* provided by the U.S. Department of Health and Human Services, is an excellent resource for both the hygienist and the patient.

Oral changes with chemotherapy   Forty percent of patients receiving chemotherapy report manifestations of oral complications. Depending on the agent used, patients report mucositis, stomatitis, and most significantly, oral bleeding resulting from bone marrow suppression. This group is also more susceptible to bacterial and fungal infections, of which candidiasis is the most common. Patient education and management is similar to that for the radiation patient. Strict oral hygiene procedures must be stressed to minimize oral complications.

Treatment phase

Surgery management   The patient managed surgically is evaluated daily by both the oral surgery team and the dental team during the hospital stay. The hygienist provides support by evaluating the patient's ability to irrigate the surgical site.

If an obturator has been placed, the patient requires instruction for irrigation of the surgical site and for care of the obturator as well. This is a particularly traumatic time for the patient. Time is needed to adjust to the new obturator as well as the new defect (stoma) (Fig. 5-9a). A bulb syringe must be used to irrigate the defect with 0.9% sodium chloride. Aseptic techniques for handling the obturator and cleaning the site should be demonstrated. Placement and removal of the obturator should also be demonstrated (Fig. 5-9b).

Following hospital release, the patient will be seen once a week by the dentist and a speech pathologist, if necessary. As the surgical site heals, the tissue constricts and the obturator requires adjusting. The hygienist can also utilize these visits to reinforce hygiene and support nutritional counseling.

Radiation management   The patient receiving radiation is seen once a week by the dentist and the hygienist. Careful evaluation of the dentition is vital to maintain optimal oral health. From the onset of radiation, the patient is highly susceptible to a severe form of osteomylitis termed osteoradionecrosis. This infection, once initiated, is very difficult to treat. Antibiotics are the drugs of choice, but are limited by the decreased vascularity of the bone resulting from the permanent effects of radiation. Bony destruction is marked and often requires the sacrifice of significant areas of bone to excise an infected area. The mandible is typically the most common site of osteoradionecrosis.

Prophylactic antibiotics may be needed prior to any major dental procedure for the lifetime of the patient who has received radiation to the head and neck regions.

The hygienist assists the dentist in careful evaluation of the patient by completing thorough dental and periodontal charts each week. With the onset of severe mucositis, the patient may need assistance in plaque control measures. Scaling procedures are often needed. If toothpaste is irritating because of the mucositis, dry brushing should be attempted. If tooth brushing itself is impossible, a soft sponge on a stick (toothette) may be temporarily substituted until sensitivity has subsided.

Chemotherapy management Patients receiving chemotherapy are evaluated prior to the course of each treatment when platelet counts are highest. Treatments are given once every 5 to 6 weeks. Length of therapy depends on the prescribed management by the team. Blood counts are evaluated frequently. The physician should always be consulted prior to any dental treatment, because these patients often need prophylactic antibiotics before dental care.

As with the patient receiving radiation treatment, careful dental evaluation must be performed. These patients are particularly susceptible to infection, and so oral antibiotic mouthrinses or lozenges are often prescribed. Antifungal agents such as nystanin rinses or chlorimazole troches are utilized to control candidiasis.

The hygienist should evaluate the patient's oral hygiene. If oral bleeding complicates brushing, the toothette sponge should be substituted temporarily for brushing. Carious lesions are usually a threat only to the patient on long-term therapy. A fluoride program should be instituted if necessary.

Posttreatment phase

An individualized recall program should be designed for all cancer patients. Routinely these patients are placed on a maximum 3-month recall program.

The routine performance of the head and neck exam is of vital importance. Communication with the patient's oral surgeon provides supportive team care. Dental radiographs should be taken judiciously for the radiation patient. Thorough dental and periodontal records should be kept to facilitate preventive care. Osteoradionecrosis is a permanent threat to radiation patients; therefore prophylactic antibiotics may be needed before major dental work. Consultation with the patient's physician should be an ongoing process.

The hygienist should perform thorough scaling and root planing at each recall visit. Selective polishing may offer a viable alternative for the patient with ongoing xerostomia. Fluoride therapy should remain a permanent part of the patient's home care program. A mouthrinse vehicle by prescription rather than an over-the-counter rinse is preferred. Nutritional counseling should continue to encourage the patient to regain weight lost prior to therapy and to maintain a balanced diet. Exercises to stretch fibrous muscle fibers (trismus) are helpful to the patient with restricted mouth opening.

The dental hygienist should be aware of the vital role she or he plays in the team management of the cancer patient. Survival rates are increasing and many of these patients are turning to the private practice dental office because of the limited numbers of hospital dental programs. As a result, it is not unlikely that many dental hygienists will have the opportunity to treat these individuals.

Systemic and localized conditions

Hormonal imbalances due to pregnancy, menopause, and the use of oral contraceptives may result in an increase in vascular proliferation and gingival bleeding (Fig. 5-10). Palliative measures may need to be employed posttherapeutically. Osteoporosis is prevalent in menopausal females and can present a severe influence on the comfortable fit of removable prosthetic appliances.

Lichen planus is a dermatologic disorder that manifests itself in the oral cavity by angulated papules. Hormonal factors may be contributory. Psychosomatic factors seem to be involved in a large percentage of clinical cases as may be dermatologic disorders. The most common lesion sites are the buccal mucosa and the facial surface of the gingiva. The lesions appear as grayish white, lace-like elevations composed of individual papules (Fig. 5-11).

Other endocrinological situations influence the etiology of periodontal disease. Hyperthyroidism and hypopituitarism have a correlation with alveolar bone and cementum pathology. Hypoparathyroidism in infancy causes enamel hypoplasia and disrupts calcification of the dentin. Hyperparathyroidism results in formation of bone cysts, giant cell tumors, and alveolar osteoporosis.

Patients who have the collagen disorder lupus erythematosus may have characteristic butterfly distri-

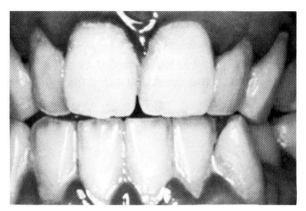

Fig. 5-10 Hormonal imbalance a contributing factor in gingivitis.

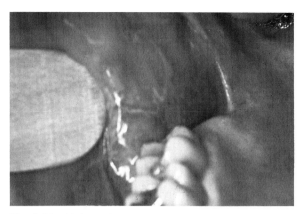

Fig. 5-11 Lichen planus.

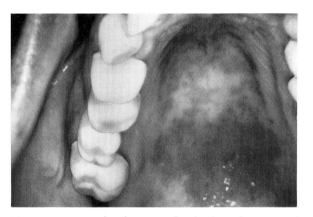

Fig. 5-12 Lesion distribution on hard palate of patient with lupus erythematosus.

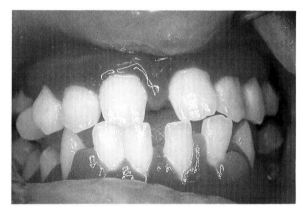

Fig. 5-13 Acute periodontal condition. (Courtesy of Dr. Anthony Gargiulo.)

bution lesions on the face and palate (Fig. 5-12). Oral manifestations are similar to pemphigus: irregular superficial or deep erosions covered with necrotic grayish pseudomembrane. These patients are light sensitive. Care should be taken because the dental light may increase skin eruptions.

Acute periodontal conditions are those that have a rapid onset and the tissue is usually red and bleeds easily (Fig. 5-13). Periodontal abscesses, acute gingivitis, pericoronitis, and acute necrotizing ulcerative gingivitis (ANUG) are those most commonly dealt with by the dental hygienist.

ANUG is an inflammatory infection of the gingiva characterized by pain, fetid odor, a whitish pseudomembrane, bleeding, ulcerated papillae, and foul metallic taste. It usually has a sudden onset (Fig. 5-14). A multitude of factors may contribute to the etiology, including poor nutrition, stress, poor oral hygiene, excessive smoking or use of alcohol, and fatigue. All factors are not present in each case, of course. The classic victim of ANUG is the college student who "burns the candles at both ends" during exam time. The use of ultrasonic scaling devices is indicated when treating the ANUG patient. Palliative use of warm water or hydrogenating agents may also be used. Antibiotic therapy may be employed during the acute phase of the infection. The techniques of therapy for all acute and chronic periodontal conditions will be elaborated in a later chapter.

Persons who abuse alcohol have oral manifesta-

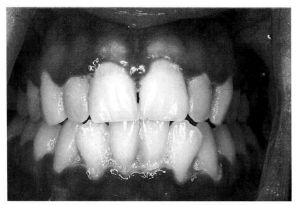

Fig. 5-14 Necrotizing ulcerative gingivitis. (Courtesy of Dr. Anthony Gargiulo.)

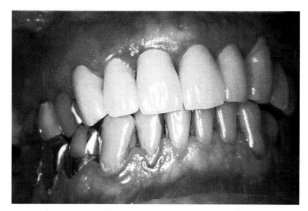

Fig. 5-15 Alcoholic patient.

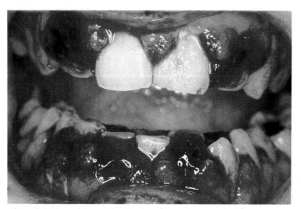

Fig. 5-16 Courtesy of Dr. Bernard Pecaro, Northwestern University, Chicago, Ill.

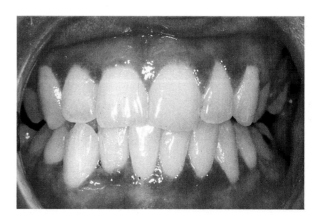

Fig. 5-17 Courtesy of Dr. Bernard Pecaro.

tions that include heavy deposits, parched lips, yellow-brown cheeks and palate, swollen parotid glands, and a red, slick tongue similar to that seen in a patient with anemia (Fig. 5-15). The characteristics of the tongue are due to malnutrition. Some of the other oral symptoms relate to the presence of liver disorders. In addition, the face of the alcoholic appears red, often with pitting edema and the presence of telangiectasia. Prolonged bleeding should be anticipated when manipulating the "beefy" red gingiva of the alcoholic patient. Wound healing will also be retarded.

With the elevated status of dentistry and dental hygiene today in the health care delivery system, medical personnel look to dental professionals to pro-

vide therapy for all types of outpatients and hospitalized patients. With new techniques and understanding, no one need go untreated.

The patient in Fig. 5-16 has a multitude of systemic complications; in fact, the patient is terminally ill. Should this patient have to spend the last 6 months of his life unable to eat, smile, or speak with his loved ones? Traditional periodontal therapies are contraindicated in this case, but the patient was treated with laser surgical techniques. The result shown in Fig. 5-17 allowed him to live out his remaining days able to converse and maintain his dignity as a human being.

If the patient has one of the systemic or localized conditions for which consultation with the physician of record is indicated, a medical consult form should be utilized.

Dental hygiene therapy phase

The classic approach to dental therapy is problem oriented. Endodontic therapy, oral surgery, and periodontal problems are therefore treated first, followed by restorative treatment. Dental hygiene therapy has usually been categorized as periodontal treatment. In reality, in the absence of an episodic crisis, it is the dental hygienist with whom the patient is first appointed. If no potential emergency and no medically compromising factors exist, the amount of deposits present, the condition of the oral tissues, and the patient's needs are used to determine the most appropriate treatment approach.

While routine dental hygiene appointments vary from office to office, typically the appointment includes radiographic survey (bite-wing or full-mouth, if indicated), oral health care instructions, health assessment or update, study models, scaling, therapeutic root planing and curettage, polishing, and the application of fluoride and/or pit and fissure sealants.

The first consideration is of the amount of calculus present and therefore the amount of subsequent instrumentation required in the mouth. If the treatment cannot be completed in one appointment because of the amount of deposits, a medically impacting factor, or the patient's intolerance of a long procedure, the

dental hygienist must determine if two or more appointments will be required. If two appointments will suffice, instrumentation should be performed to completely debride the maxillary and mandibular quadrants of one side of the mouth. If more than two appointments will be necessary, a quadrant-per-appointment approach may be established.

In the presence of significant amounts of deposit, the area being treated should be debrided completely. Use of an ultrasonic scaler to "gross scale" the entire mouth is contraindicated. Removal of the deposits that are coronal, missing small pieces of deposits apically, may result in healing occurring above the missed deposit and subsequent formation of a periodontal abscess because of the trapped infection below.

Depending on the patient's needs, the caries control and plaque control phases of the appointment may take priority. Time may need to be scheduled for educational materials such as videotapes or for discussion of pamphlets if the patient's dental condition requires restorative or periodontal therapy. The pedodontic patient may require even more preparatory time for discussion of the procedures to be employed and development of patient rapport. Fluoride therapy and emphasis of fluoride home regimens are of the utmost importance for the child patient. The use of pumice as a cleaning agent in the prophylaxis phase of the appointment is contraindicated for children as well as for patients with exposed root surfaces or gold and porcelain restorative dentistry.

References

1. Scopp, I.W. Oral Medicine. St. Louis: C.V. Mosby Co., 1973, pp. 245–248.
2. Phagan, P.A. Dental hygiene therapy for the diabetic patient. Quintessence J. 3(1):21–23, 1981.
3. Baum, B.J., and Fox, P.C. NIDR Dry Mouth Clinic Report. Bethesda: National Institute of Dental Research, 1985.
4. Brenman, H.S., Katz, P., and Schwartz, H.L. Production of saliva in patients with xerostomia by specific electro stimulation. Presented at I.A.D.R. 63rd General Session, 1985.
5. Fox, P.C., et al. Quantification of Total Salivary Mucins. Bethesda: National Institute of Dental Research, 1985.
6. Katz, S. The use of fluoride and chlorhexidine for prevention of radiation caries. J. Am. Dent. Assoc. 104(2):164–170, 1982.

chapter 6

Techniques for optimal efficiency

Dental hygiene is a profession that requires a number of skills that are repeated for each patient who is treated. Because of the level of expertise required and the close, confined area in which much of the treatment is performed, the work can easily become tedious and exhausting. While tedium may be overcome by focusing on the patient as an individual, with unique characteristics and circumstances affecting treatment, fatigue is a separate issue that can be dealt with by incorporating efficiency and motion economy into everyday practice.

Sequencing

One of the first techniques to utilize in the development of operator efficiency is the establishment of an overall pattern or routine to follow for general patient treatment. For example, always begin each appointment with a review of the medical history. Continue with the extraoral and intraoral examination, patient education, scaling, and the remaining procedures. Following a regular routine helps to assure that no important procedures are inadvertently eliminated or forgotten. There will, of course, be occasions when deviation from the pattern is both necessary and desirable, but in general a regular sequencing of tasks is the appropriate course of action.

Once the dental hygienist has established an overall pattern of treatment, a routine approach to the performance of each individual task can then be established. Again, the rationale for doing so is to avoid elimination of any component of the task. For ex-

Table 6-1 Suggested patterns for scaling procedures

Area to be scaled	Suggested pattern
Full mouth	Begin scaling tooth 32, distofacial. Proceed mesially tooth by tooth to the distofacial of tooth 17. Switch to the distolingual of tooth 17 and continue across the mandible to the distolingual of tooth 32. Follow the same sequence on the maxilla, beginning with the distofacial of tooth 1.
Half mouth	Follow the above sequence but stop at the mesiofacial of tooth 25. Scale the lingual surfaces of those teeth, then proceed to the maxillary right quadrant and follow the same sequence.
Quadrant	If only one quadrant is to be treated per appointment, several options are available: a. Scale all facial surfaces first, followed by all lingual surfaces. b. Scale two to three teeth at a time, first facial surfaces, then lingual. c. Scale each tooth completely (facial, interproximal, and lingual surfaces), one by one.

ample, when performing the extraoral and intraoral examination, the clinician might begin by examining the extraoral structures: visually inspect the head and neck area; palpate the lymph nodes in the neck, the thyroid gland, submandibular lymph nodes, temporomandibular joint; and so on. Then proceed to routinely examine the intraoral structures. The sequencing of each task involved in dental hygiene therapy may be established accordingly to individual preference.

It is especially critical to establish a definitive sequence when employing instrumentation skills, because these cannot be evaluated by visual inspection. Many clinicians find that always beginning scaling in one particular area and proceeding systematically around the dental arches is of great value in the conservation of time and motion. The individual patient's oral hygiene condition will, to a great degree, dictate the pattern to be followed. Table 6-1 lists several suggested patterns for scaling procedures. These are suggestions only, not mandates to which blind adherence is advocated.

Motion economy

Another technique that can increase efficiency is to utilize a given instrument fully before putting it down and choosing another. The instrument should be used on all appropriate tooth surfaces of the area being scaled, assuring optimum use. This will help to limit continuous reaching for various instruments during instrumentation. It also aids in concentration while working. The hygienist should also avoid constant flipping of double-ended instruments; again, a given end should be fully utilized before flipping to the instrument's opposite end.

The design of the operatory can greatly enhance or hinder efficiency. All supplies, instruments, and patient-education devices should ideally be located within arm's reach of the seated operator, thus avoiding wasted time spent with constant rising and leaving the chair to obtain needed items. Instruments that are stored on preset trays or packaged together for sterilization purposes can contribute to maximum time utilization. Planning for the usual need for instruments and supplies as opposed to the occasional or irregular need is generally considered best.

Much of the dental hygienist's day-to-day practice involves motion of all types. Efficiency can be enhanced greatly by an understanding of the system of motion classification and utilization of the most appropriate types of motions during the practice of dental hygiene. A system to classify common movements utilized in dentistry was developed following research into the subjects of motion and time. The following categorization[1] will be used in the discussion of motion economy:

Class I
Movement of the fingers only.
Class II
Movement of the fingers and wrist.
Class III
Movement of the fingers, wrist, and elbow.
Class IV
Movement of the entire arm from the shoulder.
Class V
Movement of the entire arm and twisting of the trunk.

Generally, economy of motion limits the number of Class IV and V movements as much as possible during chairside activity. These two types of movements require greater time expenditure and are substantially more fatiguing to the operator. Particularly in Class V motions, the hygienist must look away from the operating field, which is more brightly lit than the surrounding area, and refocus her or his eyes. Eyestrain and headaches can result from this constant refocusing. The design of the operatory and the storage of equipment, instruments, and supplies can substantially reduce the number of Class IV and V motions.

Positioning of the dental hygienist and patient

Efficiency is enhanced when both hygienist and patient are seated appropriately. A patient who is physically comfortable in the dental chair is more relaxed and easier to treat. The dental hygienist who is seated correctly is able to function effectively over longer periods of time and with less fatigue.

Before the patient is seated, the dental chair should be lowered completely, in an upright position, and with the chair arm lifted or adjusted so that the patient has easy access. Once the patient has been seated, the hygienist should lower or adjust the chair arm and place a patient napkin around his or her neck. The contour style dental chair usually has several buttons or control knobs located either on the back of the chair just beneath the headrest or on the side of the chair itself. A foot-control lever near the base may raise and lower the entire chair. Before the actual positioning of the patient, the dental hygienist should

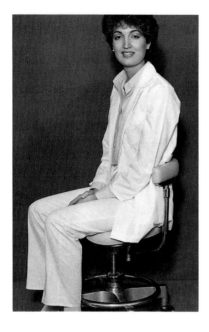 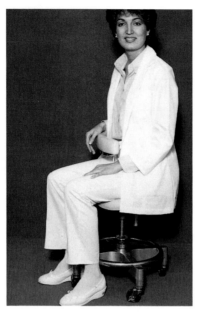

Figure 6-1a   (left)

Figure 6-1b   (right)

be seated on the operator's stool, because the amount of chair adjustment depends on the position of the operator.

The dental hygienist is seated on the middle of the stool so that her or his weight is evenly distributed over the seat (Fig. 6-1a). The feet should be flat on the floor, with the thighs parallel to the floor. Most operator stools have an adjustment knob or lever to raise or lower the seat. Some stools have an abdominal support arm; if used, this should lie just below the operator's ribs to afford support when leaning forward from the waist (Fig. 6-1b).

The operator sits astride, with the legs separated. For this reason, pants are recommended instead of skirts or dresses when treating patients. This position provides a more even distribution of the clinician's weight and less likelihood of bending, twisting, or leaning during practice. The back and neck should be straight, with the head centered over the spinal column.

While some individuals do sit with the legs together, this position tends to encourage the operator to shift her or his weight to one side, thereby allowing for uneven distribution of body weight. This in turn may cause muscle strain and increased fatigue for the operator. For this reason, this position is the less desirable and generally not recommended. If the hygienist does choose to be seated with the legs together,

however, every effort must be made to keep body weight evenly distributed, feet flat on the floor with the thighs parallel to the floor.

Once the hygienist is comfortably and appropriately seated, the patient is positioned. The entire chair is tilted back to place the patient in a supine position and settle the patient's hips in the angle of the chair. Next the back of the chair is lowered so that it lies just above the lap of the operator. The headrest is adjusted to a comfortable position. When properly positioned, the patient's head and feet should be at the same height. The entire chair may then be raised or lowered to achieve the appropriate working distance.

The patient should be positioned so that the oral cavity is at the same approximate height as the hygienist's elbows (Fig. 6-2a). The hygienist should not have either to reach up or even to lean over to reach the patient's mouth. The hygienist's elbows and upper arms should be kept close to the body while working, with the forearms parallel to the floor when the hands are in position for working (Fig. 6-2b). The distance between the patient's face and the hygienist's nose should be 14 to 18 inches. When properly positioned, both patient and hygienist should be comfortable and relaxed.

When teeth in the maxillary arch are being treated, the back portion of the chair is positioned so that it

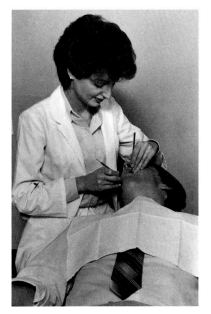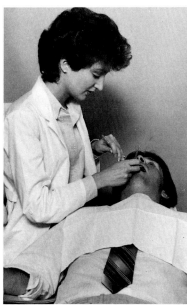

Figure 6-2a   (left)

Figure 6-2b   (right)

is level and parallel to the floor, in the complete su-pine position. The patient's feet should be slightly higher than the head. When the mandibular teeth are to be treated, the back of the chair is slightly raised and the entire chair lowered, to enhance visibility of the working area and maintain the patient's oral cavity at elbow height for the hygienist. The overhead light is adjusted to provide optimum illumination of the working area.

At times the dental hygienist may be unable to utilize the seated position when delivering patient care. Some patients may, for health reasons, be un-able to tolerate the supine position. Other patients may be confined to a wheelchair or, in the case of hospitalized or institutionalized patients, a bed or mo-bile cart. In such circumstances, the dental hygienist may be required to stand while treating the patient in order to gain access to the patient's oral cavity. The basic principles for the standing position are similar to those for the seated position: body weight should be evenly distributed on both legs, feet should be flat on the floor, and the patient should be at a height, whenever possible, to avoid excessive bending, twist-ing, or leaning by the hygienist.

Obviously, not all of these principles can be fol-lowed exactly at all times; the important point to re-member is to strive to work under conditions that resemble the ideal as often as is feasible.

Table 6-2   Operating zones

Right-handed operator		Left-handed operator
7 to 12 o'clock	Operator's zone	12 to 5 o'clock
12 to 2 o'clock	Static zone	10 to 12 o'clock
2 to 4 o'clock	Assistant's zone	8 to 10 o'clock
4 to 7 o'clock	Transfer zone	5 to 8 o'clock

Zones of operation

When the patient and operator are seated, the oper-ator assumes one of several positions in reference to the patient for actual rendering of therapy. These stan-dardized positions are referred to as operating zones, or zones of activity. With the patient in a supine po-sition, the patient's face may be imagined as the cen-ter of a clock. From this reference point, four zones have been established and are designated as shown in Table 6-2.

Generally, the hygienist remains at all times in her or his zone when providing direct patient care. De-pending on the area of the patient's mouth being treated, the hygienist will sit at a specified clock po-sition to attain optimum access and visibility.

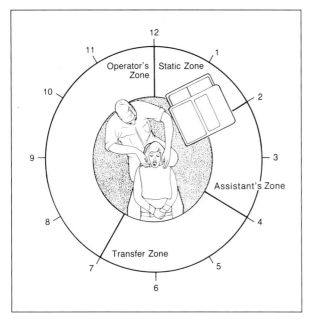

Fig. 6-3a Right-handed operator.

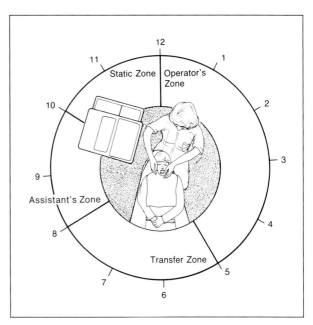

Fig. 6-3b Left-handed operator.

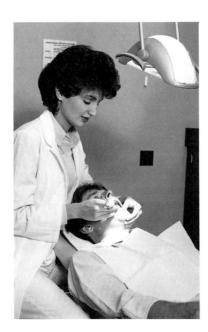
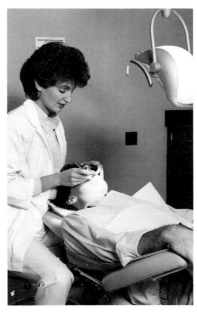

Figure 6-4a *(left)*

Figure 6-4b *(right)*

The static zone is the area in which infrequently used equipment is kept. In some equipment delivery systems, however, the dental unit itself may be located in this area, particularly if a mobile cart system is employed. The assistant's zone is the area occupied by the dental assistant. The assistant usually maintains the same position during most, if not all, dental treatment procedures—3 o'clock for the right-handed clinician, 9 o'clock for the left-handed clinician (Figs. 6-3a and b). While the dental hygienist does not usually work with a chairside assistant, often she or he will perform assisting duties when necessary.

The transfer zone is the area of greatest activity, since instruments and other dental materials are passed between assistant and operator in this zone. In many dental operatories, the dental unit itself is located here, which allows easy access to frequently utilized equipment such as air–water syringe, handpiece, evacuation system, and bracket tray for instruments. Locating the unit in this position also helps to decrease the number of Class IV and V movements on the part of the operator.

Use of the overhead dental light

Because the intraoral field of operation is both small and enclosed, visualizing all structures without the aid of an auxiliary light source is difficult. For this reason, some type of overhead lamp is utilized to illuminate the oral cavity. The light may be mounted onto the unit itself or on the wall or ceiling of the operatory. This high-intensity lamp directs light rays so that the beam is concentrated over a relatively small area, that is, the patient's oral cavity. Most overhead lamps are covered by a plastic safety shield to guard against accidental shattering of the bulb. In the majority of cases, the switch is located on the lamps themselves.

Optimum and appropriate use of the overhead light will greatly enhance the efficiency of the clinician by providing a work area that is well lit. When treating the mandibular arch, the light should be high and directed downward onto the patient's face (Fig. 6-4a). For the maxillary arch, the lamp is placed lower near the lap of the patient and directed straight into the patient's mouth (Fig. 6-4b). In addition, the light may be angled to the right or left of the patient, when necessary, to more fully illuminate a particular segment or area of the mouth. The operator should develop the habit of routinely adjusting the overhead light when the positioning of the patient is changed to assure optimum illumination of the field of operation.

References

1. Chasteen, J.E. Four-handed Dentistry in Clinical Practice. St. Louis: C.V. Mosby Co., 1978, pp. 9–10, 32–34.

chapter 7

Composition of dental deposits

Before the dental hygienist attempts to perform scaling, root planing, curettage, or polishing techniques, the type, amount, and nature of hard and soft deposits should be determined. Soft deposits include the acquired pellicle, plaque, materia alba, food debris, and stains.

Acquired pellicle

The first soft deposit to form in the oral cavity is the acquired pellicle. This deposit is an acellular, organic, amorphous mass that is derived from salivary and gingival fluids. Its composition is chiefly glycoproteins, which adhere closely to the tooth surfaces. Pellicle forms over tooth surfaces, restorations, appliances, and other existing deposits within several hours after complete deposit removal. The acquired pellicle serves as the framework, or nidus, for the development of bacterial plaque in that microorganisms selectively prefer this mode for attachment.

Pellicle is not completely removable through rinsing with water or toothbrushing; it can be removed by professional prophylaxis. It is discernable through the application of disclosing solution but will appear much lighter in color than will disclosed plaque.

Bacterial plaque

Bacterial plaque is generally considered to be the most significant of all the oral deposits and has been identified as the primary etiologic factor in the establishment of dental disease. Both periodontal disease and dental caries are prominently linked with the presence of bacterial plaque (Fig. 7-1). The primary differences among the several types of plaque are illustrated by the microbial components. Plaque may be either calculus-producing (calculogenic), periodontal disease-producing, or cariogenic in nature.

Plaque is composed primarily of bacteria that initially attach to the tooth surface via the acquired pellicle. As plaque is allowed to remain relatively undisturbed, the microorganisms begin to colonize in a thick, gel-like matrix. The actual progression of plaque formation is quite specific and the microbial composition changes as plaque matures. The specific timetable is illustrated in Table 7-1.

The overall composition of plaque is water (80%) plus organic and inorganic solids (20%). Of the solid components, the microorganisms comprise approximately 70% of the matter. The microbial content is higher in subgingival than in supragingival plaque.

The organic components of plaque consist of microorganisms, the organic matrix, by-products of microbial metabolism (acids, toxins, enzymes, endotoxins, antigens), broken down microbial cells, leukocytes, shed epithelial cells, salivary components (carbohydrates, proteins, lipids), soluble food components (particularly fermentable carbohydrates), and extracellular polysaccharides such as dextran, which are synthesized by the bacteria from sucrose. In subgingival plaque, there are also gingival sulcular fluid components.

The inorganic segment of plaque consists of calcium, phosphorous, magnesium, and fluoride. Plaque that forms in certain areas of the mouth (such as lingual surfaces of mandibular anterior teeth) will typically have a higher densification of phosphorous and calcium than other teeth. The concentration of these

124

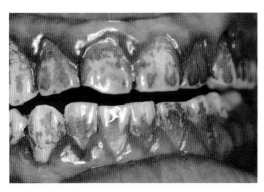

Fig. 7-1   Bacterial plaque evidenced by use of disclosing solution. (From N. Ohta, et al.: *Periodontal Therapy: Textbook for Dental Hygienists,* Quintessence Publ. Co., 1985, in Japanese.)

Table 7-1   Plaque formation timetable

Time (in days)	Microbial composition
Initial formation	Gram-positive cocci are formed (Neisseria, Nocardia, Streptococcus mutans and S. sanguis).
2 to 3	Gram-negative cocci and rods increase; filamentous forms and rods gradually replace cocci.
4 to 7	Filamentous forms and anaerobics increase (Fusobacterium, Actinomyces, Veillonella); flora is more mixed, with appearance of spirochetes and vibrios.
7 to 14	Vibrios, spirochetes, and white blood cells increase; signs of gingival inflammation begin to be observed.
14 to 21	Prevalent forms are spirochetes and vibrios, in addition to filamentous forms and cocci; gingivitis is clinically evident.

inorganic elements is generally higher in patients who form calculus very readily and heavily.

Supragingival plaque differs in several respects from subgingival plaque. Deep periodontal pockets provide shelter from oral hygiene cleaning devices, allowing the plaque to mature relatively undisturbed. The pocket also creates a different environment in which microorganisms, especially anaerobic forms, can flourish. Fusiforms, spirochetes, and *Bacteroides melaninogenicus* are more prevalent in subgingival than in supragingival plaque.

A number of research studies investigating the relationship between plaque accumulation and development of gingivitis have been conducted. When all oral hygiene measures are halted and plaque is allowed to mature undisturbed, clinical signs of gingival inflammation can be detected after 10 to 21 days. When thorough plaque removal procedures are reinstituted, gingivitis is reversed and tissues return to a healthy state.

Other studies have been conducted to determine the influence of food intake on plaque development. While the nature and consistency of the diet appear to affect the degree of plaque formation, the deposit will accumulate regardless of food availability. Increased amounts of plaque do tend to form when the diet is soft and especially if it consists of large amounts of fermentable carbohydrates. In the past, patients were routinely advised to eat "detergent" foods such as raw carrots, apples, celery, and other such foods to reduce plaque formation. Recent research has shown that plaque continues to develop along the gingival third of the teeth in spite of regular intake of these foods.

A number of chemical plaque-inhibiting substances have recently been developed and are currently being researched. Preliminary results with this modality of plaque control show promise in the future as a potentially valuable asset to control dental disease.

Materia alba

Materia alba is a white or grayish white bulky soft deposit that somewhat resembles cottage cheese in appearance. It is composed of food debris particles, salivary proteins, living and dead bacteria, desquamated epithelial cells, and disintegrating leukocytes. It is clearly visible upon clinical examination and does not require use of a disclosing solution for detection. This deposit forms over plaque and adheres loosely to the tooth surfaces. Materia alba is easily removed with oral irrigation devices or a water spray, whereas plaque must be mechanically removed.

Food debris

Loose particles of food that can be dislodged by oral

Table 7-2 Commonly observed stains

Stain type	Appearance	Etiology	Composition	Occurrence
Tobacco	Light brown; may be very dark brown or black	Smoking; chewing tobacco	Pigments from chewing tobacco; tar products	Persons who smoke cigarettes, cigars, or pipes or who use chewing or smokeless tobacco products
Yellow	Dull yellowish color	Food pigments	Discoloration of plaque	All ages, especially with poor oral hygiene
Green	Light yellowish green to darker green	Oral hygiene neglect; chromogenic bacteria; decomposed blood pigments from hemoglobin (via gingival bleeding)	Chromogenic bacteria; decomposed hemoglobin	Any age, but especially in children
Black line	Thin black line that follows gingival margin, about 1 mm above the crest	Composed of microorganisms within an intermicrobial structure	Gram-positive rods primarily; some cocci and other organisms	All ages, especially: clean mouths, women, children; most frequently on lingual and proximal surfaces of maxillary posterior teeth

hygiene aids, rinsing, or muscular action of the tongue, lips, and cheeks are known as food debris. At times, food debris may lodge between teeth, around appliances, or in plaque itself. Food particles that are highly cariogenic present particular problems, as the fermentable carbohydrates may be broken down in the mouth and begin the caries cycle.

Stains

Stains are discolorations of the teeth and restorations that may be extrinsic (occurring on the outer or external tooth surface) or intrinsic (occurring within the tooth surface itself). Extrinsic stains may be removed by scaling or polishing, or occasionally by toothbrushing, while intrinsic stains may not. Stains may also be classified by the manner in which they originate. Exogenous stains develop from sources outside the tooth structure. Such stains may be extrinsic or may become incorporated into the tooth itself, thereby becoming intrinsic. Endogenous stains develop from within the tooth structure and are always intrinsic.

Listed in Table 7-2 are the most commonly observed stains with pertinent facts about each. Other brown extrinsic stains may occur from foods such as coffee, tea, and soy sauce; from stannous fluoride

mouthrinses, dentifrices, or topical applications; and from antiplaque solutions such as chlorhexidine. In some rare instances, chromogenic bacteria may cause orange or red stains at the gingival third of tooth surfaces. Such stains are usually found on both labial and lingual surfaces of anterior teeth.

Some metals or other compounds such as drugs may cause extrinsic stains to form. Those most commonly seen are:

Color	Substance
Green, bluish green	Brass or copper; nickel (usually green only)
Greenish brown	Iron
Golden brown, yellow	Cadmium
Black	Manganese (from potassium permanganate) Iron (from iron sulfide)

Intrinsic stains may be caused by drugs such as tetracycline, by metallic ions from dental amalgam, silver nitrate cavity liners, and the breakdown of blood and pulp tissue in nonvital teeth. In some cases such staining may be lessened or eliminated by bleaching the affected tooth or teeth. In other cases, however, full crowns or bonding procedures are necessary to improve the esthetic appearance of the patient.

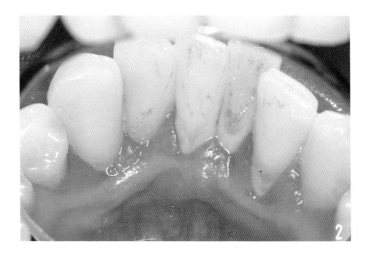

Fig. 7-2   Clinical appearance of calculus. (From Y. Takayama: *How to Select and Use Scalers,* Quintessence Publ. Co., 1985, in Japanese.)

Tooth discolorations may also result from conditions such as dentinogenesis imperfecta, amelogenesis imperfecta, hypoplasia of tooth enamel, and dental fluorosis.

Calculus

Dental calculus is basically calcified plaque. It is a hard deposit that forms on all tooth surfaces, both supra- and subgingivally, and on dental appliances. Calculus occurs in both children and adults, with more frequent occurrence in the adult population.

Clinical appearance

The clinical appearance of supragingival calculus ranges from white to creamy yellow or gray (Fig. 7-2). It may also become stained from tobacco or other foods. Subgingival calculus is usually darker in color—either dark brown, black, or dark green. Supragingival calculus is usually bulky in appearance and may form a bridge of deposit across several teeth or extend over the gingival margin. Subgingival calculus is flatter against the tooth surface and may form in a number of different manners: ledges or rings, smooth veneer, spikes or nodules, or separate individual islands.

The consistency of supragingival calculus is typically moderately hard, but can range from soft and crumbly to brittle. It is porous in nature. Subgingival calculus is comparatively much more brittle, harder, and more dense. Both types of calculus are routinely covered with a layer of plaque, and the newer layers of deposit are less dense. In the case of subgingival calculus, the newest deposits are found near the base of the pocket.

Supragingival calculus is found frequently on teeth near the ducts of the major salivary glands, that is, the lingual surfaces of mandibular anterior teeth (Wharton's and Bartholin's ducts) and the buccal surfaces of the maxillary molars (Stensen's ducts). It tends to be deposited somewhat evenly on most teeth, unless factors such as malaligned teeth, erratic personal oral hygiene techniques, or unilateral function are operational. In such instances, deposits may be much heavier in isolated areas. Distribution of subgingival calculus ranges from localized to generalized and is usually heaviest on interproximal surfaces, with lightest deposition on facial surfaces. Both types of calculus may occur separately or in conjunction with each other.

Detection of supragingival calculus is accomplished with direct or indirect vision, utilizing an intraoral mirror. Often very light deposits or thin sheets of supragingival calculus are difficult to detect visually. Use of the air syringe to dry the teeth and indirect light from the intraoral mirror can greatly aid the dental hygienist in seeing such deposits. The explorer can also assist in detection.

Subgingival calculus is usually somewhat more difficult to detect, especially for the inexperienced clinician. Because the deposit is more or less hidden from view, an explorer is generally the instrument of choice to examine the subgingival areas. At times, the hygienist will detect subgingival calculus with the probe while performing a periodontal charting. An experienced hygienist often suspects and subsequently detects the presence of calculus by observing the color change in the gingiva; at times, very dark calculus deposit may reflect through the thin marginal epithelium. Also, calculus may be directly visible at the margin itself. Use of the air syringe to deflect the free gingiva can aid in visualizing subgingival calculus, especially when the tissue is spongy, edematous, or flabby. Finally, the intraoral mirror may be employed to transilluminate anterior teeth. Both supra- and subgingival deposits will be revealed as dark opaque shadowy areas on proximal surfaces.

Formation

Two of the three phases of calculus formation have already been described. The initial step consists of formation of the acquired pellicle, followed by development of plaque colonies, which coalesce to form a unified layer. Minute centers of mineralization then form, and the third phase, mineralization, begins.

After the mineralization centers develop, they continue to expand until they touch one another. The actual process of mineralization of plaque is rapid and may begin as soon as several hours after the plaque has matured. The microorganisms in the plaque function as the organic matrix for mineral deposition. As mineralization proceeds, the composition of microbes changes from cocci to primarily filamentous rods.

The calcium and phosphorous that are deposited during the mineralization phase originate from either the saliva or from crevicular fluid for supra- or subgingival calculus formation, respectively. It should be noted that the volume of sulcular fluid increases in inflamed, diseased tissue, thereby providing a constant source of available minerals for calculus formation.

The process of mineralization consists of the establishment of crystals. The four crystals that comprise calculus are hydroxyapatite (55% of inorganic components), octocalcium phosphate (31%), whitlockite (25%), and brushite (5%). Crystal formation begins both within the intercellular matrix and on the surface of the microorganisms, and then progresses within the bacteria themselves. The actual mechanism by which the minerals precipitate out from saliva and gingival sulcular fluid and become integrated within the plaque matrix is not yet fully understood. It ap-

pears, though, that the process is similar in nature to the calcification of other body tissues such as enamel and bone.

Like plaque, calculus is composed of both organic and inorganic matter and water. The differences between the two deposits obviously lie in the percentages of the component parts. Plaque is 80% water and 20% organic and inorganic components; mature calculus, on the other hand, is 15% to 25% water and organic compounds, and 75% to 85% inorganic solids. The overall composition of sub- and supragingival calculus is comparable. Fluoride, too, can often be found in calculus, as the deposit tends to be a more porous material than enamel. The amount of fluoride present in calcified deposits is dependent upon factors such as topical application, use of dentifrices, and the amount of fluoride in drinking water.

The organic components of calculus include salivary mucins, desquamated epithelial cells, leukocytes, and nonvital microorganisms, of which the most numerous type are filaments. The inorganic portion is composed mainly of calcium and calcium phosphate salts, with calcium carbonate and magnesium phosphate occurring in minor amounts.

The timetable for the calcification process ranges from 10 to 20 days, with the average about 12 days. The rate of calculus formation, however, varies among individuals, just as does the rate of plaque formation. Other influencing factors include the patient's home care regimen and the surface texture of the teeth. Patients with inadequate plaque removal skills or rough tooth surfaces tend to develop calculus deposits more readily.

The process of calculus deposition occurs in layers that are generally parallel to the tooth surfaces. There are several means by which the deposit attaches itself to the tooth structure. The most superficial attachment is by means of the acquired pellicle; calculus that deposits by this mechanism is most often found on recently scaled root surfaces and enamel. This type of calculus is the most easily removed.

A second mode of calculus attachment is by direct contact between the calculus matrix and the tooth surfaces. When calculus attaches in this way to root surfaces, the hygienist will remove cementum during the scaling and root planing to completely remove the deposit. The calculus attachment mechanism that presents the dental hygienist with the most tenacious deposit is attachment that occurs by a physical interlocking into tiny surface irregularities on the teeth.

Cracks in the enamel, carious lesions, cemental nicks or gouges, ridges from scaling, and minute holes from loss of Sharpey's fibers are examples of such external irregularities.

Significance

Dental calculus has long been thought to be a factor in the development of gingival and periodontal disease conditions. As research evidence has accumulated, more specific information regarding the relationship of plaque and calculus to oral disease has become available. As indicated earlier, plaque has been identified as the major periodontal disease-producing entity. Because calculus is calcified plaque, its prevention is directly related to control of plaque formation. Calculus itself has a rough, porous texture that provides an ideal surface for additional plaque accumulation. Routine oral hygiene practices such as flossing and toothbrushing generally are not sufficient to completely remove plaque that forms on calculus. Plaque control is much more effective when the deposit is removed from a smooth surface rather than rough areas.

The porosity of calculus is related to disease development in that toxic waste products from plaque microorganisms are able to permeate the surface of the deposit. In turn, these toxic substances are in continuous contact with adjacent gingival tissues, thereby initiating the development of the inflammatory process. This is particularly significant in the case of subgingival calculus, because tissue inflammation results in the increased production of sulcular fluid, which leads to further calculus development. This cyclical relationship among plaque, calculus, and inflammation is an important aspect to discuss with patients when educating them about dental disease and its prevention.

Calculus deposits, especially heavy accumulations, may inhibit drainage of inflammatory products from periodontal pockets, leading to prevention of healing of the affected tissues. The likelihood of formation of periodontal and/or gingival abscesses is greatly enhanced under such circumstances.

chapter 8

The periodontal co-therapist

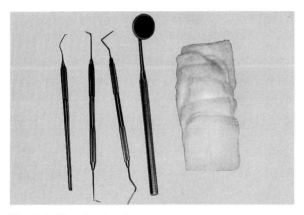

Fig. 8-1 Examination instruments.

In today's practice of dentistry, the dentist, the dental hygienist, the dental assistant, and the expanded functions dental auxiliary operate as a team to provide comprehensive preventive and therapeutic health care to patients in a variety of settings. The role of the dental hygienist varies from jurisdiction to jurisdiction and from private practice to institutional settings. In all areas, the dental hygienist's role is pivotal, the responsibilities greatly broadened from dental hygiene practice of the past.

Hand instrumentation

Many procedures of the oral prophylaxis are most often accomplished with the use of hand instruments. The dental hygienist must be familiar with the variety of hand instruments currently available and exhibit a high degree of dexterity and tactile sensitivity in their use. The five factors in instrument usage that have an important impact on removal of oral deposits—fulcrum, instrument grasp, adaptation, angulation, and stroke activation—are discussed in depth in the accompanying laboratory manual. The manual also contains detailed descriptions for the use of specific instruments for examination, scaling, root planing, and curettage. The skills necessary for the sharpening of hand instruments and the care and maintenance of motor-driven handpieces are also addressed.

Examination and detection

Three basic instruments are used routinely for examination of the teeth and gingival tissues to detect caries, tooth anomalies, and surface irregularities and to ascertain the presence of bleeding of the gingiva and to measure sulcular depth. When performing the dental and periodontal examination, the dental hygienist will utilize an intraoral mirror, explorers, and periodontal probes (Fig. 8-1).

Intraoral mirror

The intraoral mirror, used in therapeutic procedures as well as during examination, is indispensible during patient treatment. Intraoral mirrors are obtainable in a number of sizes, may be magnified or plain, and are either metal or plastic. They have four basic purposes or uses:

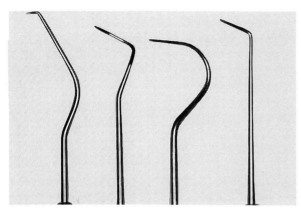

Fig. 8-2 Explorers #17, 2, 23, and 3. (Courtesy of Hu-Friedy Manufacturing Co., Chicago, Ill.)

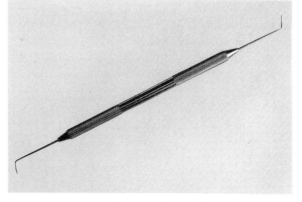

Fig. 8-3 Courtesy of Hu-Friedy Manufacturing Co.

1. Indirect vision: They are used to view tooth surfaces or areas of the mouth not otherwise seen directly, that is, lingual surfaces of anterior teeth, and the hard palate.
2. Soft tissue retraction: They are used to retract the cheeks, lips, or tongue to improve access or visibility, or to protect the tissues from trauma.
3. Indirect illumination: They are used to cast additional light onto the working area by reflecting light from the overhead lamp off the mirror head.
4. Transillumination: They are used to reflect light through the teeth to detect caries or calculus deposits.

Possibly one of the most difficult skills for the student to master is reliance on the mirror for indirect vision. By using the mirror appropriately, however, the hygienist is able to maintain correct posture and avoid much occupationally related muscle stress and strain.

When the intraoral mirror is being employed, care must be taken to avoid unintentional impingement of the soft tissue against the teeth, pressing the mirror head or handle against the teeth, or knocking the mirror head or handle against the teeth. The dental hygienist should maintain a fulcrum (or finger rest) when using this and all other instruments.

One annoying aspect of intraoral mirror usage is fogging of the mirror surface while in the patient's mouth. Several commercial preparations are available into which the mirror head may be dipped to decrease fogging. Other measures that may be taken include dipping the mirror in warm water or rubbing the reflecting surface along the buccal mucosa. Most of the time, fogging occurs because the patient is breathing through his or her mouth; requesting the patient to breathe through the nose will often correct the problem.

Explorers

Explorers are used to examine tooth surfaces for a wide variety of conditions. In addition to calculus detection, explorers are employed to identify caries; examine margins and surfaces of restorations; and detect structural defects of teeth, root surface roughness, and areas of decalcification. These instruments are used both supragingivally and subgingivally throughout the mouth.

Exploring instruments are available in a number of styles and sizes, and choice of an explorer depends upon its use and the preference of the clinician. Some explorers are more suited for the detection of carious lesions (e.g., #23), whereas others are ideal for detecting calculus and/or deep pocket exploration (e.g., #17) (Fig. 8-2).

Most exploring instruments have a handle tapering to a shank that terminates in the working end (Fig. 8-3). The shank may be straight, curved, or sharply angulated. The working end is usually a thin wire, approximately 1 mm to 2 mm in length, narrowing to a sharp point. Explorers are available as either single-ended or double-ended instruments. The double-ended instruments may be paired (for access to all tooth surfaces with a single instrument) or may have two completely different types of working ends—two explorers or an explorer paired with a probe.

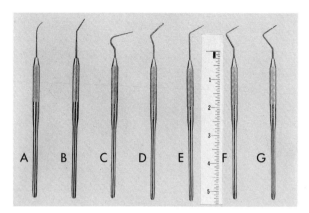

Fig. 8-4 (A) Gilmore; (B) Merritt A; (C) Glickman 26G; (D) Goldman-Fox Flat; (E) Merritt B; (F) Michigan-O; (G) Williams. (Courtesy of Hu-Friedy Manufacturing Co.)

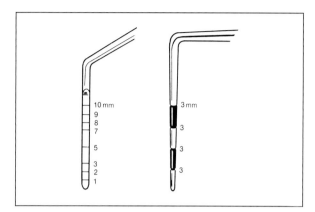

Figure 8-5

Periodontal probes

The periodontal probe is used primarily to examine the gingival tissues. The probe is utilized to measure sulci and pocket depths, perform the gingival bleeding index, measure the amount of gingival recession, evaluate the consistency of the gingiva, determine the presence of mucogingival involvement, measure the width of the attached gingiva, and detect furcation involvements.

Periodontal probes, like explorers, are available in a number of different styles (Fig. 8-4). Most probes are calibrated in millimeters, either by a color-coding mechanism or by indentations on the working end. Calibrations vary among the different types of probes, and so the dental hygienist should be familiar with the markings of the probe to be used (Fig. 8-5).

The probe consists of a handle with a straight, angulated, or curved shank. The working end has a rounded tip, which allows for insertion to the epithelial attachment without traumatizing the soft tissue. Probes are most often single-ended, although double-ended instruments are obtainable (e.g., Goldman-Fox probe paired with a Williams probe). An instrument with a probe on one end, paired with an explorer on the opposite end, is available from many manufacturers upon request.

Supragingival debridement

The instruments utilized most frequently for removal of supragingival deposits are sickle scalers. Because of their blade designs, sickles are the instruments of choice to remove calculus above the margin of the gingiva and, when tissue condition permits, slightly below the gingiva. Whenever a sickle scaler is inserted subgingivally, the hygienist must exercise great care not to traumatize either the soft gingival tissues or the root surfaces of the teeth themselves.

Sickle scalers are classified either as straight or curved, which refers to the blade design. The straight sickle has two cutting edges with a flat face on a straight blade (Fig. 8-6a). The tip of the instrument culminates in a sharp point, and the back of the blade generally tapers to an edge. In cross section, the blade is triangular in shape (Fig. 8-6b).

The curved sickle also consists of two cutting edges, but on a curved blade (Fig. 8-7a). The overall blade design of the two types of sickles is basically the same in terms of the pointed tip and tapered edge back. The cross-sectional view of the curved sickle is triangular or trapezoidal (Fig. 8-7b).

Both straight and curved sickles are obtainable with either straight or angulated shanks. As with all instruments, the straighter the shank, the more anteriorly the instrument is used. Most of the straight-shanked instruments are utilized on the anterior teeth, although in some instances the operator may be able to scale the premolars as well. Sickles with angulated shanks adapt easily to the posterior teeth. These instruments are usually paired, with the working ends mirror images of each other. One end is used on buccal surfaces, while the opposite end adapts to the lingual surfaces of a given quadrant.

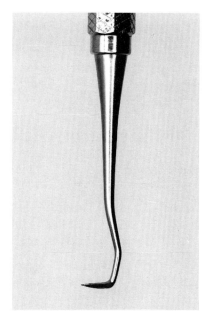
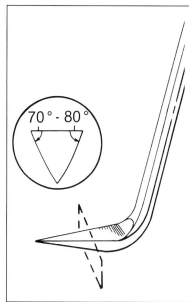

Figure 8-6a   (left)

Figure 8-6b   (right)

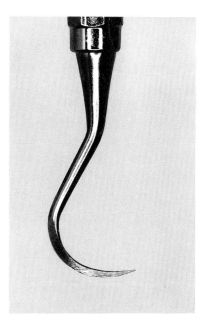
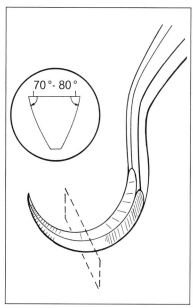

Figure 8-7a   (left)

Figure 8-7b   (right)

Interproximal supragingival calculus removal is the primary function of the sickle. Some clinicians, however, use it to remove subgingival calculus deposits both interproximally and on the facial and lingual cervical areas. Whenever the sickle is inserted subgingivally, the dental hygienist must keep in mind the instrument's blade design and take care to avoid traumatizing adjacent tissues. In addition, because of its size, bulk, and blade design, a sickle scaler cannot be considered a fine scaling instrument. Because it cannot be inserted more than approximately 2 mm below the gingiva, it is not the instrument of choice for scaling deep pockets. For removing moderate to heavy supragingival calculus, however, it is an excellent instrument because of the relative strength of the blade. Several small, thin sickles are also available

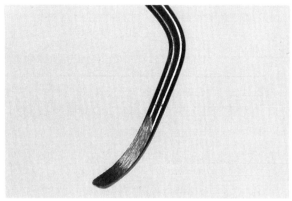

Figure 8-8a

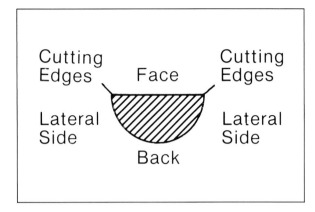

Figure 8-8b

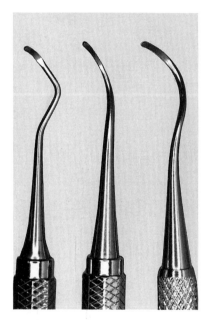

Figure 8-9 (left)

Figure 8-10 (below)

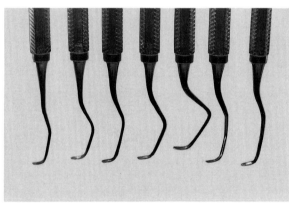

that are very good for removing thin veneer calculus on interproximal surfaces of mandibular anterior teeth, especially when these teeth are crowded or malposed.

Subgingival debridement

The instrument utilized most frequently for fine scaling, root planing, and soft tissue curettage is the curet. Curets are categorized either as universal or area specific. All curets have similar basic characteristics and design features. The choice of a particular instrument is dependent upon the amount, location, and tenacity of deposits as well as the condition of the gingival tissues.

In general, the curet blade consists of two cutting edges that terminate in a rounded tip or toe (Fig. 8-8a). Overall, the blade design is referred to as spoon shaped. The back surface of the blade is rounded. In cross section, the curet blade is a half-moon or half-circle shape (Fig. 8-8b).

The shank of the curet varies from straight to highly curved or contra-angled, depending on its intended area of use. The blade–shank relationship of the uni-

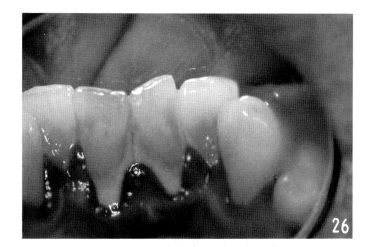

Fig. 8-11a Heavy calculus deposits. (From Y. Takayama: *How to Select and Use Scalers,* Quintessence Publ. Co., 1985, in Japanese.)

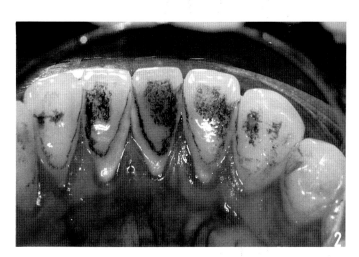

Fig. 8-11b Heavy stain. (From Y. Takayama: *How to Select and Use Scalers,* Quintessence Publ. Co., 1985, in Japanese.)

versal curet is such that the face of the instrument blade is almost perpendicular to the lower portion of the shank. Universal curets are designed so that both cutting edges are utilizable, and adaptation of the blade to all surfaces of all teeth is possible (Fig. 8-9).

Area-specific curets differ in that they are intended for use only on certain groups of teeth or particular surfaces of teeth. The Gracey series of curets is considered area specific: a full set consists of seven double-ended instruments that are designed for use only on specified teeth, with the lower numbered instruments used more anteriorly, the higher numbered ones posteriorly (Fig. 8-10). In the Gracey series only

the "lower" blade or cutting edge is used for instrumentation, and the face of the blade is offset approximately 60° to 70° to the lower shank.

Heavy deposit removal

In the contemporary practice of dental hygiene, ultrasonic scaling devices are the most often used instruments for debridement of heavy deposits of calculus and stain (Figs. 8-11a and b). Sonic scalers and three types of hand instruments also may be used for heavy calculus removal.

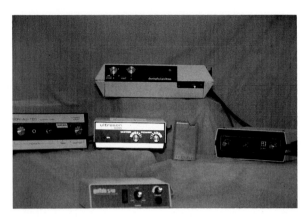

Figure 8-12

Ultrasonic scaling devices

A number of different models of ultrasonic scaling devices are available, and most operate in a similar manner (Fig. 8-12). Ultrasonic devices allow the hygienist to remove the calculus and stain quickly, efficiently, and with less operator fatigue. The saving of time is a particular benefit for both the dental hygienist and the patient. Moreover, most patients sustain less discomfort, especially if the gingival tissues are acutely inflamed, as in ANUG.

Ultrasonic scaling devices have been used for deposit removal for a number of years. The original units were large and bulky and required adjustment of the water volume, frequency, and tip inserts. Modern units are smaller and often require very little adjustment. Tip inserts are available in a variety of shapes and sizes for more thorough scaling.

Ultrasonic units are comprised of an electric generator, a handpiece, a series of tip inserts, and usually a foot control (Figs. 8-13a and b). Some models operate with the use of a finger switch control.

The generator converts electrical energy into mechanical energy, producing high frequency sound waves, which are then transmitted through the tip insert, causing very rapid vibrations of the tip (between 25,000 and 40,000 cycles per second, depending on the model). This rapid vibratory motion facilitates the fracturing of the deposits from the tooth surfaces. During the production and transmission of the ultrasonic waves, heat is produced. In order to control the heat and keep the handpiece and tip insert relatively cool, water flows through the handpiece and is expelled onto the tip either through an external tube or internally through the tip itself. The water exits either as a thin stream or, more often, as a fine spray. Concurrently, tiny vacuum bubbles collapse, which causes the release of a great deal of local pressure. This results in a lavage action to cleanse the area of blood and debris.

The tips must remain dull, as when first obtained from the manufacturer. Sharp tip inserts not only are unnecessary, because the vibratory action is what causes the removal of deposits, but also are potentially dangerous, as tooth surfaces could easily be gouged or otherwise damaged.

Ultrasonic scalers have several disadvantages or limitations. Because of the bulkiness and size of the tips, and the very light touch employed when using the device, the clinician experiences a distinct lack of tactile sensitivity and must utilize the explorer to ascertain the degree of deposit removal. Additionally, the working end of the tip cannot be inserted subgingivally so that all deposits are definitively removed; fine scaling with hand instruments must follow use of the ultrasonic scaler. The water spray, while aiding in cleansing of the working area, presents a problem for the operator when attempting to use the intraoral mirror for indirect vision; the spray tends to obscure the vision potential. The operator should be cognizant of the amount of water and the positioning of the patient in an attempt to avoid unnecessarily inconveniencing the patient with water spray to the face and neck area. A further limitation of the device is the result of patient sensitivity to the vibratory mechanism. Some individuals, especially those with very light deposits or hypersensitive areas, experience discomfort with the use of the instrument. Because the device is of limited use for patients with light deposits, the dental hygienist should discriminate among patients and utilize it appropriately.

Because of the amount of heat produced during the generation of the sound waves and the vibration of the tip, the water volume should be of sufficient level to assure cooling of the device. The hygienist must avoid prolonged contact of the tip to the tooth, keeping the instrument moving and correctly angulated to avoid potential pulp damage from excessive heat generation.

Ultrasonic scaling devices are not recommended for use on children because of potential damage to tissues that are still developing and growing. The instrument also is contraindicated for patients with

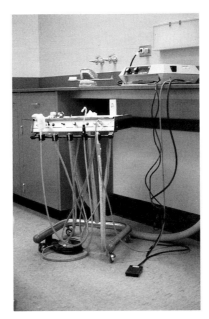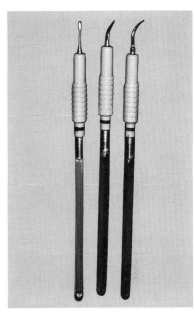

Figure 8-13a   (left)

Figure 8-13b   (right)

cardiac pacemakers because of the possibility that electromagnetic interference from the scaler may counteract the pacemaker's electronic action. The operator must note any teeth that are restored with composite resins and take care to avoid using the ultrasonic device over those restorations, because the vibration of the tip may produce leakage around the margins, with subsequent staining and loss of retention.

The ultrasonic scaler is most useful for patients with ANUG, periodontal and gingival abscesses, pericoronitis, heavy calculus, and extrinsic stains. An additional advantage of the device is its effect on the gingival tissues, in that the flushing action of the water spray removes blood and other debris, including necrotic tissue and small pieces of calculus, from the operative site.

This continual flushing action allows for better postoperative healing of the gingiva, because few local irritants remain to influence the healing process. Another therapeutic effect on the gingiva provided by use of the ultrasonic scaler is coagulation of the necrotic epithelium that lines the sulcus.

In addition to calculus and stain removal, a variety of other dental procedures may be performed, making the ultrasonic device a versatile instrument in the dental office. Excess cement from orthodontic appliances and cast restorations is easily removed with an ultrasonic device, as are overhanging margins of amalgam restorations. Other uses include root canal preparation, closed soft tissue curettage, some periodontal surgical procedures, and irrigation of periodontal abscesses. In the past, the device was used to condense amalgam. This is presently contraindicated because of the cavitation of the mercury, which presents a definitive health hazard to the operator as well as the patient.

Whenever an ultrasonic scaling device is utilized during patient therapy, the dental hygienist should be appropriately protected with safety glasses and face mask at all times. Because the device generates an aerosol, these precautions are necessary to control transmission of microorganisms and protect the operator from debris that might be splashed onto her or his face.

A detailed description of the setup and use of the unit is given in the laboratory manual. When used appropriately, the ultrasonic scaling device is a useful aid for the delivery of comprehensive periodontal therapy. Although it is only an adjunct, not a total substitute for hand instrumentation, the experienced clinician can often drastically reduce the needed amount of hand scaling and root planing through skillful use of the ultrasonic scaler.

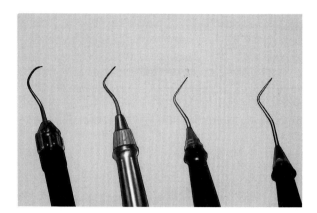

Figure 8-14

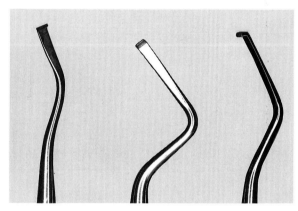

Figure 8-15a

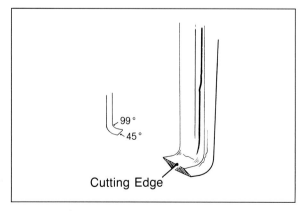

Figure 8-15b

Sonic scalers

Although ultrasonic scalers are often the preferred means of heavy deposit debridement, occasionally the device is not available or clinical circumstances will make its use difficult or impossible (e.g., for bedridden patients). In such instances, sonic scaling devices or hand instruments may be utilized.

Sonic scalers operate through attachment to the high-speed handpiece hose. They are less powerful than ultrasonic devices but are easily transported and require little or no adjustment. These scalers may be used with or without a water spray. A number of different models are available, and most have a number of different working tips from which to choose (Fig. 8-14). Because they operate at a lower frequency (approximately 2000 cycles/second), many hygienists feel that calculus and stain removal is not unduly enhanced by their use. They are, however, useful in certain situations and may perform adequately.

Hoe scalers

The hoe scaler is designed primarily for supragingival debridement of calculus, especially large tenacious pieces. Because of its blade design, it has very limited use subgingivally. Generally, the instrument may be inserted only 2 mm to 3 mm below the margin of the gingiva, and then only if the tissue is spongy and easily distensible.

The hoe has a single blade with a straight cutting edge, which is offset from the shank at an angle of approximately 100° (Fig. 8-15a). The cutting edge is beveled at an angle of 45° to the end of the blade (Fig. 8-15b). The shank portion may be straight or angulated, depending upon the area of its intended use. The instrument itself may be single ended or double ended.

When using the hoe, the clinician must be cognizant of the very sharp edges on either side of the blade that can easily gouge root surfaces. One approach to avoid this is to round off the pointed edges with a sharpening stone. Moreover, the concept of two-point contact, in which both the cutting edge and a portion of the shank are in contact with the tooth, helps to stabilize the instrument and employ the entire cutting edge during the working stroke (Fig. 8-16).

Chisel scalers

The chisel is an instrument with a blade that is continuous with a slightly curved shank. It has a single straight cutting edge, with the end of the blade flat and beveled at a 45° angle (Fig. 8-17). This instrument is generally used only when very heavy calculus deposits are apparent, specifically on the mandibular anterior teeth. If a heavy bridge of calculus has deposited on the lingual surfaces of these teeth, and the patient no longer has interdental papillae in the area, the chisel is useful to dislodge this deposit by pushing the instrument horizontally from the labial aspect to break the calculus into smaller pieces. Occasionally, this instrument is also used to remove calculus from exposed proximal surfaces of premolars, but only if the patient's lips and cheeks have sufficient flexibility to allow for adequate retraction.

Like the hoe, the chisel's blade has very sharp corners, and so precautions apply to this instrument as well. When the chisel is used, the entire width of the blade's cutting edge should be employed.

Periodontal files

Files are best described as instruments with multiple hoe blades; a number of cutting edges are lined up on a base that is either round, rectangular, or oval in shape (Fig. 8-18). Also similar to the hoe, the file's shank design ranges from straight to angulated. The instrument may be single ended or double ended.

Files are most useful to crush heavy calculus deposits, to smooth roughened cementum and other tooth surfaces (i.e., at the cementoenamel junction), and to obtain a smoother surface on overhanging or rough margins of amalgam restorations. Because of the file's bulky working end, the clinician's tactile sensitivity is diminished and it has limited definitive use in deep periodontal pockets. While some clinicians use only files for root planing, most available evidence suggests that files should be followed by curets to obtain the smoothest possible surface.

Therapeutic root planing

In conjunction with the scaling procedures, root planing should be performed for removal of calculus, debris, and irregularities on the root surfaces of the teeth. Failure to remove residual deposits and irregularities in the cementum results in continuation of the inflammatory process in the adjacent soft tissues and accumulation of more deposits on the rough root surface.

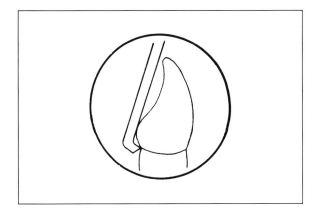

Figure 8-16

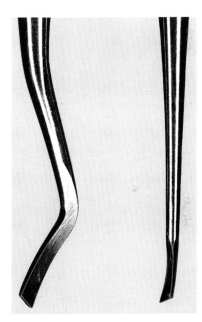

Figure 8-17

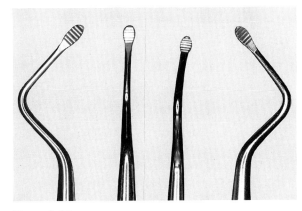

Figure 8-18

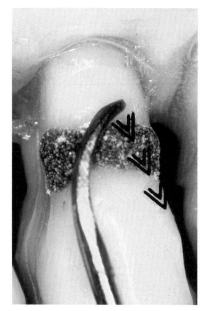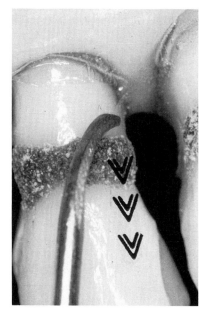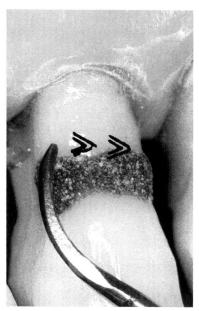

Figs. 8-19a to c From B. Wasserman: *Root Scaling and Planing: A Fundamental Therapy,* Quintessence Publ. Co., 1986.

Because of the differences in the characteristics of the cementum of the root and the enamel of the tooth, some variations in technique when performing therapeutic root planing as compared to scaling are indicated. Root planing is more of a continuous shaving of the root surface. Less pressure is required than for the scaling procedure.

Coronal, diagonal, or circumferential strokes may be employed (Figs. 8-19a to c). Gradually reducing the depth of the cutting stroke will elicit a smoother surface by making smaller and smaller scratches. The depth of the cut is reduced by gradually closing the angle of the blade, reducing the applied pressure, and lengthening the stroke.

In this procedure of continuous shaving, the curet or file sometimes causes a "washboard effect" in the cementum. This may be detected by tactile sensitivity or by a "clatter" heard as the instrument goes over the indentations. The more the operator tries to smooth the surface, the more it "clatters." The solution is to change the direction of the stroke. If the planing procedure was begun with coronal strokes, circumferential strokes will remove the indentations by addressing several of the ridges with each stroke rather than going over them one by one. Alteration in the direction of the stroke may be indicated again before the objective of a smooth root surface free of debris and altered cementum is achieved[1] (Figs.

8-20a to d). Thorough root planing contributes to a reduction in inflammation and in debris accumulation and facilitates subsequent calculus removal from the surfaces.[2,3]

Various solutions such as citric acid have been used as an application to root surfaces that are planed or nonplaned. Acid causes exposure of collagen fibrils in the dentin matrix because of demineralization and thus provides a nidus for splicing with new fibrils during the healing process. Most of the research indicates the application of citric acid is beneficial only in terms of promotion of cell attachment and growth when applied to root-planed roots.[3–6]

Thorough scaling and root planing is a time-consuming task. When it is coupled with the additional components of preventive appointments, the average periodontal maintenance patient visit requires 52.6 minutes.[7] Appointments of 1 hour in length, then, would seem to be most appropriate for providing optimum care.

Gingival curettage

Gingival curettage is sequenced in the treatment plan following complete debridement of the tooth surfaces and the root planing procedure. The term gingival curettage may refer to several procedures. In state

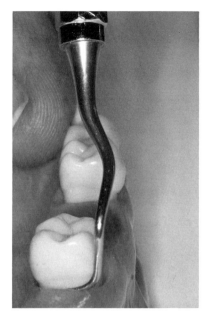

Fig. 8-20a (left) From B. Wasserman: *Root Scaling and Planing: A Fundamental Therapy,* Quintessence Publ. Co., 1986.

Fig. 8-20b (below) From B. Wasserman: *Root Scaling and Planing: A Fundamental Therapy,* Quintessence Publ. Co., 1986.

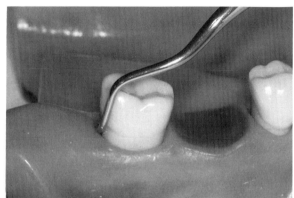

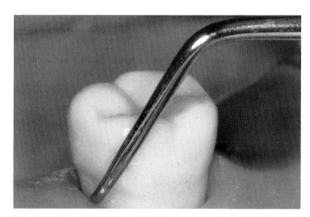

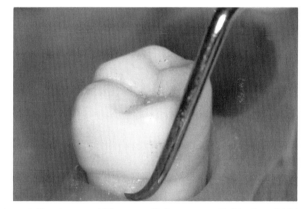

Figs. 8-20c and d   From B. Wasserman: *Root Scaling and Planing: A Fundamental Therapy,* Quintessence Publ. Co., 1986.

dental practice acts the term most often used to describe the therapy provided by the dental hygienist is *closed soft tissue curettage.* This is a definitive procedure to remove the ulcerated epithelial lining, the inflammatory tissues from the gingival pocket wall, and also the immediately subjacent diseased connective tissue. If the state practice act allows it, the dental hygienist may also be involved in *open-flap curettage.* This procedure utilizes a surgical flap to gain access to the diseased tissue so that it can be excised.

The procedure of gingival curettage is determined to change a chronic wound to an acute surgical

wound. The resultant shrinkage of the edematous tissue and wound healing within the pocket contribute to pocket reduction. The preponderance of research findings indicates that, although open flap curettage procedures are the most desirable method of attaining pocket reduction and in some cases pocket elimination, routine closed soft tissue curettage provides long-term results that may modify or eliminate the need for surgical intervention.[8,9]

Although some inadvertent curettage occurs in the pocket wall during thorough scaling and root planing procedures, definitive curettage should be planned

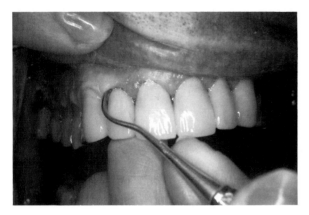

Figure 8-21a

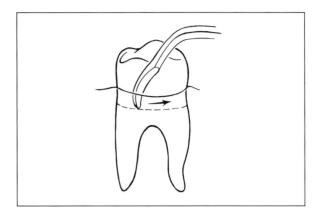

Figure 8-21b

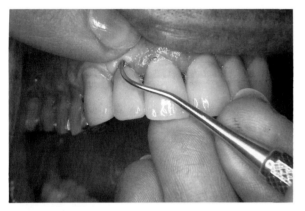

Figure 8-21c

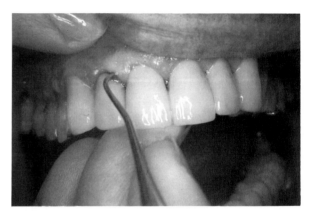

Figure 8-21d

when tissues exhibit signs of persistent inflammation or when shallow, suprabony pockets or spongy, rolled tissue are present.

Conditions that contraindicate definitive curettage procedures are:

- Dilantin hyperplasia.
- Firm fibrotic tissues, either from chronic periodontal conditions resulting in noninflammatory altered repair process or naturally fibrotic tissue areas such as the palate or the retromolar pads.
- Infrabony pockets.
- Complications associated with frenum attachments.
- Mucogingival involvements and insufficient attached gingiva.

The technique for closed soft tissue curettage usually involves the administration of a local anesthetic agent. For some areas, topical anesthetic application may suffice. The first step in treatment should be to probe. This will enable the hygienist to familiarize herself or himself with unusual anatomical conditions and the configuration of the soft tissue attachment of the area involved.

If a universal curet is employed, the cutting edge of the blade to be used for the procedure is the open blade, the opposite edge of that used for scaling. The Gracey series of curets have one cutting edge; therefore the opposite end of the instrument would be used for curettage. The curets used for gingival curettage should not be the same instruments used for scaling and root planing because they may have minute nicks in the blade from calculus and residual cementum removal. Curets should be very sharp to facilitate the complete removal of the necrotic tissue and to maximize patient comfort during the procedure.

The blade is inserted against the pocket wall with the toe of the blade directed apically (Figs. 8-21a and b). The toe of the blade is moved apically until the tension of the soft tissue at the base of the pocket is felt (Fig. 8-21c). The blade is then activated with a horizontal continuous stroke around the full circumference of the facial or lingual surface of the tooth (Fig. 8-21d). The diseased pocket epithelium will be visible on the face of the blade as it is removed from the sulcus (Fig. 8-21e). Spontaneous bleeding will occur (Fig. 8-21f). Placement of the index finger of the opposite hand over the area being curetted may facilitate the procedure by providing stability and support (Fig. 8-21g). The procedure is repeated until no more diseased soft tissue breaks away from the healthy tissue; usually two to four strokes will complete the operation. In interproximal areas a combination of the horizontal stroke followed by vertical strokes is employed.

The area is flushed with water and pressure is applied with a 2 × 2 gauze. Periodontal dressing may be used to protect the area after curettage. Most of the current research suggests that the use of periodontal dressings, because of their tendency to promote bacterial colonization, does not accelerate the healing process. In more extensive periodontal therapies such as an apically repositioned flap, dressings may prevent coronal displacement, but for curettage they are probably unnecessary and potentially contraindicated.

The use of antibacterial mouthrinses poses a more contemporary solution. Recently accepted for prescription use in the United States, chlorhexidine seems to have great potential in this area. It is bactericidal against a wide range of both gram-positive and gram-negative organisms, although the gram-positive bacteria are the most sensitive. Chlorhexidine was initially used to clean surgical sites and as a root canal antiseptic. More recently there has been widespread interest in the compound as a plaque prevention agent. The side effects are an unpleasant taste; transient loss or reduction of taste sensation; and most notably discoloration of teeth, restorations, and the dorsal surface of the tongue (Fig. 8-22). Research is currently being conducted on chlorhexidine rinses and pastes by the American Dental Association and other institutions.

Because a surgical wound has been created, the gingiva will be hemorrhagic in appearance immediately following curettage. Blood clotting will have

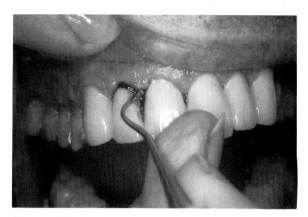

Figure 8-21e

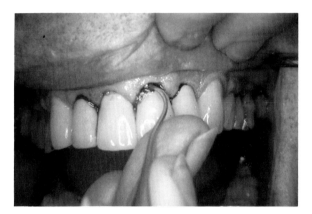

Figure 8-21f

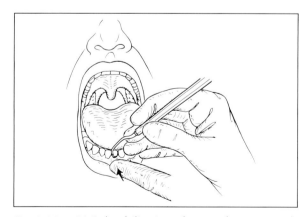

Fig. 8-21g   Digital stabilization of area to be curettaged.

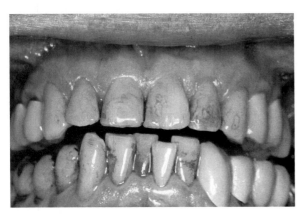

Fig. 8-22 Stain resulting from the use of chlorhexidine mouthrinse.

begun and be apparent at the margin of the gingiva. In the next day or two, the tissue will have signs of edema and blood clots will still be present. Four days postoperative the edema and the redness will have dissipated. Follow-up probing should not be conducted this early, because bleeding will be elicited. Shrinkage will continue and the gingiva should appear normal in color and texture in 10 days. Complete keratinization of the gingiva and connective tissue maturation will not occur for approximately 4 weeks postoperatively.

The use of ultrasonic devices for soft tissue curettage has been proposed. The inserts are special curet inserts (Dentsply* EWPP, EWPT, WWP10) and they are used with a sparse water lavage. In this way the necrotic tissues are cauterized and the debridement completed by the water lavage. The technique for instrumentation use is the same as for scaling.

The use of sodium hypochlorite acid solution (Antiformin) or a combination sodium hypochlorite and citric acid solution have been projected as an approach to chemical curettage and root treatment.[10] Adequate debridement and root planing are necessary as with other approaches. The medicament is placed with the use of a medicament loop or a curet (Figs. 8-23a and b). The sodium hypochlorite is applied for 60 seconds, followed by citric acid solution application for neutralization for 2 to 3 minutes. Complete irrigation to remove the chemicals is followed by cu-

*Dentsply Equipment, York, Pa.

rettage of the necrotic sulcular tissues with an instrument. Thorough rinsing and application of firm pressure with a gauze follows. Periodontal dressing may or may not be used.[10]

Experiments show that advantages to this technique include reduced bleeding, enhancement of visibility, and more comfort to the patient because use of an anesthetic is not required. Plaque is destroyed by the bactericidal effects of the solutions. The demineralization to the tooth surface exposes the dentinal tubules and may therefore increase the healing process. Some researchers propose that this technique is very thorough with less effort than the traditional approach.[6,10] The use of the solutions must, of course, be carefully monitored. Improper isolation and protection of the soft tissues may result in chemical burns. In the presence of extensive inflammation, the effect of the solution may be altered due to crevicular exudate, blood, bacteria, and debris.

Postoperatively, the curettage patient should be instructed as to the clinical signs of the histological conditions of wound healing. Oral hygiene procedures should be altered initially for patient comfort but the importance of plaque control should be reiterated. The patient should be encouraged to return to his or her full personal oral hygiene regimen within a few days. Initially acidic foods or fruit juices may cause some discomfort for the patient. Hypertonic saline solutions or oxygenating agents are palliative measures that the hygienist may consider recommending initially.

Monitored Modulated Therapy

As a periodontal co-therapist, the dental hygienist may practice in an office that subscribes to the Monitored Modulated Therapy approach to periodontal maintenance. Dr. Paul Keyes, the developer of the technique, was associated with the National Institute of Dental Research for more than 25 years. Keyes' approach stems from a philosophy that periodontal disease is caused by bacteria and should therefore be treated by antibacterial agents.[11] The technique employs scaling and root planing followed by home application of hydrogen peroxide, baking soda, and salt solutions in the sulci. The standard mixture is ½ capful of 3% hydrogen peroxide mixed with 1 tablespoon of baking soda. The mixture is used as a dentifrice and manipulated into the sulcus area with a rubber

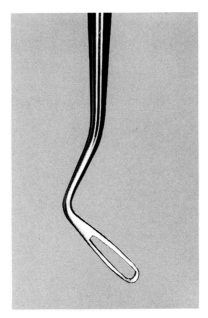

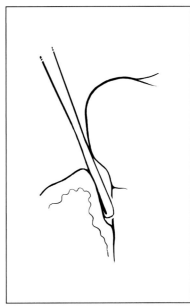

Figure 8-23a   (left)

Fig. 8-23b   (right) Courtesy of Diane Roberto, R.D.H., Chicago, Ill.

tip stimulator or a toothbrush and floss.[11,12] Tetracycline prescription may also be utilized. The patient's progress is monitored by periodic microscopic examination of plaque and material from the mouth. The microscope is pivotal in the Keyes' approach because of the ability to identify sites of active disease earlier than through radiography or clinical examination techniques.

However, much controversy surrounds the MMT approach.[13–18]

The greatest criticism is a lack of scientifically controlled studies with subsequent hard data on the results of the therapy. The American Academy of Periodontology's position paper released on the subject states:

The Academy is in favor of any method of treatment that has been demonstrated, through properly designed and executed research studies, to be beneficial to patients with periodontal disease. Historically, bacterial plaque control has been the cornerstone of periodontal therapy. From its very inception, the academy has advocated strongly the concept of personal oral hygiene as a vital part of the prevention and treatment of periodontal disease. Studies reported in the dental literature support that effective oral hygiene is important to periodontal health. It is the policy of the American Academy of Periodontology not to take a position on the effectiveness of any treatment method unless it has been supported by sufficient evidence on which to base its judgment. To date, neither Dr. Keyes nor other investigators have provided data which would serve as an adequate basis for judgment of the technique advocated by Dr. Keyes to treat periodontal disease.[19]

The dental hygienist's involvement in this therapeutic approach to periodontal disease would include microscopic monitoring for the presence of motile bacteria, spirochetes, and white blood cell levels; recording of bleeding points, deep scaling, and root planing; application of the antibacterial pastes; irrigation of sulci; and providing the patient with explicit instructions for home care.

References

1. Toews, S.E. Root topography following instrumentation: a SEM study. Dent. Hyg. 59(8):350, 1985.

2. Kieser, J.B., and Davies, R.M. The removal of root surface deposits. J. Clin. Periodontol. 12(2):141–152, 1985.

3. Cogen, R.B., Garrison, D.C., and Weatherford, T.W. Effect of various root surface treatments on the viability and attachment of human gingival fibroblasts. J. Periodontol. 55(5):277, 1983.

4. Stahl, S.S., and Froum, S.J. Human clinical and histological repair response following the use of citric acid in periodontal therapy. J. Periodontol. 48(5):261, 1977.

5. Garrett, J.S., Crigger, M., and Egelberg, J. Effects of citric acid on diseased root surfaces. J. Periodontol. 13(2):155, 1978.

6. Lasho, D.J., O'Leary, T.J., and Kafrawy, A.H. A scanning electron microscope study of the effects of various agents on instrumented periodontally involved root surfaces. J. Periodontol. 54(4):210–219, 1983.

7. Dodson, L.E. Periodontal maintenance therapy. II. Dent. Hyg. 58(5):208–215, 1984.

8. Hirschfeld, L., and Wasserman, B. A long term survey of tooth loss in 600 treated periodontal patients. J. Periodontol. 49(5):225, 1978.

9. Lightner, L.M., et al. Preventive periodontic treatment procedures: results over 46 months. J. Periodontol. 42(9):555, 1971.

10. Kalkwarf, K.L., Tussing, G.L., and Davis, M.J. Histologic evaluation of gingival curettage facilitated by sodium hypochlorite solution. J. Periodontol. 53(2):63, 1982.

11. Keyes, P.H. Microbiologically modulated periodontal therapeutics: an introduction. Quintessence Int. 13:1321, 1982.

12. Chace, R., and Keyes, P.H. Salt, soda and hydrogen peroxide, is it enough? Yes. Fla. Dent. J. 52(2):12–13, 1981.

13. Wolff, L.F., et al. Microbial interpretation of plaque relative to the diagnosis and treatment of periodontal disease. J. Periodontol. 56(5):281–284, 1985.

14. Fletcher, P. Keyes approach to periodontics. N. Y. State Dent. J. 48:284, 1982.

15. Weatherford, T.W. A new (?) treatment for periodontal disease. Ala. J. Med. Sci. 19:462, 1982.

16. Scheffler, R.M., and Ravin, S. Preventing and treating periodontal disease with the Keyes technique: a preliminary assessment. Prevent. Med. 11:677, 1982.

17. Finkleman, E.S., and Crompton, S. The Keyes method of alternative periodontal therapy. Dent. Hyg. 59(7):302, 1985.

18. Report of the Special Committee on NIH. NIDR study on periodontal therapy. Presented to the General Assembly of the American Academy of Periodontology, September 1984.

19. A position paper: the American Academy of Periodontology's view on the prevention and treatment of gum disease, 1981.

chapter 9

Treatment modalities for the postsurgical patient

The dental hygienist often sees the patient at the first periodontal postoperative appointment. After removal of the dressing if one was utilized, suture removal should follow if directed by the surgeon's treatment plan.

Periodontal dressing manipulation

Periodontal dressings may typically be categorized as those that contain eugenol and those that do not. Some recent studies have shown that eugenol dressings are more irritating to the tissues than noneugenol dressings. Typically, they contain 40% to 50% eugenol but the set material contains some free eugenol that tends to increase in amount as the zinc eugenate decomposes. In addition, eugenol-containing dressings leave an undesirable taste in the patient's mouth.

If a eugenol dressing is used, approximately 1 teaspoon of powder to 10 drops of liquid are mixed together with a tongue blade or spatula, a small amount at a time (Fig. 9-1). After all of the liquid has been incorporated, the material should be rolled with the fingers into appropriate lengths for the treated site (Fig. 9-2). One advantage of the use of this type of dressing is that it may be made in advance and frozen until needed.

The roll of dressing is placed at the surgical site after all blood, debris, and saliva have been removed. Pressure is applied with the finger or cotton swab to force the material interproximally (Fig. 9-3). A

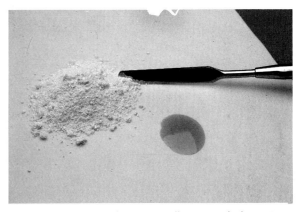

Fig. 9-1 Courtesy of Nancy Balkema Nichols, R.D.H., Chicago, Ill.

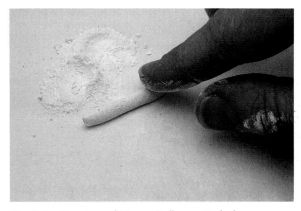

Fig. 9-2 Courtesy of Nancy Balkema Nichols.

147

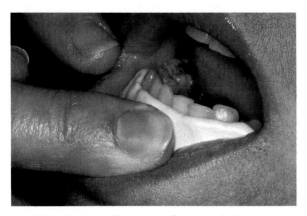

Fig. 9-3 Courtesy of Nancy Balkema Nichols.

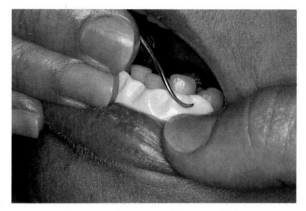

Fig. 9-4 Courtesy of Nancy Balkema Nichols.

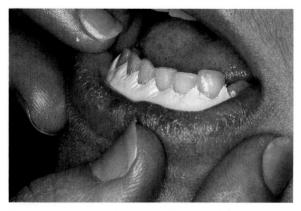

Fig. 9-5 Courtesy of Nancy Balkema Nichols.

universal curet is then used to ensure retention interproximally and to contour the dressing where necessary for optimal esthetics (Fig. 9-4), freedom of musculature, and avoidance of interference with the occlusion (Fig. 9-5).

If a noneugenol dressing such as Coe-Pak* or Peri-pac† is used, both components are in paste form (Fig. 9-6). One of the most commonly used pastes, Coe-Pak contains zinc oxide, an oil (for plasticity), a gum (for cohesiveness), and lorothidol (a fungicide). Peri-pac contains liquid coconut fatty acids thickened with colophony resin and chlorothymol as a bacteriostatic agent. Equal amounts of the two pastes are mixed together on a paper pad with the use of a tongue blade until no streaks of the original contrasting colors remain (Fig. 9-7). The fingers are lubricated with water or vaseline in order to roll the dressing into the desired lengths. The use of hot water followed by cold water facilitates setting of the material and attainment of the correct consistency in order to manipulate it more quickly. The application procedure is the same as for a eugenol dressing (Figs. 9-8 and 9-9).

The patient should be instructed to follow his or her usual oral hygiene regimen in other areas of the mouth but to avoid brushing in the area of the dressing. Antimicrobial or palliative rinses may be recommended.

There is currently a great deal of controversy in the literature as to the advisability of using periodontal dressings.[1] Patient comfort may be an advantage of the use of such dressings. Promotion of bacterial colonization and no apparent positive correlation to healing appear to be disadvantages.

Suture removal

Suture materials may be absorbable or nonabsorbable. Examples of absorbable sutures are plain gut, which is prepared from the submucosa of sheep intestines, and synthetic, chromic gut. Surgical silk, cotton, linen, synthetic, and wire sutures are nonabsorbable.

Common forms of suturing in periodontal surgery are the interrupted, the continuous, the cross-mattress, and the simple mattress techniques. For the interrupted suture each stitch is taken and tied sepa-

*Coe Laboratories, Inc., Chicago, Ill.
†de Trey Freres S.A., Zurich, Switzerland.

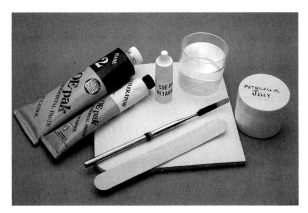

Fig. 9-6 Courtesy of Nancy Balkema Nichols.

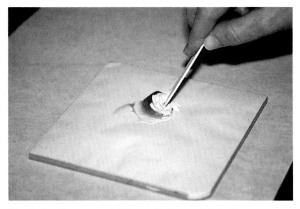

Fig. 9-7 Courtesy of Nancy Balkema Nichols.

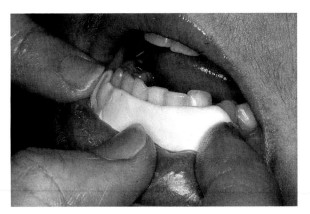

Fig. 9-8 Courtesy of Nancy Balkema Nichols.

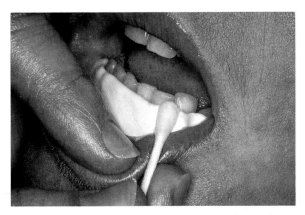

Fig. 9-9 Courtesy of Nancy Balkema Nichols.

rately. This is a common technique employed in the interproximal area (Fig. 9-10). Continuous sutures are a long series of sutures tied only at one end (Fig. 9-11). This technique is employed for periodontal flap surgery. The simple mattress, secured on the proximal ends with single interrupted sutures, is used for small periodontal flaps (Fig. 9-12). The cross mattress suture, which is secured on both ends by a single interrupted suture, is used to stabilize detached flaps to firm tissue (Fig. 9-13).

Sutures aid in healing by maintaining continuity of the tissues, by preventing dry sockets through maintenance of the initial blood clot, and by protecting the site from foreign debris and trauma. Before the sutures are removed, the tissue should be cleansed and the patient's surgical record checked to ascertain the number of sutures placed.

When interrupted sutures are removed, cotton pliers are used to pull gently on the knot (Fig. 9-14). Suture scissors are used to cut the suture between the knot and the tissue. The knot should never be drawn through the tissue. An infectious response may result from this approach. The knot end is held with the cotton pliers and the suture gently pulled out (Fig. 9-15). Each suture must be placed on the bracket table so that the number of sutures removed may be checked. A missed suture may cause granulation tissue to develop at the wound site.

When continuous sutures are removed, the sutures are cut between the knot and the tissue (Fig. 9-16). All vertical loops of sutures are then cut where they enter the tissue in each papillary area (Fig. 9-17). The portion of suture material is drawn from each site. The same procedure is followed for the lingual flap.

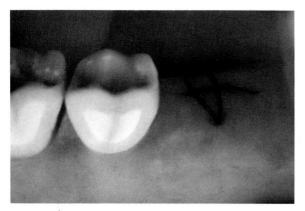

Fig. 9-10 Courtesy of Nancy Balkema Nichols.

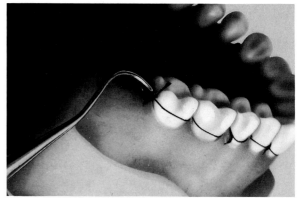

Fig. 9-11 Courtesy of Nancy Balkema Nichols.

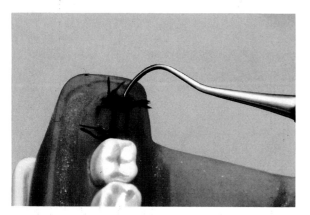

Fig. 9-12 Courtesy of Nancy Balkema Nichols.

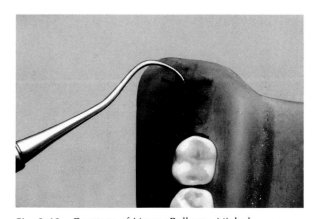

Fig. 9-13 Courtesy of Nancy Balkema Nichols.

A continuous suture must not be removed by drawing it through the length of the surgical site.

The patient should be instructed to rinse with hydrogen peroxide or diluted mouthrinse. The patient's personal home care regimen should be adapted for the surgical site with instructions on how to return to the normal regimen.

Hypersensitivity control

One of the most common complaints of patients undergoing periodontal therapy is that the therapy has made their teeth sensitive. Hypersensitivity of teeth after root planing procedures is due to the exposure of new dentin. Also, newly exposed root surfaces after surgery may be very sensitive to extrinsic factors such as temperature changes, foods, and plaque control

implements. In most cases, if the patient follows a stern regimen of plaque control, hypersensitivity is transient. Although the patient has difficulty being thorough in the plaque control program when the sensitivity is present, he or she must be educated as to the direct correlation between the presence of plaque and an increase in sensitivity of the teeth.

If the hypersensitivity persists, a number of chemical approaches exist to make the patient more comfortable. Fluorides are often employed for this purpose following thorough debridement and root preparation. Fluoride pastes and rinses may be used at home by the patient. In addition, in-office fluoride treatments to the affected areas may be beneficial. Fluoride may be administered by tray, paint-on technique, or iontophoresis. Iontophoresis utilizes a machine that elicits a direct electrical current through a paintbrush handpiece. The manufacturers propose that this

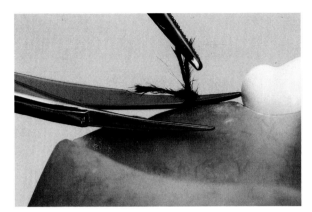

Fig. 9-14 Courtesy of Nancy Balkema Nichols.

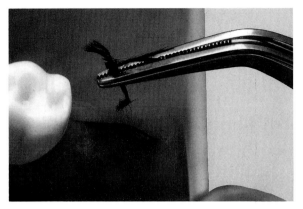

Fig. 9-15 Courtesy of Nancy Balkema Nichols.

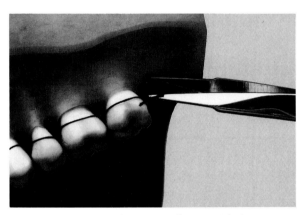

Fig. 9-16 Courtesy of Nancy Balkema Nichols.

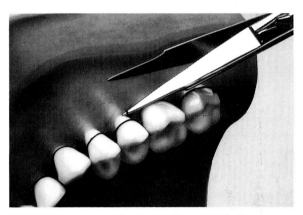

Fig. 9-17 Courtesy of Nancy Balkema Nichols.

mechanism more efficiently integrates the negatively charged fluoride ions into the tooth surface. Ionto-phoresis toothbrush devices are also available for home use.

Products containing sodium fluoride, silicofluoride, and fluoride in combination with other materials are used in the office as hypersensitivity therapies. When these medicaments are used, care must be taken to isolate the teeth so that the material does not come in contact with the gingival tissues or the mucosa, because a chemical burn may result. Explicit directions should be followed for the use of these products. Typically two or three subsequent applications are needed at 1-week intervals. Application may be achieved by use of cotton pellets or swabs, a porte polisher, or a dental instrument.

Corticosteroid compounds used previously for sensitivity during preparation for restorative dentistry are currently being marketed for dentin hypersensitivity. The agent is applied in the same manner as the fluoride agents. The corticosteroid agent decreases sensitivity by inhibiting the inflammatory reaction within the pulp.

Commercially available dentifrices are indicated for hypersensitivity. Some contain strontium chloride, formalin, and sodium monofluorophosphate.[2] The Council on Dental Therapeutics of the American Dental Association has rendered its approval on some of these pastes; some are still being researched. Some products work to desensitize the dentition but have other undesirable properties such as a high abrasitivity index. The dental hygienist should investigate all the dentifrice products available so as to provide the best direction for her or his patients. Complete information may be obtained by contacting the American Dental Association.

References

1. Sachs, H.A., et al. Current status of periodontal dressing. J. Periodontol. 55(12):689, 1984.

2. Collins, J.F., et al. Reducing dentinal hypersensitivity with strontium chloride and potassium nitrate. Gen. Dent. 32(1):40–43, 1984.

chapter 10

Polishing
mechanisms

The removal of plaque, materia alba, and extrinsic stains from tooth surfaces by polishing has been a component of routine dental hygiene therapy for a significant amount of time. Many patients still consider polishing an important aspect of the prophylaxis and expect that it will be routinely employed following scaling and root planing. Recent evidence, however, suggests that polishing all teeth in the patient's dentition after each prophylaxis, regardless of stain deposition, may not be in the patient's best interest.[1] Rather, prior to polishing, all pertinent factors should be considered and discussed with the patient, including the relatively recent concept of selective polishing, before a decision is made to polish all teeth.

Selective polishing[2–4] involves a decision-making process that results in polishing only the teeth from which extrinsic stains were not removed during scaling and toothbrushing. Stains are not considered etiologic agents in the initiation of dental diseases in and of themselves, other than to provide a roughened surface that may encourage plaque formation. Esthetically, however, stains are undesirable to most patients and should therefore be removed during the prophylaxis appointment.

Because the concept of selective polishing represents a substantial procedural change to most patients, the patient must be involved in the decision to selectively polish. Most patients, when presented with information about the effects of polishing, tend to accept the idea of selective polishing with little hesitation.

Effects of polishing procedures

Although previously thought to be an inconsequential procedure, a number of deleterious effects of polishing have been identified.[5] These factors must be considered, along with the individual needs of patients, prior to polishing.

The tooth structure itself may be affected when an abrasive pumice paste is utilized during polishing. Some studies have shown that up to 4 μm of surface enamel may be removed. This can be a significant loss if the teeth are polished regularly over a number of years. Loss of the outer layer of enamel is of particular importance when treating pedodontic patients, because newly erupted teeth are not fully mineralized.

Harsh abrasives are also damaging to cementum and dentin, which are softer tissues than enamel, and therefore more susceptible to structural loss. Areas of decalcified enamel are another type of tooth structure that may be easily damaged with coarse abrasive polishing agents. Because loss of tooth structure is so easily accomplished, abrasive polishing procedures should be avoided in these areas. Cervical tooth surfaces should also be avoided during polishing because the enamel may be very thin or the cementum exposed. In such cases, the patient may exhibit hypersensitivity of these areas, and abrasive polishing may increase the amount of discomfort.

Another factor to consider is the fluoride content of the enamel itself. Because the outer layer of enamel contains the highest concentration of fluoride, loss of this layer removes the most caries-resistant surface of the tooth. Although many commercial prophylaxis pastes contain fluoride, the uptake by the enamel is slight and is not to be considered a replacement for the lost fluoride. If polishing is performed, a topical fluoride replacement mechanism should be employed.

Use of the rubber polishing cup and bristle brush attachments can generate heat that is potentially dangerous to the pulp of the tooth. Certainly the heat produced may cause the patient discomfort or actual pain. Care must be taken to utilize proper techniques when polishing is performed.

The gingival tissues may be damaged through incorrect use of the handpiece and polishing attachments. Removal of epithelium from the free gingiva can occur when the handpiece is used at high speed and the bristle brush or rubber cup is held against the tissue for an extended length of time. The resulting wound is at an increased risk of continued inflammation because patients tend to avoid brushing and flossing sensitive areas with the result that plaque may form more easily and further irritate the tissues.

Effects on the hygienist

The dental hygienist faces potentially deleterious effects during polishing procedures unless appropriate precautions are taken. Splatter of the polishing pastes is unsanitary in general and may cause serious damage to the eyes. Protective eyeglasses should always be worn for all dental hygiene procedures, especially instrumentation and polishing.

Another hazard is the production of aerosols during the use of the handpiece and the air–water syringe. Because airborne contaminants may transmit diseases, the hygienist should routinely wear a face mask for protection. If a patient has a communicable disease, the use of any aerosol-producing instrument should be avoided.

Effects on the patient

The most significant effect polishing has on the health of the patient is the bacteremia that can be produced. Use of the rubber cup can cause bleeding of the gingiva, especially when the tissues are inflamed. Microorganisms can then be introduced into the patient's bloodstream. If the patient has a medical history for which antibiotic prophylactic premedication is indicated, this should be provided prior to any tissue manipulation.

Polishing usually has a positive effect on the patient in terms of a clean feeling in the mouth, with tooth surfaces feeling smoother and appearing more esthetically pleasing. Smooth surfaces are easier to keep plaque-free; however, the acquired pellicle deposits very quickly following complete plaque removal. The value of polishing for these purposes only is therefore questionable. Motivation of the patient to attempt to replicate the plaque-free feeling regularly through home care procedures may be accomplished, at least in part, by polishing the tooth surfaces. If polishing is performed, the clinician should always use the least abrasive agent possible.

Conditions that warrant polishing

Polishing should be employed primarily to remove extrinsic stains that were not removed either during scaling procedures or the patient's personal toothbrushing technique. As much stain as possible should be removed when scaling and root planing to reduce the amount of polishing needed.

Polishing has also typically been employed prior to the application of topical fluorides and pit and fissure sealants. The value of abrasive polishing prior to applying topical fluoride solutions and gels is questionable, because current research indicates that the uptake of fluoride by the enamel surface is not inhibited by the presence of the acquired pellicle. In addition, fluoride uptake appears to be comparable in tooth enamel that is abrasively polished or that is brushed by the patient. For the application of pit and fissure sealants, the preparation of the tooth surfaces generally involves thorough cleaning with a fine pumice slurry. Prophylaxis pastes containing oils and other agents such as fluoride that may interfere with the soundness of the sealant should not be used.

The third circumstance in which polishing procedures are utilized is in the polishing of amalgam restorations. Polishing hinders corrosion and tarnish, and prolongs the life of the restoration.

Conditions for which polishing is contraindicated

Contraindications for polishing include recently erupted teeth; exposed root surfaces; areas of decalcification; restorations made of gold, porcelain, and other easily scratched materials; and gingival tissues that are soft, spongy, and bleed easily. Polishing should not immediately follow deep scaling, root planing, or curettage because of the likelihood of particles from the polishing agent being forced into the epithelium and contributing to continued inflammation. Lastly, teeth that do not exhibit extrinsic stains generally should not be polished.

Polishing agents

Polishing agents consist of abrasive particles similar to those used in commercial dentifrices but at a higher abrasivity. The movement of these particles across the surface of the tooth produces microscopic scratches via frictional rubbing or grinding action. The abrasivity of a given agent is determined by the size, shape, hardness, and number of abrasive particles incorporated. As size, hardness, and number of particles decrease, and as particle shape is less irregular, less tooth surface abrasion occurs.

Commonly used abrasive products include silex (silicon dioxide), zirconium silicate, recrystallized kaolinate, calcium carbonate, pumice, and tin oxide. Pumice and tin oxide are more often used in dental hygiene practice. Each of these agents may be purchased alone or as a component of commercially prepared prophylaxis pastes.

Although polishing agents may be classified as fine, medium, or coarse, no universal standard exists among manufacturers to assure uniformity. Each company categorizes its products according to individual criteria. The dental hygienist should become familiar with the ingredients and abrasivity of the various pastes.

Prophylaxis polishing pastes can be purchased as bulk powders and self mixed or as commercially prepared products ready to use. Self-mixed pastes may be prepared in advance and stored in a closed container and are relatively inexpensive. The disadvantage of the self-prepared agents is the time spent in preparation and cleanup afterward and, more important, in regulating the abrasivity of the paste, which is controlled by the amount of liquid added to the powder.

Self-mixed polishing pastes are prepared by combining the abrasive powder with a lubricant. The lubricant facilitates particle movement across the tooth surfaces and helps to reduce frictional heat. Liquids that may be used include water, flavored mouthwash, and hydrogen peroxide. The latter is particularly helpful in the removal of tenacious extrinsic stain. Preparation of the paste involves placing the lubricant in a dappen dish, adding the dry agent to the saturation point, and stirring. The consistency of the paste should be as liquid as possible and still be transportable between the dappen dish and the teeth without dripping.

Commercially prepared polishing pastes are available in both jars and individually premeasured packets. Premeasured packets have the advantages of a longer shelf life, of remaining moist for a longer period, and of being more sanitary. The cost tends to be higher than when purchased in jars. Most commercially prepared polishing agents consist of an abrasive, which is the main ingredient (50% to 60%), water (10% to 20%), a humectant (20% to 25%) to retain moisture and stabilize the ingredients, a binding agent (1.5% to 2%) to prevent separation and splatter, and sweetening and flavoring agents.

When a polishing paste is selected, both the abrasiveness of the paste and the amount, type, and tenacity of the stain should be considered. A fine-grade paste with mild abrasivity and high polishing abilities is used to remove light stain and soft deposits. This type of paste is most appropriate for pedodontic and periodontal recall patients. A medium-grade paste is recommended for moderate stain and soft deposits covering one third to two thirds of the teeth. Coarse prophylaxis paste is indicated when heavy brown, black, or tobacco stain is present on two thirds or more of the teeth.

Methods of polishing

Motor-driven polishing is the most widely used method in dental hygiene practice. Air polishing and manual polishing are also utilized. Each of these techniques including the necessary equipment, is described here. The polishing procedure is discussed more fully in the laboratory manual.

Motor-driven polishing

Motor-driven polishing is accomplished by the use of a handpiece with a prophylaxis angle attachment to which rubber polishing cups or bristle brushes are affixed (Fig. 10-1). The handpiece operates from a power source in the dental unit and is driven by compressed air or a belt or cable. Handpieces may be categorized according to revolutions per minute (rpm):

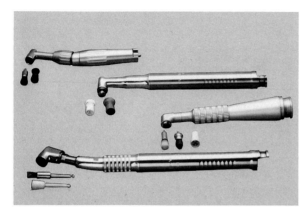

Figure 10-1

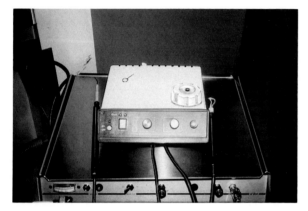

Figure 10-2

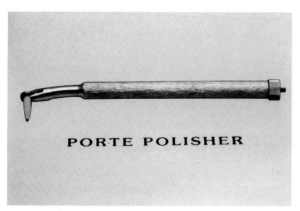

Figure 10-3

1. Low speed: under 20,000 rpm.
2. Intermediate speed: between 20,000 and 100,000 rpm.
3. High-speed (ultraspeed):
   Class A—greater than 160,000 rpm.
   Class B—100,000 to 160,000 rpm.

When natural surfaces are polished, the low-speed handpiece should be operated at the slowest possible rpm to accomplish the procedure.

The prophylaxis angle may be either a right-angle or contra-angle device that attaches directly to the handpiece. Its function is to hold the polishing cups and brushes. A wide variety of prophy angles are manufactured, usually of stainless steel, although other materials including plastics have been employed.

The attachment devices that fit on to the prophylaxis angle are a variety of rubber polishing cups and bristle brushes. These devices may either screw into or snap on over a small protruding knob on the angle or they may fit into the angle with a mandrel and locking mechanism. The cups are made of natural or synthetic rubber and may be ribbed, webbed, or have bristles inside. Polishing cups are used to remove stains and soft deposits and to polish restorations.

Bristle brushes are made of natural or nylon bristles. The brushes may be flat or pointed, with textures ranging from soft to very stiff. Brushes are used to remove stains from deep grooves, pits, or fissures of occlusal surfaces as well as some stains of labial or lingual surfaces well away from the gingival margin. Care must be taken when using brushes to avoid exposed cementum, because they can easily damage such tissues. Brushes are also used in the beginning phase of amalgam polishing.

The use of motor-driven instruments for polishing has the disadvantages of some loss of tooth structure when used with an abrasive agent, trauma to the gingiva when improperly used, and pain or discomfort from frictional heat that can result from excess speed or extended application of the rubber cup.

Air polishing

Air polishing[6-8] is a relatively new form of polishing that employs an abrasive system of sodium bicarbonate–water slurry under air pressure to remove soft deposits and stains (Fig. 10-2). The air pressure ranges from 500 to 1,000 pounds per square inch, and water pressure is from 10 to 50 pounds per square inch.

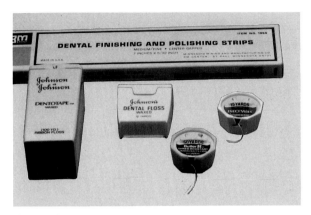

Figure 10-4

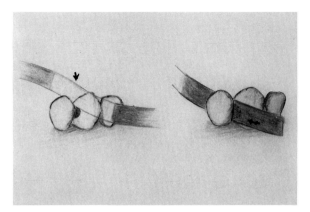

Figure 10-5

The temperature of the water is thermostatically controlled at approximately 37.7°C (100°F). The unit has a handpiece with a contra-angled nozzle through which the slurry is propelled by activation of a foot control pedal. The device has been shown to be quite effective in the removal of plaque and stains.

Air polishing has a number of advantages. Less time is required for the polishing procedure than for more traditional means, fatigue is reduced for both the operator and the patient, decreased gingival marginal redness and bleeding occur, and the operator has better visual access to the area being treated. Patients who object to the taste of commercial pastes may find the sodium bicarbonate flavor less noxious. Use of an air polisher usually generates less noise than a motor-driven handpiece, resulting in greater comfort for both patient and operator.

Disadvantages of the system include the initial cost of the device, possible gingival laceration if the slurry is aimed directly at the soft tissues, and patient complaints of discomfort and a stinging sensation. Use of the device is contraindicated for patients with histories of hypertension because of the sodium bicarbonate.

The research to date indicates that air polishing is a safe and effective means of removing plaque and stain from the teeth. Because the technique is relatively new, the dental hygienist should be alert to new evaluations.

Manual polishing

Manual polishing is performed using a porte polisher, which has a thick handle with a straight shank slightly angled from the handle. The working end is designed to accept variously shaped orangewood points (Fig. 10-3). The orangewood points are either wedge- or cone-shaped and are of several lengths and widths. They may be cut or trimmed to specification, packaged, and sterilized prior to use.

Because the time involved in polishing an entire dentition is considerable, the porte polisher is impractical for routine use in dental hygiene therapy. On a limited basis, and for certain types of patients, however, it can be very useful. It is completely portable and can be used when electricity or motor-driven equipment is unavailable. Porte polishing provides a gentle massage to the marginal gingiva, which can be beneficial. The device can be adapted more easily than motor-driven equipment to difficult-to-reach areas such as malpositioned teeth. It produces very little if any frictional heat and no noise. This can be highly beneficial for children, handicapped individuals, and other patients who are disturbed by excess noise. The porte polisher is easily cleaned and sterilized, making it desirable from an aseptic point of view. Possibly the greatest advantage of the porte polisher, and its most contemporary use, is in the application of desensitizing agents to exposed cementum and dentin.

Obvious disadvantages of the use of the porte polisher include operator fatigue and excessive amounts of time required to polish the dentition.

Polishing proximal surfaces

Deposit removal on proximal tooth surfaces is accomplished by dental floss, dental tape, and polishing strips (Fig. 10-4). Floss and tape are made of nylon or spun silk and are obtainable in waxed or unwaxed forms.

Unwaxed floss is used to polish interproximal surfaces, especially prior to application of topical fluoride. The wax coating on floss has several purposes: it assists in moving the floss or tape through the contact areas, prevents shredding, provides a degree of protection to the tissues, and prevents excessive moisture absorption. It also may leave a light layer of wax on the tooth surface following use. For this reason, the use of waxed floss or tape prior to a topical fluoride application is not recommended, because the fluoride may not uniformly contact the entire enamel surface.

Polishing or finishing strips are thin, flexible strips made of linen or plastic. One part of the strip is smooth, the other embedded with an abrasive agent. Some strips have a small segment that is smooth on both sides, to allow inserting the strip through the contact area without undue abrasion of the enamel (Fig. 10-5). Finishing strips are available in four widths—extra-narrow, narrow, medium, and wide—and in extra fine, fine, medium, and coarse grits.

Polishing strips are useful to remove stains from proximal surfaces of anterior teeth but should be used only if other polishing techniques fail to remove the stain. Only narrow or extra-narrow fine grit strips should be used, and then only as necessary. Discretion must be employed in their use because the abrasive side of the strip can remove tooth structure, especially cementum. The use of strips should be restricted to enamel only. During use, care must be taken to avoid accidental trauma to gingiva and other soft tissues, because the edge of the strip is sharp and capable of cutting soft tissue if used carelessly or improperly.

References

1. Walsh, M.M., et al. Effect of a rubber cup polish after scaling. Dent. Hyg. 59(11):494–498, 1985.
2. Cross, G.N., and Carr, E.H. Patients' acceptance of selective polishing. Dent. Hyg. 57(12):20, 1983.
3. Hassel, B.L., and Kohut, R.D. Survey on selected polishing. Dent. Hyg. 55(9):27–30, 1981.
4. Rohleder, P.V., and Slim, L.H. Alternatives to rubber cup polishing. Dent. Hyg. 55(9):16–20, 1981.
5. Putt, M.S., Kleber, C.J., and Muhler, J.C. Enamel polish and abrasion by prophylaxis paste. Dent. Hyg. 56(9):38, 40–43, 1982.
6. Lehne, R.K., and Winston, A.E. Abrasivity of sodium bicarbonate. Clin. Prevent. Dent. 5(1):17–18, 1983.
7. Vande, V.F., et al. Clinical, histological and scanning electron microscopy evaluation of the prophy-jet in vivo and in vitro. Rev. Belge Med. Dent. 37(4):153–157, 1982.
8. Williman, D.E., Norling, B.K., and Johnson, W.N. A new prophylaxis instrument: effect on enamel alterations. J. Am. Dent. Assoc. 101(6):923–925, 1980.

Preventive dentistry and oral
health maintenance

chapter 11

The control of
dental disease

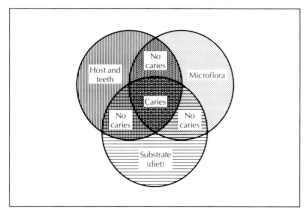

Fig. 11-1 Keyes' diagram.

Control of dental disease became possible once the causative agent, bacterial plaque, was identified. In addition, nutritional factors such as the use of fluorides and the elimination of sucrose in the diet have had an impact on the dental caries process. A considerable amount of time and energy has been devoted to the eradication of dental caries, and the dental profession can indeed be proud of its efforts in caries reduction. Current evidence indicates, however, that 20% of children in the United States still have high caries rates.[1]

The primary responsibility of the contemporary dental hygienist is to assist patients in attaining and maintaining optimum oral health. Patients increasingly tend to seek out health care providers who do not assume sole responsibility for decisions related to their health. Rather, they seek education regarding health and disease states and choose health professionals who provide instruction on how to develop the skills and understanding necessary for maintenance of their own health.

This chapter will present a broad spectrum of approaches to the preventive dentistry aspect of the patient's total treatment. The emphasis of health care practitioners in general in recent years has focused on prevention and health maintenance. Because the dental hygiene profession was established solely in this interest, the dental hygienist is uniquely suited to assume a role of leadership in today's practice of dentistry.

Cariology

The interplay of microorganisms, the teeth, and the substrate (food) that leads to dental caries is demonstrated by the Keyes' diagram[2] (Fig. 11-1). The susceptibility of an individual to caries depends upon tooth structure, saliva, and plaque environment. Genetics, nutrition, the use of medications, and oral hygiene behaviors all have an impact.

Plaque

Plaque is a complex mixture of dense microbial elements enmeshed within a gel-like matrix of salivary products plus bacterial polysaccharides. The by-products of plaque cause demineralization of the tooth structure by providing a period of low pH values resulting from the fermentative activities of ingested sugars. Also, by its thick nature, plaque prevents diffusion of the acidic products into the saliva where natural buffering would occur. The primary cariogenic organism that has been isolated from destruc-

Table 11-1 Interpretation of results of the Snyder Test

	Incubation period		
24 hours	48 hours	72 hours	Caries susceptibility
Green	Green	Green	Little or none
Green	Light green	Yellow	Slight
Green	Yellow	–	Moderate
Yellow	–	–	Marked

tive plaques is *Streptococcus mutans*.[2] In addition, other strains of oral streptococci (faecalis, mitis, salivarius, and sanguis) have been implicated in the caries process.

Caries activity testing

Caries activity tests may be utilized to aid in identifying patients who may be at an increased risk of developing caries. In addition, visual results of such tests can serve as patient education and motivational tools and can also easily be used as a component of nutritional counseling.

The Snyder Test measures the ability of salivary microorganisms, specifically lactobacillus organisms, to form acids by fermenting the sugar contained in the agar medium. For the test the patient chews a stick of paraffin to stimulate the flow of saliva, which is then collected in a sterile test tube. The Snyder agar is melted in a second test tube and inoculated with 1 cc of the saliva. This tube is checked daily for 3 days and the color change, if any, noted. The color of the test agar after incubation suggests the degree of caries activity. The significance of color results can be found in Table 11-1.

The agar medium has an acidity level (pH 4.8 to 5.1) that inhibits all acid-producing bacteria except lactobacilli. The pH indicator in the agar medium, brom-cresol-green, changes color from blue-green to yellow as acidity increases. The speed with which the culture changes determines the degree of caries susceptibility. The test is inexpensive, easy to perform, and yields results in a relatively short period of time.

The *Lactobacillus acidophilus* count is a quantitative test of caries activity. Saliva is collected in a

Table 11-2 Interpretation of the results of the *Lactobacillus acidophilus* count

Colonies	Caries susceptibility
0 to 1,000	Little or none
1,000 to 5,000	Slight
5,000 to 10,000	Moderate
10,000 to 50,000	Marked
More than 50,000	Rampant

sterile test tube and diluted to specific concentrations with saline. The diluted mixture is spread on a series of agar plates containing Ragoso's lactobacilli selective medium. The plates are incubated for 72 hours at 37°C. The number of bacterial colonies is then counted to determine the patient's susceptibility to caries. An interpretation of the results is given in Table 11-2. The *Lactobacillus acidophilus* count correlates well to the Snyder test because it measures the presence of lactobacilli. It was the first caries activity test used by practitioners but, because of its complicated methodology, the usefulness of this test is limited and its accuracy is questionable.

Actinomyces bacteria have been associated with the development of root surface caries in the elderly patient population. Selective media for cultivating *Actinomyces* in plaque and saliva samples are available but not yet widely in use.

Nutritional counseling

Carbohydrates constitute the fuel for the dental caries process. Carbohydrates the patient eats become the

Table 11-3 The basic-four food guide

Group	Daily amounts
Milk milk, cheese, ice cream, yogurt, cottage cheese	Children, 3 cups Teenagers, 4 cups Adults, 2 cups* Pregnant women, 3 cups or more Nursing women, 4 cups or more
Meats meats, fish, eggs, beans, peas, legumes	2 servings
Vegetables and fruits	4 servings
Breads and cereals	4 servings

*Two servings from the milk group provides approximately 800 mg of calcium, which may not be adequate for women.[4]

substrate for bacterial metabolism. Foods containing monosaccharides or disaccharides are converted into lactic acid, which contributes to the demineralization of enamel via the bacteria of plaque.[2] Frequent intake of retentive carbohydrates, especially sucrose, is the most cariogenic food habit. The retentiveness of the carbohydrate to the tooth surface and the frequency of the exposure to sucrose are more critical factors than total sugar consumption.

Nutritional analysis and counseling related to dental disease prevention and dental health maintenance have in many instances become part of the repertoire of the dental hygienist. The frequency of dental recall appointments provides an opportunity to become aware of dietary changes that may have an impact on dental health and may lead to general health concerns. The dental hygienist should be trained to provide basic dietary analysis and prescription and to recognize dietary behavior problems that may require the expertise of other health professionals in the nutritional field.

Food diary

Food intake data must be secured, analyzed, and evaluated relative to nutritional adequacy and sucrose consumption. The patient should be instructed to record in a food diary, usually for a 5-day period, the foods and the amounts ingested. Ideally the 5-day period would include a weekend so that a broader representation of the patient's dietary behaviors is elicited.

The basic-four food groups analysis is employed in many dental practices to evaluate basic daily food patterns. Although the RDA (Recommended Dietary Allowances) of the National Academy of Sciences is the appropriate standard to apply in complete evaluation of nutrient consumption, the basic-four approach provides a convenient mechanism for dietary counseling within the limitations of time and expertise in the dental office environment.

The basic-four guide groups food according to major nutrient components contributed to the diet on a daily basis (Table 11-3). General quantities are addressed relative to the number of servings recommended for different population groups (i.e., children or pregnant or lactating women).[3]

Evaluation of the nutrient consumption as recorded in the patient's diary may be done by use of a nutritional analysis sheet elaborating each food group, the deficiencies or over-consumption of each, and an explanation of the nutrient contribution of each.[3] Alternatively, evaluation may be indicated directly on the diary through the use of colored pencils to represent each of the food groups or a code utilizing initials to calculate satisfaction of the daily recommendation for each group. A discussion with the patient about the role of the various nutrients and their relationship to health of the teeth and oral tissues may be a motivational tool during this phase of the procedure.

The use of a red pen to circle sucrose exposures or "insults" is commonly employed as the next step in the analysis. The significance of the red circles is in their impact on the patient when the quantity is multiplied by a factor of 20. The figure 20 represents approximately the number of minutes that an acid condition conducive to the caries process continues after ingestion of fermentable carbohydrates.[5] This is a convenient mechanism for counseling, although some foods may affect acid production much less or much more than 20 minutes. In addition, foods that are not traditionally considered cariogenic in composition may adversely affect the pH so that an acid condition occurs. As a tool for motivation however, demonstrating to the patient the total minutes of acid condition per day—120 minutes, as an example—is very useful, particularly when counseling the child patient and the parent. Because of the hidden sugar content of many foods, this aspect of the dietary counseling is usually a significant learning experience for the patient.

The dental hygienist should then involve the pa-

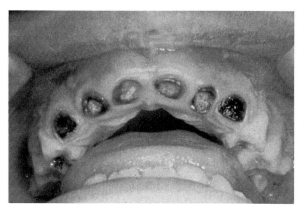

Fig. 11-2 Baby bottle tooth decay.

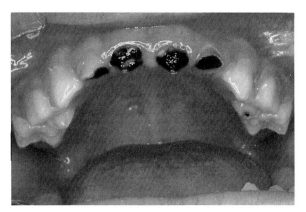

Fig. 11-3 Baby bottle tooth decay.

tient in identifying foods to be eliminated or adaptations to be made in the daily diet. A participatory approach is more likely to meet with success in dietary behavioral changes, as with any attempt to elicit long-term behavioral changes.

Nursing bottle caries

A dietary impact on infants that is currently receiving a lot of attention is nursing bottle caries. At a 1985 meeting of the Oral Health Subcommittee of the Healthy Mothers/Healthy Babies Coalition, the disease was renamed Baby Bottle Tooth Decay. It was felt by the federal agency committee that this term would be better understood by the general public.[6] Several studies show the prevalence to be approximately 10%, with a greater prevalence of the condition among those of lower socioeconomic status.[6]

This phenomenon is related to infants and very young children who have experienced extensive dental caries of their teeth as a result of prolonged drinking of liquids, particularly sucrose-containing liquids, during the sleeping hours. The condition is characterized by the destruction of the maxillary anterior teeth and the interproximal and labial surfaces of the first primary molars (Fig. 11-2). The destruction of the teeth is usually extensive, and often entire clinical crowns are destroyed (Fig. 11-3). Sugar water, juices, and syrupy vitamin concentrations are the major offenders, but even milk should not be given to a child in a bottle to be taken to bed. If a child needs the comfort of a bottle at night, a bottle with water or a pacifier may be utilized.

Patient education

The role of the dental hygienist in patient education is to initiate a personalized program for each patient by evaluating his oral hygiene needs and suggesting appropriate methods of oral physiotherapy. Oral physiotherapy is defined as procedures practiced by the patient for the purpose of maintaining oral hygiene. These procedures, such as brushing, flossing, and gingival stimulation, must be achieved without causing trauma to either the teeth or gingival tissues. The employment of agents for plaque reduction and inhibition may also be recommended. The dental hygienist reevaluates the patient's oral hygiene needs at subsequent appointments and may suggest modifications to the program that will contribute to the patient's continued long-term success.

The goal of most patient education programs is to produce long-term behavioral changes that will result in an optimum state of oral health. Most research, however, indicates that at best only 50% of patients comply with regular toothbrushing and flossing regimens and that two thirds of patients who leave preventive programs do so within 90 days.[7] One reason may be that many dental personnel still approach the providing of home care instruction in an authoritarian manner, acting simply as the dispenser of knowledge. The patient is then expected passively to comply with the instructions given. Any self-care behaviors previously or currently practiced by the patient are, as a rule, not considered relevant.[7]

Recent trends in health care delivery emphasize the active role of the patient. Dental hygienists should

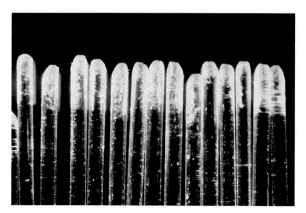

Fig. 11-4a Polished, rounded bristle tips.

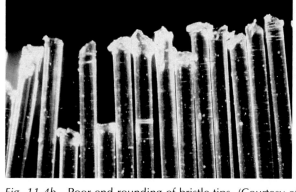

Fig. 11-4b Poor end-rounding of bristle tips. (Courtesy of Oral-B Laboratories.)

recognize that a high percentage of patients already practice oral hygiene procedures to some degree. By recognizing and helping to refine already existing self-care patterns, the hygienist may enable patients to exhibit higher long-term rates of cleansing activities.[7]

A major factor in successful patient behavior change is appropriate problem ownership. Too often, the dental hygienist or dentist makes the decision that the patient has a problem. The patient may not perceive any problem at all and, in fact, may believe that he or she is already controlling plaque to an acceptable level. If the patient does not agree that a problem exists or does not wish to make a change, the dental hygienist can do little.[7]

Too often techniques for plaque control are provided at the initial appointment, frequently at its commencement. Little or no time is allowed for eliciting and understanding the patient's needs or for developing a rapport. As a result, the description of preventive techniques sounds rote and "canned." In contemporary society, with computerization replacing personal contact in so many instances, it becomes increasingly important for health care professionals to relate to patients as individuals. The way to motive them is to show interest and concern, listen, and then provide information.[7]

Patients usually judge concern by the length of time the practitioner spends listening and discussing their health and concerns. The knowledge provided need not be scientific, but it must be relevant. Dental professionals often provide more technical information than patients want or need, thinking that they require a course in oral microbiology.[7] Effective

listening[8] may be one of the most important skills in the dental hygienist's repertoire.

Since the identification of plaque as the etiologic agent of dental disease, numerous devices and mechanisms have been developed for its control. With so many gadgets and agents available, the hygienist may be tempted to inundate the patient with every device, every mouthrinse and toothpaste, and every therapeutic treatment available, in the belief that something is bound to work. The mistake in this approach cannot be overemphasized. These aids require differing levels of psychomotor skill development as well as a commitment of time. When too little instruction with a wide variety of oral hygiene devices is provided to a patient who may not perceive a problem in the first place, frustration and lack of compliance are inevitable. A more successful approach is to provide instruction in small steps: teach the use of one plaque control aid until it has been mastered; have the patient concentrate his or her efforts toward cleaning specific areas of the mouth. If allowed to experience success, the patient is more likely to continue with the program.

A critical aspect of long-term behavior change is adequate follow-up on the part of the practitioner, which includes ongoing assistance in the management of the behavior.[8] Too many patients revert to old habits when they feel that the dental hygienist or dentist is not caring or interested enough to aid in continuously motivating them over long periods of time. Behaviors that a patient has practiced for a number of years cannot and will not dramatically change overnight, with rare exceptions. Rather, the rebuilding

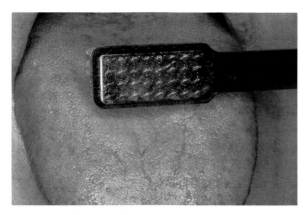

Fig. 11-5a Brushing the tongue.

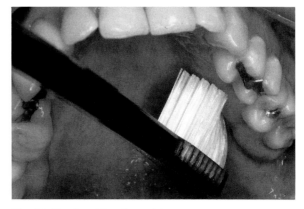

Fig. 11-5b Brushing the palate.

of habit patterns requires time and effort on the part of both the patient and hygienist, with constant reinforcement and encouragement.

Manual plaque control modalities

In addition to interpersonal skills, the dental hygienist has numerous devices to provide patients to control plaque and maintain oral health.

Manual toothbrush

The toothbrush is traditionally considered the basic tool of oral physiotherapy. It is designed to promote oral cleanliness by removing soft deposits on the tooth surfaces from the occlusal–incisal edge to just below the gingival margin. In addition, the toothbrush may be used to stimulate the gingiva. The one most often recommended for the adult patient is composed of nylon bristles with rounded and polished ends (Figs. 11-4a and b). The brush should be of a soft texture to allow the bristles to flex and adapt to tooth contour. The variety of toothbrushes available is great enough for all patient conditions and uses. Determining the patient's primary need for a toothbrush will aid the dental hygienist in recommending the most appropriate style.

Different toothbrushing methods have been designed to meet individual patient's specific needs for removal of soft deposits or for gingival stimulation. To assure that all teeth are cleaned without omission, a pattern for toothbrushing should be established. The

tongue and hard palate should be brushed to remove food debris, plaque, and to give the mouth a refreshed feeling (Figs. 11-5a and b).

Rolling stroke method   The purpose of the rolling stroke method is to remove soft deposits and debris from the tooth surfaces and gingiva and to stimulate the gingiva. It is often used in conjunction with other methods. Bristles are directed apically at a 45° angle to the long axis of the tooth. Bristle tips are placed on the attached gingiva. Lateral pressure is applied so that bristle tips and sides flex against the attached gingiva, causing the gingival tissue to blanch (Fig. 11-6).

The bristles are rolled over the gingiva and tooth surfaces in an incisal–occlusal direction. Moderate speed and adequate pressure maintained throughout the stroke allow bristles to reach the interproximal and cervical areas. The brush is replaced in the initial position and the stroke repeated five to ten times.

The rolling stroke method is indicated for individuals with healthy gingiva and well-aligned teeth, children and adult patients with limited dexterity, and patients requiring gingival massage and stimulation.

Modified Stillman's method   The modified Stillman's method is intended to massage and stimulate the gingiva and to remove soft deposit and debris from the cervical areas of tooth surfaces. This technique adds a rolling stroke to the conventional Stillman's method to achieve a more thorough cleaning and massage.

Bristles are directed apically at a 45° angle to the

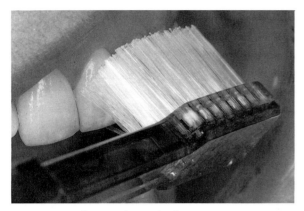

Fig. 11-6 Rolling stroke method.

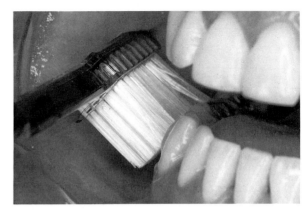

Fig. 11-7 Modified Stillman's method.

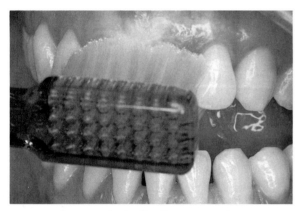

Fig. 11-8a Bass (sulcular brushing) method.

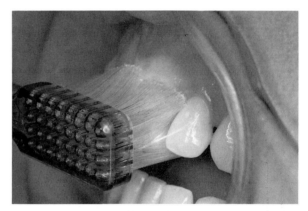

Fig. 11-8b Bass (sulcular brushing) method.

long axis of the tooth. Bristle ends are placed on the attached gingiva. Lateral pressure is applied so that most of the bristle ends are on the attached gingiva, causing the gingival tissue to blanch. Some of the bristle ends and particularly the sides of the bristles should be at the cervical and interproximal marginal gingiva and tooth areas (Fig. 11-7).

With moderate pressure, the bristles are vibrated back and forth or in a small circle while keeping the bristle ends in position for a count of 8 to 10 seconds. This action is followed with a roll stroke in an incisal—occlusal direction. The brush is replaced in its initial position and the vibration and rolling stroke repeated five to ten times before moving to the next position.

The modified Stillman's method is indicated for individuals with average to good dexterity; patients with spongy, hemorrhagic, or enlarged gingiva; and patients with receded gingiva, especially in interproximal areas.

Bass method/sulcular brushing technique Sulcular brushing has been shown to be the most effective toothbrushing method for plaque removal at and just below the gingival margin. Because this area is prone to collecting dental plaque that may lead to gingival and periodontal disease, sulcular brushing is the method of choice for most adult patients, particularly those who have undergone periodontal surgery. Because the bristles are directed into the gingival sulcus, only a soft toothbrush with rounded bristle tips should be used.

Bristles are directed apically at a 45° angle to the long axis of the tooth: bristle ends are placed at the cervical area so that the row of bristles closest to the tooth is directed into the sulcus with the remaining rows directed over the free and attached gingiva (Fig. 11-8a). Lateral pressure is lightly applied to allow the bristles to enter the sulcus and flex against the gingiva in the cervical and interproximal areas, causing gingival tissue to blanch. The sides of the bristles should be contacting the facial or lingual tooth surfaces and interproximal areas (Fig. 11-8b).

With light pressure, the bristles are gently vibrated back and forth or in a circular motion for a count of 8 to 10 seconds. This method may be modified by following the vibrating action with a roll stroke in an incisal–occlusal direction (modified Bass method). The roll stroke will help to clean the remainder of the tooth surface and interproximal areas and to stimulate the attached gingiva. Following five to ten rolling strokes, the brush may be moved to the next area, repeating the vibratory and rolling motions.

Charters' method   The Charters' method of toothbrushing has been indicated for individuals who have open interdental spaces with missing papillae and exposed root surfaces and for those wearing a fixed partial denture or orthodontic appliances. Its purpose is to remove soft deposits as well as to stimulate the gingiva. Because this method does not promote cleansing of the gingival sulcus, it should be used in conjunction with other methods that cleanse this area.

Bristles are directed incisally–occlusally at a 45° angle to the long axis of the tooth. Bristle ends and sides of bristles are placed on the cervical and proximal portions of teeth. Moderate lateral pressure is applied to flex the bristles against the teeth and to force the bristle ends between the teeth. The sides of the bristles press against the gingival margin (Fig. 11-9).

The Charters' method is indicated for patients who have had periodontal surgery, patients with moderate gingival recession, particularly interproximally, and patients with a fixed partial denture or orthodontic appliances.

Placement for cleansing orthodontic appliances
Bristles are directed incisally–occlusally at a 45° angle to the long axis of the tooth. Bristle ends are placed on the edge of the orthodontic appliance near the gingiva (Fig. 11-10a). Pressure is applied, allowing the bristles to cleanse the appliances (Fig. 11-10b). For cleaning the opposite edge of the appliance, the

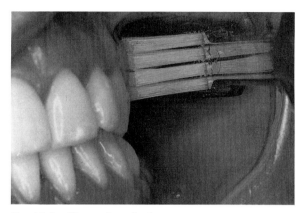

Fig. 11-9   Charters' method.

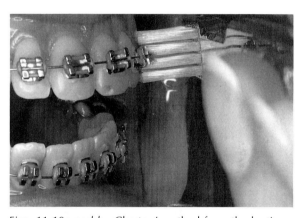

Figs. 11-10a and b   Charters' method for orthodontic appliances.

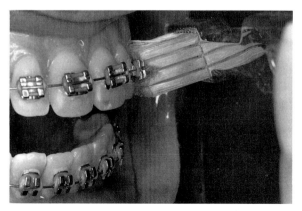

Figure 11-10b

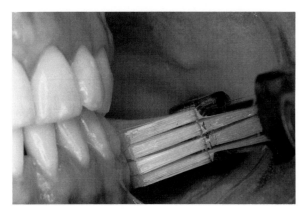

Fig. 11-11 Circular method.

bristles are placed on the apical side of the bands, brackets, and wires. A gentle back and forth or circular motion is used, maintaining the bristle ends in position for a slow count of 8 to 10 seconds. A roll stroke is added to this action (five to ten times) before moving to the next area in order to provide a thorough cleaning.

Circular method   The circular method of brushing is often recommended for young children because it is easy to learn and does not employ a complicated technique. Because it could cause damage if used too vigorously, a soft toothbrush should be used.

With teeth closed in occlusion, the brush is placed at a 90° angle to the long axis of the teeth to be brushed. With a light circular motion, the brush is moved under the buccal surfaces of posterior teeth and gingiva of both maxillary and mandibular arches (Fig. 11-11). Anterior teeth should be in end-to-end contact as they are brushed. Lingual surfaces are to be brushed in the same manner; however, maxillary and mandibular arches are brushed separately with the mouth open.

Patients for whom this technique is indicated include small children, physically or emotionally handicapped individuals, and patients who lack the dexterity for a more technical brushing method.

Automatic toothbrush

The automatic toothbrush is similar to the manual toothbrush in purpose and basic structural design. It differs in several aspects, however, including its han-

dle design, shank length, number of parts, and size. The brush attachment consists of a shank, which fits into a spike at the end of the handle, and a brush head that extends from the shank. The brush attachment and head are much smaller than that of a manual toothbrush and can be either in the same plane as the handle or at an angle.

Some individuals may lack the ability to thoroughly brush with a manual toothbrush. Because the automatic toothbrush has a large handle circumference, and because it provides motion for the bristles, it may be an appropriate alternative for patients who have limited manual dexterity. This group of individuals may include the elderly, physically disabled and those with arthritis in their hands, wrists, and arms. Small children who are unable to grasp the small handle of a manual toothbrush or unable to control the bristle placement and motion may also benefit from using the automatic toothbrush.

Dental floss

Dental floss is used to remove plaque and debris from the proximal surfaces of teeth, including the contact and sulcus areas. Because the toothbrush is unable to reach these areas, dental floss is the oral hygiene aid of choice.

Dental floss is a thin thread-like material made of either nylon or silk thread (Fig. 11-12). Depending on the manufacturer, floss may be either bonded or nonbonded. Bonding prevents the fibers from spreading apart when used on a tooth surface. The fibers may or may not have a waxed coating. Waxed dental floss is often used for flossing between teeth with tight contacts or rough margins of restorations because it is less likely to shred than unwaxed floss. Dental flossing should be done at least once each day prior to brushing to ensure that the plaque-free proximal surfaces receive the maximum benefits of a fluoride dentifrice.

As with toothbrushing, using dental floss in a systematic pattern around the mouth is recommended. A strand of dental floss approximately 18 inches in length is needed (Fig. 11-13). A small amount is wrapped around the middle finger to secure the end. The remainder is wrapped around the middle finger of the other hand (Fig. 11-14a). The floss is held between thumbs and index fingers of both hands, leaving about a half to an inch between the two thumbs (Fig. 11-14b). It is directed gently through the contact

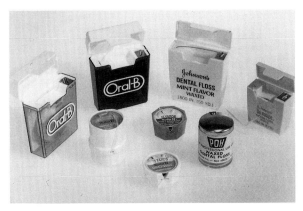

Fig. 11-12   Commercially available types of dental floss.

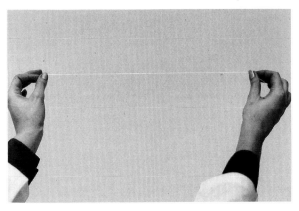

Fig. 11-13   Correct length of dental floss.

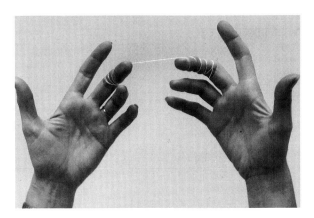

Figs. 11-14a and b   Securing the floss for proper utilization.

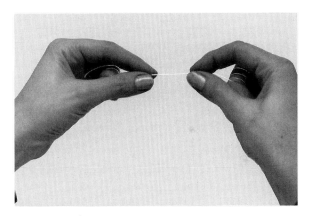

Figure 11-14b

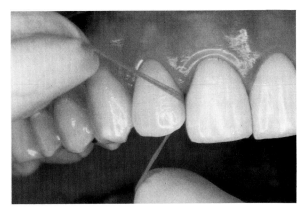

Figs. 11-15a and b   Placement of floss.

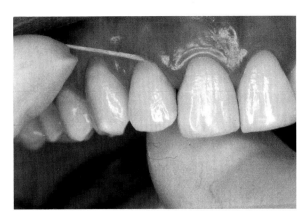

Figure 11-15b

area, using a back-and-forth motion. Maintaining control with the thumbs and index fingers will prevent the floss from snapping through the contact and damaging the gingiva. Once the dental floss is through the contact area, it is curved in a C-shape and wrapped firmly around the proximal surface of the tooth (Fig. 11-15a).

The floss is gently guided apically into the sulcus until resistance is felt, indicating that it has reached the base of the sulcus (Fig. 11-15b). The floss is slid into the sulcus and back to the contact several times in an up-and-down motion—until the surface feels clean.

Without being removed from the contact, it is gently slid over the interdental papilla, and the proximal surface of the adjacent tooth is flossed.

When both adjacent tooth surfaces are plaque-free, the floss is snapped out through the contact area. If contacts are extremely tight or restorations have rough or open margins, the floss may shred upon removal. If this is anticipated, the floss should be held beneath these areas and pulled out in a facial direction. For each contact area that is cleaned, a fresh section of floss should be obtained by unwinding the floss from the fingers.

Proximal cleaning aids

Floss holder A dental floss holder is a plastic device recommended for patients who are unable to manipulate and hold floss in their own hands. Essentially, a floss holder replaces the hands in holding floss in position for cleaning the proximal surfaces of the teeth.

The design of floss holders varies with the manufacturer. All types, however, include a handle, two prongs to support and guide the floss, and an anchor to secure the floss in place (Fig. 11-16). A key consideration in assembling any type of floss holder is to securely anchor and firmly stretch the floss across the prongs so that it has enough tension to remove plaque from proximal tooth surfaces.

When using the floss holder, the handle is firmly grasped and the holder is moved back and forth in a buccal–lingual direction, working the floss through the contact area. Pressure is applied against the surface so that the floss curves around the proximal surface (Fig. 11-17). The floss holder is moved gently up and down, sliding the floss into the sulcus and coronally to the contact. This motion is repeated until

the proximal surface is clean. The floss is moved up and over the interdental papilla, and the proximal surface of the adjacent tooth is flossed.

Patients who may benefit from the use of a floss holder include those who lack coordination or dexterity to floss some areas of the mouth by hand; those who lack the motivation to floss by hand; small patients with extremely large hands, who may find the floss holders easier to use, especially in posterior areas; and parents of small children and those who care for another individual.

Floss threaders A floss threader, used with dental floss, is useful for patients with fixed partial dentures, orthodontic appliances, and splints. It enables the floss to be slipped beneath the appliance so that proximal surfaces of natural teeth may be flossed and loose debris collecting around the appliance may be removed. Several types of floss threaders are available in a variety of widths. All types are made of either plastic or wire and have a slit, loop, or hole at one end through which the floss is passed.

The threader is assembled by obtaining an 18-inch strand of floss and threading the floss through the opening, pulling approximately 2 inches through. Remaining floss should be pulled alongside the 2-inch piece to prevent it from slipping out of the opening. If a patient has difficulty keeping the floss in the threader, the floss may be tied to the threader to secure it. The threader and floss are gently inserted from buccal to lingual beneath the fixed partial denture or appliance to be flossed and pulled through (Fig. 11-18a). The floss is grasped on either side of the tooth, adapting it to the proximal surfaces of the natural teeth and flossing as described in the previous section (Fig. 11-18b). If a fixed partial denture is being flossed, the dental floss is also guided under the pontic to loosen and remove debris.

Gauze strip Gauze strips may be used to clean proximal surfaces of widely spaced teeth or teeth adjacent to edentulous areas. Unlike dental floss, its use is confined to the clinical crowns of teeth. The strip is prepared by folding it in half or in thirds, lengthwise. The fold of the strip is positioned at the cervical area next to the gingival margin. The strip is formed in a C shape around the proximal surface of the tooth and worked in a back-and-forth motion several times (Fig. 11-19). A clean portion of the gauze is used for each area to be cleaned.

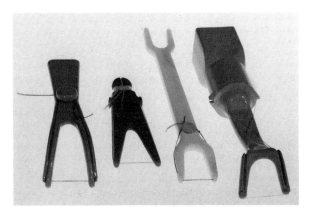

Fig. 11-16   Types of dental floss holders.

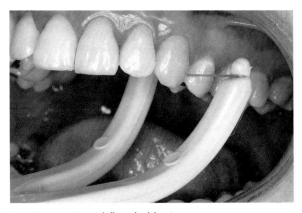

Fig. 11-17   Dental floss holder in use.

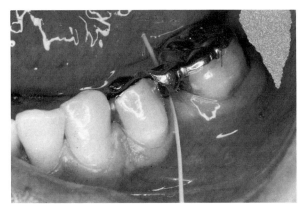

Figs. 11-18a and b   Use of the floss threader.

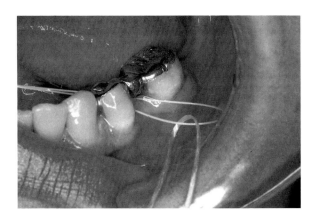

Figure 11-18b

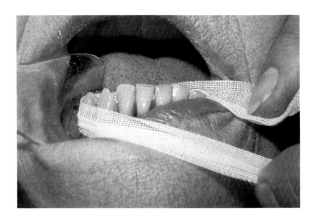

Fig. 11-19   Use of gauze strip.

Gauze strips are most useful for patients with exposed proximal surface where there are large spaces between the teeth, particularly those with missing or blunted interdental papillae, and for tooth surfaces adjacent to edentulous areas. Sometimes they may enable an elderly patient living in an extended care facility to maintain independence in his or her plaque control regime rather than necessitating involvement of the nursing staff to brush and floss the patient's teeth.

Interproximal brush

An interproximal brush is used to clean exposed furcation areas and proximal surfaces of teeth with open embrasures or large spacing between the teeth (Fig. 11-20). For devices that must be assembled, the wire end of the brush attachment is inserted through the hole in the handle until the bristles on the brush meet the handle (Fig. 11-21a). The wire is bent so that it fits in the slot on the back of the handle. The ring is twisted up and over the slot to the bristle to hold the brush firmly in place (Fig. 11-21b). Some interproximal brushes are manufactured with the brush in place in the handle when purchased. The entire device is disposable.

In use, the brush is placed perpendicular to the long axis of the tooth. With the side of the brush kept against the tooth as much as possible, the tip is moved in a facial–lingual motion (Figs. 11-22a and b). Care must be taken not to abrade tooth or gingival tissues with the wire point of the brush.

The interproximal brush is indicated for patients who have exposed furcation areas that cannot be thoroughly cleaned with a toothbrush and for patients with large open embrasures or large spacing between the teeth. It is an ideal cleaning aid for patients who have undergone periodontal therapy and patients who have difficulty brushing the distal surfaces of the most posterior teeth.

Perio-Aid

The Perio-Aid®* is used to clean plaque and debris from furcations and roots that cannot be easily reached with a brush and floss. It may also be used to clean proximal, facial, and lingual tooth surfaces along the gingival margins.

A round-end toothpick is inserted through the hole located at one end of the Perio-Aid® handle so that a half to an inch is pushed through. The ring is tightened until it meets the toothpick. The excess toothpick on the long end is broken off and the ring tightened to further stabilize the toothpick (Fig. 11-23a and b). The tip of the toothpick is moistened with water and placed perpendicular to the long axis of the tooth surface. The side of the tip is kept against the tooth while the tip is moved along the gingival margin with a firm lateral pressure (Fig. 11-24).

The Perio-Aid® is recommended for patients having exposed furcation areas and root surfaces, usually after periodontal surgery, and patients with exposed root surfaces apical to crown margins.

Superfloss

Superfloss®* is a spongelike variation of dental floss. One end of a strand of Superfloss® is stiff so that it may be inserted above the contact area. The middle portion is sponge-like. Because of its thickness and roughened texture, this portion of the floss is useful for gaining access to and removing plaque from proximal tooth surfaces where there are open interdental areas. The remaining portion of the strand is regular dental floss and may be used for normal interproximal cleaning (Fig. 11-25).

Superfloss® is an extremely effective tool for plaque removal in patients with large embrasure spaces from periodontal disease and surgical intervention (Fig. 11-26). Periodontal dental hygienists also often employ Superfloss® as a vehicle for carrying fluoride or other bactericidal agents subgingivally and interproximally.

Aids for gingival stimulation

Gingival stimulation is performed to increase the circulation of spongy, edematous gingiva. For patients with traumatized or diseased tissue, the stimulator massages the gingiva, increases blood flow, and aids in recontouring the interdental papilla area. Gingival stimulation is particularly recommended for those patients who have undergone periodontal surgery.

---

*Marquis Dental Co., Aurora, Colo.

*Oral-B Laboratories Inc., Redwood City, Calif.

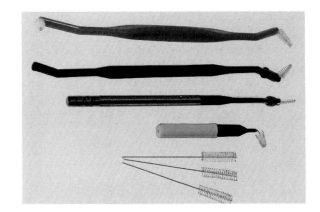

Fig. 11-20   Variety of interproximal brushes.

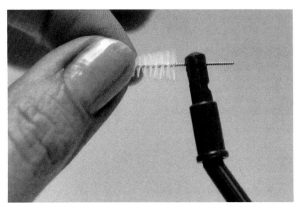

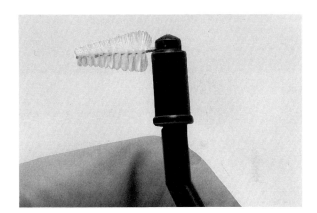

Figs. 11-21a and b   Assembly of the interproximal brush.

Figure 11-21b

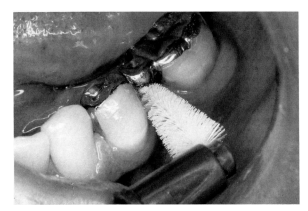

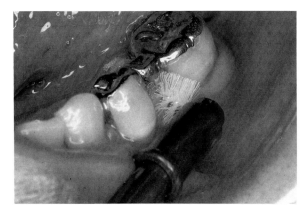

Figs. 11-22a and b   Use of the interproximal brush.

Figure 11-22b

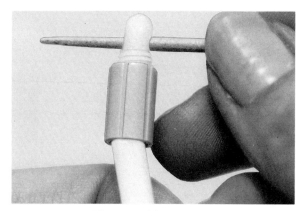

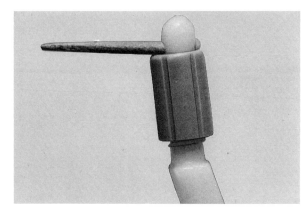

Figs. 11-23a and b Assembly of the Perio-Aid.®

Figure 11-23b

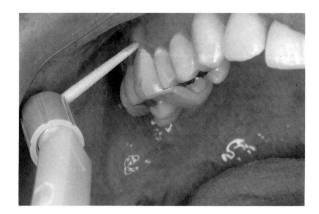

Fig. 11-24 Perio-Aid® in use.

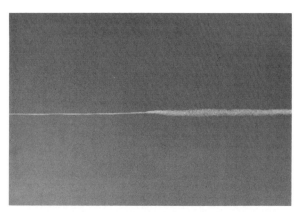

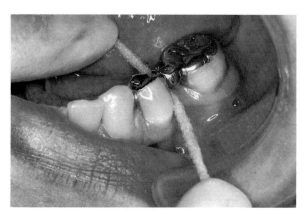

Fig. 11-25 Superfloss®: dental floss on the left, sponge area on the right.

Fig. 11-26 Use of Superfloss® to cleanse beneath a fixed partial denture.

Rubber tip stimulator

The rubber tip stimulator is used for stimulation of the interdental gingival tissues. It is also recommended for reshaping gingival tissues after periodontal surgery (Fig. 11-27).

The tip is inserted into the interproximal area so that the point is wedged between the gingiva and the contact. It is angled so that it adapts to the contours of the gingiva (approximately 45° to the interdental gingiva). The tip is pressed against the gingiva and moved with a gentle pumping motion across the papilla approximately ten times (Figs. 11-28a and b). It is then moved to the next area.

Balsa wood wedge

The balsa wood wedge is a triangular piece of balsa wood used to stimulate the interdental gingival tissue (Fig. 11-29). The tip of the wedge is moistened with saliva and inserted into the interdental area so that the base of the triangle is against the gingiva, with the apex directed incisally (Fig. 11-30). The wedge is angled so that it adapts to the contours of the gingiva (approximately 45° at the interdental gingiva). It is moved gently in and out of the interdental area in a pumping motion approximately ten times. The wedge is then moved to the next area or replaced with a fresh wedge if it has become soft and lost its shape.

Balsa wedges are indicated for patients needing stimulation of interdental gingiva and who have embrasure spaces wide enough to accommodate the wedge.

Irrigation devices for plaque control

Until recently, oral irrigating devices were at best considered adjunctive instruments in a patient's overall oral physiotherapy regime. They were typically recommended for specific types of patients, that is, orthodontic and postperiodontal surgical patients, for removal of materia alba and stimulation of the gingival tissues. Patients were cautioned that oral irrigators were not capable replacements for brushing, flossing, and other more traditional means of plaque removal.[9]

Current research into the role of plaque as the initiator of dental disease has led to a better understanding of the microbiology of the plaque itself. Plaque is a highly structured, complex microbial system that can vary significantly in nature depending on its location in the patient's mouth. The periodontal disease

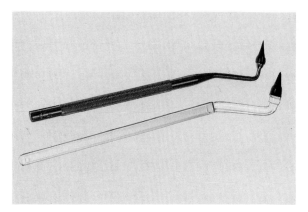

Fig. 11-27 Types of rubber tip stimulators.

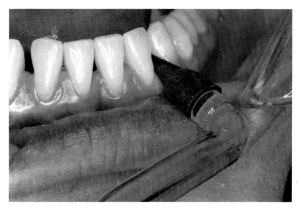

Figs. 11-28a and b Use of the rubber tip stimulator from both buccal and lingual aspects.

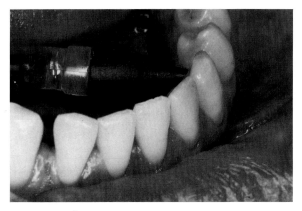

Figure 11-28b

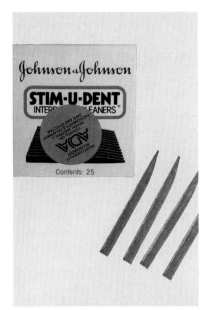

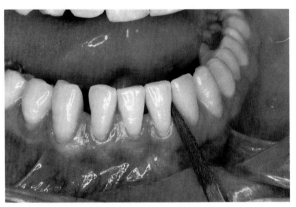

Fig. 11-29 (left) Balsa wood wedges.

Fig. 11-30 (below) Balsa wood wedge in use.

process has also been studied in more depth, leading to a better understanding that periodontal destruction occurs in cycles of exacerbation and remission. Traditional home care methodologies have been shown to be effective in pockets with depths of 3 mm or less.

Because of these factors, the patient may not be able to control plaque solely by mechanical means. As a result, the oral irrigation device is enjoying a resurgence in popularity as a potential plaque control device via the use of antimicrobial agents. The term plaque control thus takes on a much broader meaning, referring to a wide range of mechanisms to both remove and interfere with the metabolic activity of plaque.

Oral irrigation is a general term that actually refers to two different activities. As most commonly used it refers to irrigation of supragingival areas, with very limited access to subgingival sulci/pockets. Subgingival irrigation involves the use of a specialized syringe with a blunt tip to deliver antimicrobial solutions directly into the sulci/pockets. Subgingival irrigation is performed by the dental hygienist or dentist in the dental office: it is not performed by the patient himself (Fig. 11-31).

Several recent studies[10-17] have shown that patient's use of an oral irrigator with antimicrobial solutions (e.g., stannous fluoride or chlorhexidine) can inhibit or disrupt plaque development to a substantial

degree, leading to an improved state of periodontal health. One of the limitations of the use of the traditional oral irrigator, however, is its restricted ability to subgingivally deliver liquid solutions. Varying depths of penetration occur in shallow pockets as compared to intermediate and deep periodontal pockets.[18-19]

Newer oral irrigation devices have tip attachments that will permit the patient to subgingivally irrigate his or her own mouth at home (Fig. 11-32). Because of the potential for damage if used incorrectly, the patient must be thoroughly instructed in the appropriate use of such a device prior to its routine incorporation into the plaque control program.

Use of oral irrigating devices has been shown to produce bacteremia in some patients.[20-21] Because of this, patients with medically compromised histories may require prophylactic antibiotic coverage prior to the use of an oral irrigator. For those at-risk patients, consultation with the physician is advised prior to recommending the use of oral irrigating devices.

Aids for edentulous or partially edentulous patients

Denture and partial clasp brushes A denture brush is used to clean both complete dentures and the synthetic tooth and tissue portion of a partial denture. A clasp brush is used to clean clasps or precision attachments of a partial denture (Fig. 11-33). The bristles of a denture brush are arranged in tufts that are much thicker and stiffer than those of a manual toothbrush. This allows for better adaptation to different parts of the denture. The bristle texture is usually hard.

The partial clasp brush is shaped similarly to a small bottle brush. It is designed to fit the inner surfaces of the clasps that anchor the partial denture in the mouth. The bristle texture is usually hard. Neither brush is intended for intraoral use on natural teeth.

The denture brush is used by grasping the brush with one hand and holding the denture firmly in the palm of the other hand. All areas of the denture are brushed with moderate, even pressure until all debris is removed. The denture is rinsed under running water until the loosened debris is flushed away.

A partial clasp brush is used by holding the partial denture firmly in one hand and taking care not to exert pressure on the clasps. The brush is applied to the clasp area, inside and out, and adapted to the clasp's contours. The prosthesis is thoroughly rinsed under warm water. Both complete and partial dentures should be cleaned over a sink lined with a towel or filled with water to avoid breakage of the prosthetic appliance if dropped.

Cleansing solutions   Complete and partial dentures may be cleaned by immersing them in a special cleansing solution to remove loose debris. This method is not always effective for removal of all deposits and should therefore be accompanied by brushing. The effectiveness of immersion is dependent on the type of chemical cleaning solution used.

Commercial preparations (oxygenating agents) are available in tablets or premeasured packets of powder. The cleansing effect of these agents comes from the mechanical action of the bubbles created by the release of oxygen. Immersion time is 10 to 15 minutes.

White vinegar may be used as a cleansing agent. When diluted with water, this solution is capable of removing calculus from the denture. It should not be used on a routine basis because it is too corrosive. Immersion time will depend on the amount and tenacity of the deposit; in some cases, overnight immersion for complete removal may be necessary. One to two teaspoons of vinegar are added to 8 ounces of warm water. The appliance is immersed and allowed to remain until the debris has loosened.

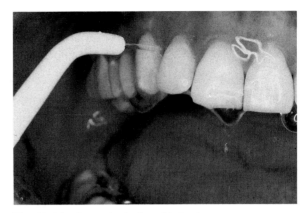

Fig. 11-31   Supragingival oral irrigation.

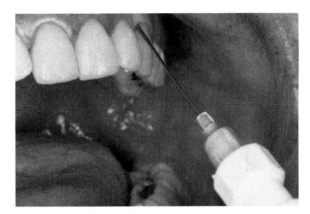

Fig. 11-32   Subgingival irrigation.

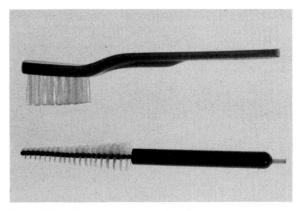

Fig. 11-33   Clasp and denture brushes.

A hypochlorite solution can be made with Calgon, liquid bleach, and water. This solution is used for removal of stain and calculus but may be too corrosive for routine use; immersion time should be no longer than 15 minutes. For mixing the solution the proportions are 1 teaspoon bleach, 2 teaspoons Calgon, and 4 ounces warm water.

Toothpaste, denture toothpaste, or a baking soda and warm water mixture may also be used to clean removable denture appliances. Cleansing agents such as household cleaners should be avoided because they are too abrasive and will scratch the prosthetic appliance.

Disabled patients

The primary goals in the delivery of oral hygiene instruction for disabled patients are optimal dental health care and the highest degree of independence possible regarding self-care for the patients. As with all patients, motivation of the disabled patient is of critical importance. On occasion, other individuals may be needed to assist with the patient's oral hygiene practices—for example the parent, nurse, attendant, or whoever acts as the primary care provider (caretaker). The dental hygienist must plan educational strategies that will suit both audiences.

Before oral hygiene instruction is planned, the following factors should be assessed:

1. The handicapping condition: type of condition, when it occurred (i.e., at birth or later in life), prognosis and potential for recovery, medications taken, and current dental health condition.
2. Attitude and knowledge of target audience(s): reasons for seeking dental care, educational level and training of the patient, and the attitude of the caretaker toward the patient and oral hygiene.
3. Degree of manual dexterity: motor skills currently possessed by the patient and the potential for improvement and training.

After the initial assessment and evaluation, oral hygiene education can be planned and plaque control aids and/or adaptation mechanisms can be selected. Although approaches for oral hygiene care are discussed in terms of groups, not all handicapped patients fit easily into any one group nor will all patients necessarily remain within the same group. Each patient, disabled or not, must be evaluated on an individual basis and reassessed periodically according to changes in ability, skills, and independence.

Self-help Patients in the self-help group can brush and floss alone with limited need for adaptations. They may require assistance in structuring a home care routine as well as encouragement and some degree of supervision. These individuals include paraplegic and hemiplegic patients and some geriatric and medically compromised patients (e.g., diabetics and cancer patients). Recommended oral hygiene aids include disclosing tablets, soft toothbrush, floss with a floss holder, and intraoral mirror to better visualize areas of plaque retention.

Partial help Patients requiring partial help can perform some oral hygiene procedures on their own but may require supervision. Their total understanding of oral hygiene concepts may be limited, so that additional training for these individuals may be necessary. Adaptations for plaque removal devices may also be needed. Patients in this category include cerebral vascular accident (stroke) victims; cerebral palsy, arm amputee, and arthritic patients; and some mentally disabled individuals. Suggested aids include floss holders, electric toothbrushes, and adapted toothbrushes.

Total help Patients who require total assistance because they are unable to personally perform oral hygiene procedures include spinal cord injury, head trauma, quadraplegic, profoundly mentally retarded, and comatose patients as well as recent stroke victims. Adaptations necessary to treat these persons include several unconventional approaches such as mouth props or tongue depressors to keep the mouth open and irrigating syringes for rinsing. The comatose patient requires additional measures such as petroleum jelly to lubricate the lips and wiping of the teeth with moist gauze squares.

Positioning and stabilization

In order for the plaque to be properly removed from the teeth, good visibility is important. For those individuals requiring partial or total help from a parent or guardian, the following positions can be utilized:

1. The patient sits on the floor with his or her head

tipped back in the lap of the parent or guardian.
2. The patient lies down on a sofa or bed with his or her head in the lap of the parent or guardian.

When patients are uncooperative or have uncontrolled movements that make toothbrushing and flossing difficult, restraining positions can be utilized. The individual's head can be locked in between the knees of the parent or guardian for better support. Mouth props may be selected as a means of obtaining an open work area. A second individual may be required to assist in stabilization of the patient. Some have suggested a beanbag chair for small children. Regardless of the technique selected, both the patient and the caretaker must have enough space to ensure a safe and comfortable environment for plaque removal. The bathroom is usually the least preferred area for toothbrushing and flossing because of the many potential obstacles in the way of the patient's uncontrolled movements.

Adaptations of aids

For individuals unable to use conventional oral hygiene aids, adaptations can be devised based on the patient's disability. In the following circumstances, adjustments can be made to preexisting materials:

1. Loss of motion at a joint (arthritis patient). Elongating the handle of the toothbrush will help to compensate for the limited motion. A common approach is to tape tongue blades, plastic rods, or other toothbrush handles together. Toothbrush handles can also be bent by warming the plastic in hot water (Figs. 11-34a and b).
2. Loss of muscle strength (stroke, spinal cord injury, or multiple sclerosis patients). Patients have difficulty holding or grasping the toothbrush. A holder with an opening for the patient's hand to slip through and grip the brush handle would increase stability. Velcro strips can be added around the toothbrush handle (Fig. 11-35). Toothbrushes and floss holders can also be placed in a universal cuff. Occasionally, a brush handle will require enlargement. This can be accomplished by reinforcing the handle with acrylic, foam rubber, a bicycle handle, rubber or plastic ball, can, or any other innovative material (Fig. 11-36). Toothbrush heads can be bent and angled for improved access.

3. Loss of coordination (i.e., cerebral palsy, head trauma, and stroke patients). Attempts should be made to stabilize the toothbrush to compensate for shaking or rocking movement by the patient. Adhesive fabric can be added to the handle to prevent slippage.
4. Loss of a limb (i.e., arm amputee). Stabilization will be necessary. Techniques may be employed similar to those for patients with loss of muscle strength or coordination.
5. Loss of motion below the neck (i.e., quadraplegic patient). Specific adaptations may include additions of plastic tubing to a toothbrush. Toothbrushes mounted on the wall can provide the necessary stabilization so that patients can use them by adjusting their head positions (Fig. 11-37).

Dentifrices Screw-on caps of toothpaste tubes can be difficult to open for many disabled individuals. New pump devices are practical alternatives. Other suggestions include removal of the cap and insertion of a pin through the top for easier opening and closing. Dentifrices must be recommended cautiously because the foaming action may cause excessive gagging and drooling. In quadraplegic and cerebral palsy patients, toothpastes are contraindicated. Each patient must be individually evaluated before dentifrices are suggested.

Fluoride Application of fluoride at home through gel tray, brush on, or mouth rinse will require supervision and monitoring by the parent or caretaker. The dental needs of the disabled are extensive, not because of caries prevalence but because of inadequate dental care. Infrequent and sporadic dental services result in greater needs. Fluoride therapies are a means of decreasing some of the dental problems of the disabled.

Visually impaired patients

Some patients treated in the dental office may have varying degrees of blindness or other visual impairment. A significant percentage of these individuals are age 65 or older. With the increasing numbers of geriatric patients, the likelihood of providing care for this type of patient is substantial.

No single approach is appropriate for all visually impaired patients. Other considerations include the patient's intellectual capacity, hearing, attitude to-

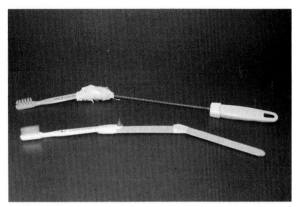

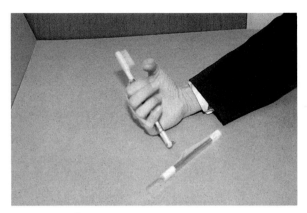

Figs. 11-34a and b   Adapting toothbrushes by elongating handles.

Figure 11-34b

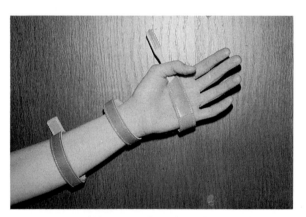

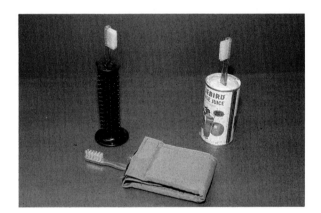

Fig. 11-35   Stabilization of toothbrush with Velcro and toothbrush enlargements.

Figure 11-36

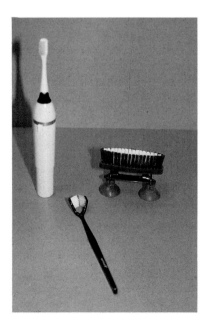

Fig. 11-37   Adaptations for quadraplegic patients.

ward dentistry and dental health, prior education and training, and degree of visual limitation. The dental hygienist should be aware that the patient's other senses may not be actually heightened, but the patient may have been trained to more extensively utilize them. Specific references to sight and seeing should be avoided. Some visually impaired individuals may have residual vision, but most are accustomed to following verbal instructions.

When greeting the patient, the dental hygienist should identify herself or himself by name and offer an arm to escort the patient to the operatory. Some patients will take the hygienist's arm; others will prefer to walk alone, using a cane or seeing-eye dog. Obstacles should be removed from the patient's path. The hygienist should verbalize the direction to be taken and indicate any steps, stairs, carpeting, and other changes the patient will encounter. If the patient is with a companion, parent, or friend, care should be taken to speak to the patient, not the other person.

Appointments should be of short duration whenever feasible. Other office personnel should be introduced to the patient and described in as much detail as possible. All procedures to be undertaken should also be thoroughly explained. The hygienist should alert the patient before placing instruments in his or her mouth or using compressed air and should allow the patient to touch and manipulate the objects to be used during the appointment. The types of sensations that will be felt, such as the vibration of the handpiece should be described. The patient should be allowed to utilize other senses when appropriate—for example, smell and taste fluoride gel or prophylaxis paste. A variety of terms should be used when discussing and describing procedures.

When providing home care instructions, the hygienist should demonstrate in the mouth, allowing the patient to feel and place the implements. Placement can be guided with the hand. The patient should feel the sensation of a clean tooth surface. In this, plastic models or dentecs may be helpful. Braille pamphlets are available, and audio tapes are of great assistance. If the patient has some sight, written materials with large print should be selected.

Hearing impaired patients

When dealing with hearing impaired patients, the hygienist should remember that deafness reduces the ability to communicate more than does blindness. Especially if the patient has been deaf since birth, natural absorption of social values and abstract concepts contained in language is a difficulty.

Diagrams and simple demonstrations may be helpful. Few of the deaf population (26%) can communicate by reading lips. A normal volume and relationship of the words should be used when speaking. Sign language is a skill that many dental hygienists have chosen to add to their repertoire. Body language and gestures are also important.

The deaf patient wants to see what is happening. The dental hygienist should demonstrate procedures and verbalize as much as possible during treatment. Pamphlets and forms the patient must fill out should be geared to low-level reading skills. If the patient has a hearing aid, which may amplify sounds such as those from the high speed handpiece, he or she may want to readjust it.

Chemical plaque control approaches

Assisting patients in behavioral modification that results in long-term, acceptable personal oral hygiene techniques has always been a challenge for the dental hygienist. As with other health issues, patients often ask their dental hygienist if there is an easier approach to plaque inhibition, one that requires less time and less skill than the traditional manual plaque control techniques.

Recently, much investigation and speculation has centered on the control of plaque by chemical means. The success of a chemical agent in the control of plaque requires that it affect a broad range of microorganisms. An important determining factor in a compound's antiplaque action appears to be retention on the tooth surface so that slow release of the agent prevents bacterial colonization (substantivity).[22]

Antibiotics

For many years various antibiotics and antiseptics have been examined for their effectiveness as antiplaque agents. Spiramycin,* vancomycin, kanamycin, metronidazole, and erythromycin have all been the subject of research efforts.[22] The value of all these

*Ives Laboratories, New York, N.Y.

Table 11-4 Periodontal disease: etiologies and antibiotics for noncompromised patients

Disorder	Bacteria implicated*	Antibiotics of choice†‡
ANUG	Spirochetes, gram-negative anaerobes	Penicillin, metronidazole, tetracycline¶
Periodontal abscess	Gram-negative and gram-positive anaerobes	Penicillin, erythromycin, tetracycline¶
Gingivitis	Gram-positive	None, unless streptococcal in origin; then, a penicillin or erythromycin
—early	Gram-negative	
—established		
Juvenile periodontitis	Gram-negative capnophiles	Tetracycline
Periodontitis	Gram-negative anaerobes	Tetracycline?

*Implicated by cultural and/or clinical studies. Other groups of bacteria and specific pathogens likely to be discovered.
†When more than one drug is listed, the choice is ordered.
‡Without specific knowledge of resistant or susceptible organisms from laboratory testing.
¶If local debridement is not successful or is painful.
Source: M.P. Newman and A.D. Goodman (eds.) Guide to Antibiotic Use in Dental Practice. Chicago: Quintessence Publ. Co., 1984.

Table 11-5 Topical agents for plaque control listed in order of effectiveness

1. Chlorhexidine gluconate (0.2%), alexidine (0.035%)
   Mouthrinse twice daily
   Bitter taste
   Brown staining of anterior restorations
   Plaque reduction >85%
2. Stannous fluoride (0.1%)
   Mouthrinse twice daily
   Bad taste
   Brown staining of anterior restorations
   Plaque reduction approximately 50%
3. Stannous fluoride (1.64%)
   Subgingival irrigation
   Reduction in motile bacteria and spirochetes
   Further research required
4. Cetylpyridinium chloride (1:2,000)
   Mouthrinse twice daily
   Plaque reduction <40%
5. Baking soda, table salt, hydrogen peroxide
   Possible clinical effectiveness
   Further research required

Source: Adapted from M.G. Newman and A.D. Goodman (eds.) Guide to Antibiotic Use in Dental Practice. Chicago: Quintessence Publ. Co., 1984.

antibiotics has been found to be limited in long-term plaque control.[23] Tetracycline and older antibiotics have been shown to be useful in the treatment of certain forms of periodontitis (Table 11-4).

Antiseptics

Antiseptic mouthwashes, which contain essential oils, may reduce the development of plaque mass and pathogenic activity.[24] Research indicates that the use of an antiseptic mouthwash twice daily reduces the accumulation of plaque and the development of gingivitis.[25]

Herbal extract composition rinses and pastes have been extensively studied. Oral rinses containing sanguinaria extract have shown antiplaque activities in humans.[26] Sanguinarine appears to have a retentive property in plaque. Rinses containing the extract have had a demonstrable effect on overnight plaque formation. Therefore, recommendation of such rinses at bedtime may be effective in a home care regimen.[27]

Antimicrobials

Chlorhexidine gluconate has proven to be highly effective in dental plaque reduction[22] (Table 11-5). Animal and human tests have indicated the use of chlorhexidine to be safe, although typical side effects include an unpleasant taste, staining of the teeth and tongue, and some loss of taste sensation.[28] Chlorhexidine has recently been approved for intraoral use by the Food and Drug Administration, and extensive investigation is currently being conducted on the compound by governmental, institutional, and academic bodies.

Quartenary ammonium compounds commonly found in mouthwashes have been shown to reduce plaque and gingivitis. Benzalkonium chloride and cetylpyridinium chloride are two that have been the subject of research.[22]

Fluoride is bacteriostatic or bactericidal depending on its concentration. Baking soda, table salt, and hydrogen peroxide combinations are utilized in the Monitored Modulated Therapy approach to the control of periodontal disease. All of these compounds and uses are discussed elsewhere in this text.

Dentifrices

Dentifrices are by far the most common topical agents used in patients' personal plaque care regimens. Many types of dentifrices are available with diverse components, abrasivity levels, and degrees of effectiveness. New dentifrices appear on the market frequently, many with claims of plaque, caries, and periodontal disease reduction capabilities. The contemporary dental hygiene practitioner must be knowledgeable about new products in order to answer patients' questions appropriately and provide guidance to individuals establishing a personal plaque control program.

Toothpastes may contain whiteners, brighteners, binding agents, humectants, flavoring agents, abrasive products, various drug substances for therapeutic effects, detergents, and even tube corrosion inhibitors.[30,31] Some pastes are marketed for particular population groups such as smokers or people with extrinsic stain or hypersensitivity.

The most common therapeutic additive to commercial toothpastes is fluoride. Research on its effectiveness in caries reduction is extensive, and the collective body of data suggests that sodium fluoride is most effective.[1-11] The utilization of a fluoride paste is an important component of all patients' personal oral hygiene programs.

Other components of toothpastes may assist in caries reduction and periodontal disease prevention by bacteriostatic activity that results in the inhibition of plaque. Enzyme-containing pastes, and pastes that contain botanical herbal extracts, antiseptics, and aloe, represent a sampling of the dentifrices available.

Studies suggest that a dentifrice containing soluble pyrophosphates in a fluoride compound inhibits the ordinary development of calculus deposits in adults.[24] Soluble pyrophosphates are crystal growth inhibitors that interrupt the transformation of amorphous calcium phosphate in dental calculus.[24]

The Council on Dental Therapeutics of the American Dental Association monitors dental products, including dentifrices. Commercial products are examined by the council and then classified as accepted, provisionally accepted, or unacceptable. Accepted products include those for which there is adequate evidence of safety and effectiveness. They are listed in *Accepted Dental Therapeutics* and may use the Seal of Acceptance or an authorized statement, unless otherwise provided.[33]

Provisionally accepted products include those for which reasonable evidence of usefulness and safety exists but that lack sufficient evidence of dental usefulness to justify acceptance. These products meet the other qualifications and standards established by the Council on Dental Therapeutics. The council may authorize the use of a suitable statement to define specifically the area of usefulness of a product classified as provisionally accepted. The council's initial consideration of products that may be eligible for provisional acceptance is influenced favorably by the knowledge of further investigations in progress. The council reconsiders products each year on the basis of new evidence that may be produced in their support. Classification as provisionally accepted is not ordinarily continued for more than 3 years.[33]

Unaccepted products include those for which the council has found no substantial evidence of usefulness or for which a question of safety exists.[33]

The council also provides a comparison of abrasivity of dentifrices and categorization into specific groups so that dental professionals may refer to information on these products.

The United States Food and Drug Administration has jurisdiction over the safety and purity of toothpastes. The regulations are different for toothpastes claimed to have stain removal and whitening (cosmetic) properties and those claimed to have antiplaque remineralization (therapeutic) benefits.[22] Fluoride toothpastes are categorized as therapeutic agents, as are desensitizing toothpastes. Therefore, they are subject to over-the-counter drug regulations related to labeling of ingredients and directions.

Pit and fissure sealants

A relatively recent addition to the field of preventive dentistry is the development of materials to seal the pits and fissures of posterior teeth to prevent carious lesions. First described in 1967,[34] sealants have undergone a number of adjustments to increase their efficacy. Most of the sealant products currently available are similar in composition, based on the bisphenol A-glycidyl methacrylate formulation (BIS-GMA). The major differences occur in their methods of polymerization.

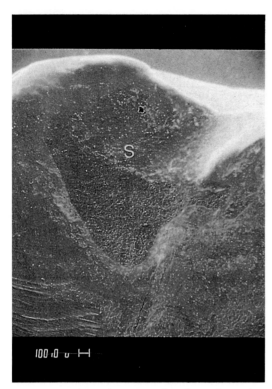

Fig. 11-38 SEM of an enamel surface after etching for 60 seconds with 30% phosphoric acid. (From R. Simonsen: *Clinical Applications of the Acid Etch Technique,* Quintessence Publ. Co., 1978.)

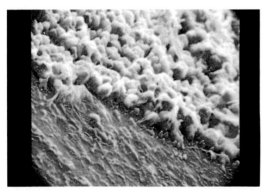

Fig. 11-39 SEM of resin base tags. (From R. Simonsen: *Clinical Applications of the Acid Etch Technique,* Quintessence Publ. Co., 1978.)

Sealants are polymerized by three basic mechanisms.[35] In the chemically cured, or autopolymerized, system, two resin compounds are mixed and then set after a short time period, usually 60 seconds. In the second type, polymerization is by means of exposure to an ultraviolet light source. The third and most recent system utilizes visible light to set the sealant. A high-intensity white-light source is used to polymerize the material. No long-term research studies have yet been conducted to determine the retention and caries reduction rates for the visible light system.

A number of clinical studies, some lasting as long as 7 years, have attested to the preventive benefits of sealant usage.[36-43] Sealant retention rates of 56% to 82% after 5 years have been observed, along with reductions in carious lesions of more than 90% on teeth with fully retained sealants. Even partially retained sealants provide protection benefits.[36]

Protection offered

Sealants may be either colorless or colored, depending on operator preference and the product utilized. The colored types may be white or tinted a light pink or yellow. The advantages of using a colored sealant are several: explanation of the concept of sealants is easier, because the patient or parent can more readily see the sealant; less examination time is required at recall appointments to determine retention of the sealant; and a more accurate assessment of retention is possible.[35]

Sealant materials provide protection by a bonding action between the resin and the enamel tissue.[35] This bonding is achieved after first etching the enamel surface with an acid solution (Fig. 11-38). Phosphoric acid is the primary agent currently used. Pyruvic, lactic, and citric acids have also been used, but a less satisfactory bond is produced with these agents. During the acid etch phase, a shallow layer of enamel (about 10 μm in depth) is removed, along with plaque and surface and subsurface pellicles. Application of the acid solution results in a porous enamel surface into which the resin will flow and mechanically bond with the enamel (Fig. 11-39). Additionally, removal of chemically inert mineral crystals in the surface enamel results in an enhanced chemical union between the resin and enamel surface.[35]

Sealant retention on primary teeth is generally poorer than with permanent teeth.[44,45] Varying theories exist as to the reason for this, but it appears that

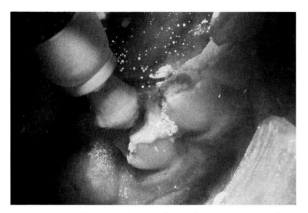

Fig. 11-40 Cleaning the tooth surface prior to etching. (Courtesy of Johnson & Johnson, East Windsor, N.J.)

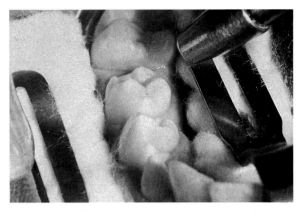

Fig. 11-41 Isolation with cotton rolls. (Courtesy of Johnson & Johnson.)

a longer etching period for primary teeth (2 minutes instead of 1 minute) could provide similar etching patterns to those produced with permanent enamel.[46,47]

A major consideration in the profession's general acceptance of sealants has related to the supposed increased susceptibility of etched enamel to caries in the event the sealant was lost. A number of research studies have been conducted to investigate this question, and findings clearly indicate that exposure of the etched surface to saliva results in remineralization of the enamel surface,[48,49] even to the point that the surface becomes more resistant to formation of caries.[35]

One of the most significant causes of sealant failure is contamination of the etched surface with saliva prior to application of the resin.[35] It has been shown that surface coating of the etched surface occurs as quickly as 1 second following salivary contamination, and that the coating is not removed by the washing procedure.[50] As a result, if any contamination occurs during the procedure, the surface must be re-etched before the resin is placed. The air–water syringe is another potential source of contamination if the air line contains oil or water. The system should be checked prior to use.[35]

Another factor that has affected the adoption of sealants as a routine preventive service is the fear that sealing an undetected carious lesion would result in progression of the caries process to such a degree that the vitality of the tooth would be threatened. A number of studies[51–56] have shown that placement of a

sealant over an incipient lesion results in a decrease in the viable bacteria count by eliminating the source of nutrients, and therefore rendering a dormant lesion.[57] As a result, sealant use can actually arrest the development of tiny, incipient, clinically undetectable carious lesions.

The caries preventive effect of sealants has been increased through the incorporation of fluoride into the material. The intent was to effect a slow diffusion of fluoride into the oral cavity, thus providing continuous levels of fluoride to the teeth. In order for the fluoride ions to diffuse freely through the resin, the sealant must be fairly porous in nature. As a result, the physical barrier protection aspect of the sealant was diminished. Additional studies are necessary to determine the effect of incorporating fluoride into the more permanent types of sealant resins used today.[58]

Procedure for placement

The basic methodology for placement of sealants is described below.[59] Although certain variations do occur, such as in the mechanism for isolation of the teeth and the actual sealant system employed, the step-by-step procedure is generally the same. It is fairly simple and easily delegated to the dental hygienist if the state practice act allows it. Success in sealant retention is dependent upon the operator's technique. Contamination of the etched surface, a major cause of sealant failure, is totally operator controlled.

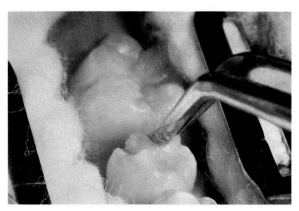

Fig. 11-42   Etching the enamel surface. (Courtesy of Johnson & Johnson).

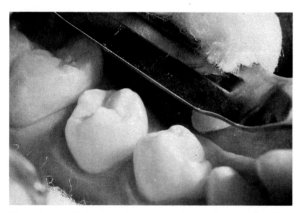

Fig. 11-43   Frosted appearance of etched enamel. (Courtesy of Johnson & Johnson.)

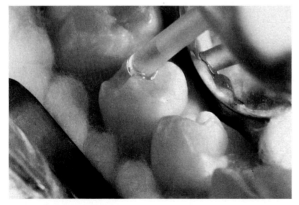

Fig. 11-44   Applying the sealant. (Courtesy of Johnson & Johnson.)

Selection of teeth to be sealed   Patients who have teeth with deep pits and fissures, and who may have had previous episodes of occlusal caries, are candidates for placement of sealants.

Cleaning the surface   Prior to etching, the surface(s) to be sealed must be thoroughly cleaned with a pointed bristle brush and pumice–water slurry (Fig. 11-40). Prophylaxis pastes and other products containing fluoride or an oil base are contraindicated. Following the cleaning procedure, an explorer tip can be dragged across the developmental grooves to further debride the area. The area should be thoroughly rinsed with water.

Isolation   Appropriate isolation of the teeth, which is possibly the most critical step, is the best assurance of success and sealant retention (Fig. 11-41). Although isolation ideally employs the rubber dam, cotton rolls may also be used and may be a more practical approach. Sufficient cotton rolls should be used to maintain a dry field. Fresh ones are placed on top of saturated rolls and the used ones removed from beneath. In the lingual areas especially, several cotton rolls may be required. Cotton roll holders pose a particular threat to maintenance of a dry field if replacement of the cotton rolls is attempted.

Etching   Following isolation, the teeth should be completely dried to remove any saliva remaining on the surface. Next, the phosphoric acid solution is dabbed onto the surface, using either a small sponge or a cotton pellet (Fig. 11-42). After the entire surface is covered with the acid etchant, the timer is set for 60 seconds. The operator continues dabbing the acid onto the tooth to keep it moist and circulate fresh acid to the enamel. The solution must only be dabbed, *not rubbed,* onto the enamel. Rubbing the acid with the cotton pellet may damage the porous etched enamel.

Washing   Complete removal of the phosphoric acid following the etching is another critical step in successful sealant retention. The area should be flushed with water alone for at least 5 seconds using the air–water syringe. For at least 15 to 20 additional seconds washing continues using the spray. A saliva ejector or, preferably, high-speed evacuation should be used to remove the water. The etched surface will appear frosted (Fig. 11-43).

Re-isolation   After the washing procedure the cotton rolls are replaced. Protecting the etched surface at this point from salivary contamination is extremely important. Should the surface become contaminated, the etching–washing phase must be repeated prior to sealant placement.

Drying and mixing   After the area has been re-isolated, it is thoroughly dried. This also is a critical step, because any moisture on the surface will prevent penetration of the resin into the enamel. At least 15 seconds of air drying for a single tooth (25 seconds for a quadrant) should be performed up to the point of actual resin application. While the drying is being performed, an assistant can mix the resin material.

Application of sealant   A brush on a manufacturer-supplied carrier or special applicator is used to gently apply the resin to the etched surface (Fig. 11-44). Brushes are preferred over sponges or cotton pellets for application because they are less likely to damage the enamel surface or to produce bubbles. The resin may be absorbed into the cotton material, causing the operator to apply pressure to the enamel in order to dispense the resin, which is contraindicated. The sealant is applied in a fairly thick layer. For the autopolymerizing systems, it is allowed to harden (1 to 3 minutes). For light-cure systems, the light is applied directly over the resin for the length of time specified by the manufacturer. After the sealant has polymerized, the surface is wiped with a piece of gauze to remove the film that appears. The film results from the lack of polymerization of the outer layer of resin, because the presence of oxygen inhibits the set. Removing the film will minimize any unpleasant taste the patient may experience.

The total time required from initial isolation through application should be approximately 3½ minutes for one tooth, slightly more for a quadrant. Sealing all four quadrants at a single appointment should not take longer than approximately 20 minutes.

Sealants placed properly are effective caries-preventing agents. Research has shown that, even 18 months after application, little wear occurs (Figs. 11-45a to c).

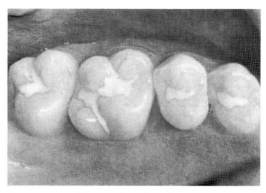

Fig. 11-45a   Six months after placement. (From R. Simonsen: *Clinical Applications of the Acid Etch Technique,* Quintessence Publ. Co., 1978.)

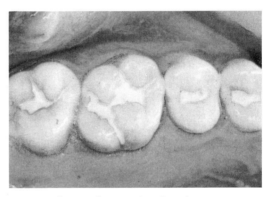

Fig. 11-45b   Twelve months after placement. (From R. Simonsen: *Clinical Applications of the Acid Etch Technique,* Quintessence Publ. Co., 1978.)

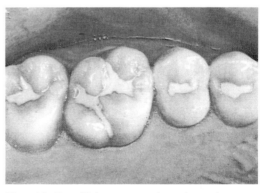

Fig. 11-45c   Eighteen months after placement. (From R. Simonsen: *Clinical Applications of the Acid Etch Technique,* Quintessence Publ. Co., 1978.)

References

1. Bales, D.J. Oral health status in the United States: the prevalence of dental caries. J. Dent. Ed. 49(6):352–353, 1985.

2. Pollack, R.L., and Kravitz, E. (eds.) Nutrition in Oral Health and Disease. Philadelphia: Lea & Febiger, 1985, pp. 119–127.

3. Williams, S.R. Essential Nutrition and Diet Therapy. St. Louis: C.V. Mosby Co., 1974, pp. 137–139.

4. Dairy Nutrition Council. Calcium: A Summary of Current Research for the Health Professional. Rosemont, Ill.: National Dairy Council, 1984, p. 13.

5. Nizel, A.E. Nutrition in Preventive Dentistry: Science and Practice. Philadelphia: W.B. Saunders Co., 1981, pp. 372–373.

6. U.S. Public Health Service. Statement of Purpose. Bethesda: Department of Health and Human Services, November, 1985, pp. 1–3.

7. Weinstein P., Getz, T., and Milgrom, P. Oral Self Case: Strategies for Preventive Dentistry. Reston, Va.: Reston Publishing Co. 1985, pp. 1–10.

8. Geboy, M.J. Communication and Behavior Management in Dentistry. Baltimore: Williams and Wilkins, 1985, pp. 29–43.

9. Hugoson, A. Effect of the Water Pik® device on plaque accumulation and development of gingivitis. J. Clin. Periodontol. 5:95–104, 1978.

10. Boyd, R.L., et al. Effect of self-administered daily irrigation with 0.02% SnF_2 on periodontal disease activity. J. Clin. Periodontol. 12(6):420–431, 1985.

11. Lang, N.P., and Räber, K. Use of oral irrigations as vehicle for the application of antimicrobial agents in chemical plaque control. J. Clin. Periodontol. 8(3):177–188, 1981.

12. Lang, N.P., and Ramseier-Grossman, K. Optimal dosage of chlorhexidine digluconate in chemical plaque control when applied by the oral irrigator. J. Clin. Periodontol. 8(3):189–202, 1981.

13. Derdivanis, J.P., Bushmaker, S., and Dagenais, F. Effects of a mouthwash in an irrigating device on accumulation and maturation of dental plaque. J. Periodontol. 49(2):81–84, 1978.

14. Wolff, L.F., et al. Phase contrast microscopic evaluation of subgingival plaque in combination with either conventional or antimicrobial home treatment of patients with periodontal inflammation. J. Periodont. Res. 17:537–540, 1982.

15. Aday, J.B. An evaluation of an oral irrigating device's ability to quantitatively reduce the bacterial count of spirochetes, filaments, fusiforms and motile bacteria from subgingival plaque. Thesis. Department of Periodontics. Kansas City: University of Missouri, 1982.

16. West, B.L. An evaluation of an oral irrigating device's ability to reduce the microbial count of subgingival plaque at six millimeters in depth. Thesis. Kansas City: University of Missouri, 1983.

17. Gamoa, R.M., et al. Effect of pulsating water lavage on the microorganisms of the periodontal pocket. Thesis. Los Angeles: University of Southern California, 1980.

18. Eakle, W.S., et al. Pocket penetration with irrigation. J. Clin. Periodontol. September, 1985.

19. Selting, W.J., et al. Water jet direction and periodontal pocket debridement. J. Periodontol. 43:569, 1972.

20. Felix, J.E., Rosen, S., and App, G.R. Detection of bacteremia after the use of an oral irrigation device in subjects with periodontitis. J. Periodontol. 42(12):785–787, 1971.

21. Roamns, A.R., and App, G.R. Bacteremia, a result from oral irrigation in subjects with gingivitis. J. Periodontol. 42(12):757–760, 1971.

22. Newman, M.G., and Goodman, A.D. (eds.) Guide to Antibiotic Use in Dental Practice. Chicago: Quintessence Publ. Co., 1984, pp. 58–66.

23. Löe, A., et al. Experimental gingivitis in man. III. The influence of antibiotics on gingival plaque development. J. Periodont. Res. 2:282–289, 1967.

24. Fine, D.H., Letizia, J., and Mandel, I.D. The effect of rinsing with Listerine antiseptic on the properties of developing dental plaque. J. Clin. Periodontol. 12(8):660–666, 1984.

25. Gordon, J.M., Lamster, I.B., and Seigir, M.C. Efficiency of Listerine antiseptic in inhibiting the development of plaque and gingivitis. J. Clin. Periodontol. 12(4):697–704, 1985.

26. Southard G.L., et al. Sangiunarine, a new antiplaque agent: retention and plaque specificity. J. Am. Dent. Assoc. 108(3):338–341, 1984.

27. Yankell, S., et al. Overnight plaque formation. J. Prev. Dent. 6:313–315, 1980.

28. Tonelli, P.M., Hume, W.R., and Kenney, E.B. Chlorhexidine: a review of the literature. J. West. Soc. Periodontol. 31(1):5–10, 1983.

29. Zacherl, W.A., Pfeiffer, H.J., and Swancar, J.R. The effect of soluble pyrophosphates on dental calculus in adults. 5(110):737–738, 1985.

30. Allen, C.E., and Nunez, L.J. A look at toothpaste ingredients. Gen. Dent. 33(1):58–60, 1985.

31. Stallard, R.W. A Textbook of Preventive Dentistry. Philadelphia: W.B. Saunders Co., 1982, p. 171.

32. Stookey, G.K. Are all fluoride dentrifices the same? pp. 105–131. In S.H.Y. Wei (ed.) Clinical Uses of Fluorides. Philadelphia: Lea & Febiger, 1985.

33. ADA Council on Dental Therapeutics. Provisions for

Acceptance of Products by the Council on Dental Therapeutics, 1985.

34. Cueto, E.I., and Buonocore, M.G. Sealing of pits and fissures with an adhesive resin: its use in caries prevention. J. Am. Dent. Assoc. 75(1):121–128, 1967.

35. Silverstone, L.M. The current status of fissure sealants and priorities for future research. I. Compend. Cont. Ed. 5(3):204–214, 1984.

36. Horowitz, H.S., Heifetz, S.B., and Poulsen, S. Retention and effectiveness of a single application of an adhesive sealant in preventing occlusal caries: final report after five years of a study in Kalispell, Montana. J. Am. Dent. Assoc. 95:1133–1139, 1977.

37. Doyle, W.W., and Brose, J.A. A five-year study of the longevity of fissure sealants. J. Dent. Child. 45:23–25, 1978.

38. Houpt, M., and Sheykholeslam, Z. The clinical effectiveness of Delton® fissure sealant after one year. J. Dent. Child. 45:26–28, 1978.

39. Bojanine, J., et al. Effectiveness of pit and fissure sealants in the prevention of caries. J. Prev. Dent. 3:31–35, 1976.

40. Mertz-Fairhurst, E.J., et al. Seven-year clinical evaluation of two pit and fissure sealants. J. Dent. Res. 61:298 (Special Issue A): IADR Abstr. 1076, 1982.

41. Thylastrup, A., and Poulsen, A. Retention and effectiveness of a chemically polymerized pit and fissure sealant after two years. Scand. J. Dent. Res. 86:21–26, 1978.

42. Simonsen, R.J. Five-year results of sealant effects on caries prevention and treatment costs. J. Dent. Res. Abstr. 1380, March, 1982.

43. Tonn, E.M., and Ryge, G. Three-year clinical evaluation of four sealants in Los Altos, California. J. Dent. Res. Abstr. 1379, March, 1982.

44. Ripa, L.W., and Cole, W.W. Occlusal sealing and caries prevention: results 12 months after a single application of adhesive resin. J. Dent. Res. 49:171–173, 1970.

45. Buonocore, J.G. Caries prevention in pits and fissures sealed with an adhesive resin polymerized by ultraviolet light: a two year study of a single adhesive application. J. Am. Dent. Assoc. 82:1090–1093, 1971.

46. Silverstone, L.M., and Dogon, I.L. The effect of phosphoric acid on human deciduous enamel surfaces in vitro. J. Int. Assoc. Dent. Child. 7:11–15, 1976.

47. Silverstone, L.M., et al. Variation in the pattern of acid etching of human enamel examined by scanning electron microscopy. Caries Res. 9:373–387, 1975.

48. Silverstone, L.M. Fissure sealants: the susceptibility to dissolution of acid-etched and subsequently abraded enamel in vitro. Caries Res. 11:46–51, 1977.

49. Silverstone, L.M., and Featherstone, M.J. Remineralization of acid-etched surfaces in vivo. J. Int. Assoc. Dent. Child. Accepted for publication.

50. Silverstone, L.M., Hicks, M.J., and Featherstone, M.J. Oral fluid contamination of etched enamel surfaces: an SEM study. J. Am. Dent. Assoc. 110:329–332, 1985.

51. Handleman, S.L., Buonocore, M.G., and Heseck, D.J. A preliminary report on the effect of fissure sealant on bacteria in dental caries. J. Prosthet. Dent. 27:390–392, 1972.

52. Handleman, S.L., Buonocore, M.G., and Schoute, P.C. Progress report on the effect of a fissure sealant on bacteria in dental caries. J. Am. Dent. Assoc. 87(5):1189–1191, 1973.

53. Handleman, S.L. Microbiolic aspects of sealing carious lesions. J. Prev. Dent. 32:29–32, 1976.

54. Handleman, S.L., Washburn, F., and Wopperer, P. Two-year report of sealant effect on bacteria in dental caries. J. Am. Dent. Assoc. 93(5):967–970, 1976.

55. Jeronimus, D.J., Till, M.J., and Sveen, O.B. Reduced viability of microorganisms under dental sealants. J. Dent. Child. 42:275–279, 1975.

56. Going, R.E., et al. The viability of microorganisms in carious lesions five years after covering with a fissure sealant. J. Am. Dent. Assoc. 97(a):455–462, 1978.

57. Simonsen, R.J. Selection criteria for pit and fissure sealant in a private practice. Compend. Cont. Ed. 5(4):289–294, 1984.

58. Silverstone, L.M. The current status of fissure sealants and priorities for future research. II. Compend. Cont. Ed. 5(4):299–306, 1984.

59. Simonsen, R.J. Clinical Applications of the Acid Etch Technique. Chicago: Quintessence Publ. Co., 1978, pp. 19–23.

chapter 12

Fluoride therapies

Fluoride has been the single most effective factor in the area of preventive dentistry. Studies have demonstrated that optimum results are obtained with a fluoride program that combines a variety of approaches. Education of patients by dental hygienists as to the health and financial benefits of a life-long combined fluoride therapy program can have far-reaching and significant effects on the oral health of the population as a whole. The previous notion that fluoride was beneficial only for children is outmoded and unsubstantiated in the light of recent evidence that the caries demineralization process is histologically identifiable up to 3 years prior to radiographic appearance of a lesion.[1-3] As a result, fluoride is therapeutically indicated for all age groups, from the pediatric to the geriatric patient.

Early in the study of fluoride it was determined that a caries reduction benefit existed. Physiologically, fluoride affects enamel solubility by promotion of the conversion of hydroxyapatite crystals in the tooth enamel to fluorapatite, which strengthens the tooth structure against acid attack. Although not a complete explanation of the mechanism of fluoride's action, this was the basis for the establishment of fluoride treatments as a part of the routine preventive dental services regimen of dental practice.

More recent research has determined that one of the major mechanisms by which fluoride affects dental caries is through remineralization. Cariologists utilizing polarizing light and scanning electron microscopy have found that low concentrations of fluoride utilized at frequent intervals literally reverse the caries (demineralization) process.[1,2] Cariologists have identified four zones of the carious lesion: the surface zone, which is a thin layer of healthy enamel; the body of the lesion (Fig. 12-1); the dark zone; and the translucent zone, which is adjacent to the unaffected enamel (Fig. 12-2). In experimentation, as tooth sections with carious lesions are exposed to acidified gel containing fluoride, new enamel crystal development is stimulated. The dark zone, which is an area of remineralization, becomes broader and darker (Fig. 12-3a); the surface zone begins to return to the composition of sound enamel (Fig. 12-3b); the translucent zone begins to remineralize; and therefore the lesion is reduced in size.

The body of the lesion, the largest part of the demineralized area, actually stores fluoride (Fig. 12-3c). This phenomenon of the body of the lesion acting as a reservoir for fluoride leads to a tooth more resistant to future caries progression. Enamel crystals in the remineralized areas are actually larger than those found in some enamel.[1-3] These results are obtained not from high concentrations of fluoride but rather from frequent use of low levels of fluoride. The concept of fluoride treatments provided to patients every 6 months in the dental office is obviously not the optimal approach to providing comprehensive fluoride therapy. A combination of systemic fluoride, frequent professional fluoride applications, and home care regimens that utilize fluoride products is a more complete approach to the prevention of dental caries.

In addition to all of the new information related to fluoride and cariology, fluoride is being recognized as an adjunctive therapy for periodontal disease control. When present in high concentrations, fluoride is bactericidal and, in lower concentrations, bacteriostatic, which can then affect the microorganisms in plaque.

In periodontal disease, there is an increase in subgingival levels of bacteria that require carbon dioxide, as well as specific anaerobic bacteria. Preliminary studies have led to irrigation with fluorides (Fig. 12-4), salt, baking soda, and hydrogen peroxide com-

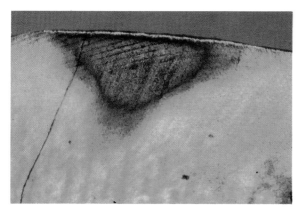

Fig. 12-1 Zones of the carious lesion. (Courtesy of Dr. Leon Silverstone, University of Colorado, Denver, Colo.)

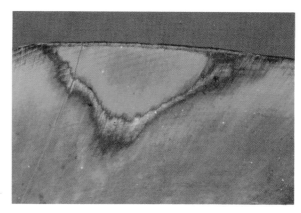

Figure 12-2

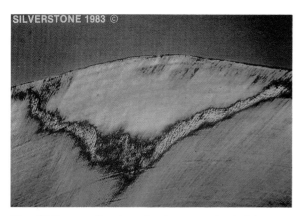

Figs. 12-3a to c Remineralization occurring in laboratory-induced caries. (Courtesy of Dr. Leon Silverstone.)

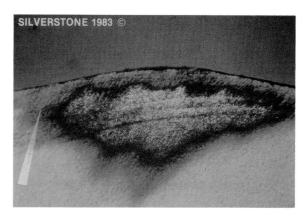

Figure 12-3b

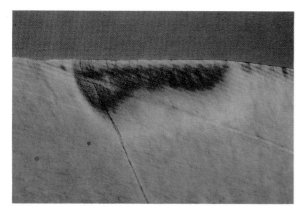

Figure 12-3c

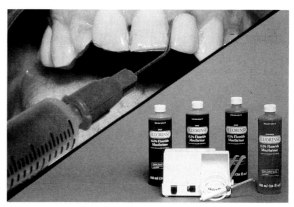

Fig. 12-4 Subgingival irrigation. (Courtesy of Oral-B Laboratories, Palo Alto, Calif.)

binations and the use of antibiotics in an attempt to shift the bacterial composition of periodontal pockets.[4,5] Many dental practices are employing this type of approach in conjunction with frequent debridement and root planing at the recall appointment in order to control periodontal disease progression.

Fluoride is utilizable via two basic mechanisms: systemic ingestion and topical application. The mode of action is different for each. The benefits to the teeth are substantial, especially with combined programs of fluoride therapy.

Systemic fluoride modalities

Fluoride, once ingested, is circulated to all body tissues by the bloodstream. Benefits to the teeth occur during the calcification phase prior to eruption, after calcification but prior to eruption, and after the teeth have erupted into the oral cavity. Deposition of fluoride into the enamel matrix occurs during the calcification phase of tooth development, with the result that the fluoride incorporates as fluorapatite. In cases of excess fluoride consumption, the ameloblastic activity may be hindered, causing a defective enamel matrix to form. The resulting condition is known as fluorosis.

After the teeth have calcified, but have not yet erupted, the surface enamel continues to receive fluoride at the surface level. This fluoride is available from the adjacent tissue fluids. As a result, the outer enamel surface is much more fluoride-rich than are the inner layers.

Following eruption, fluoride continues to deposit on the surface enamel throughout life. Available sources include saliva, food, drinking water, and fluoride products such as dentifrices and topical applications. The uptake of the mineral is highest during the years immediately following eruption, but teeth continue to accept the deposition of fluoride into adulthood.

Recent evidence suggests that ingestion of fluoride during the years in which the teeth are developing may cause the teeth to mature at a more rapid rate.[6] Newly erupted enamel has areas of incomplete mineralization. Fluoride appears to increase the rate of mineralization in these hypomineralized areas. In addition, these areas are likely to contain more fluorapatite than enamel that was fully mineralized upon eruption.

Fluoride may cause changes in tooth morphology as well. Some research suggests that fluoride tends to make teeth slightly smaller and make the fissures somewhat shallower.[6] Because pits and fissures are highly susceptible to caries development, this feature could be significant in caries prevention.

Of the several mechanisms for the delivery of systemic fluoride, the most effective to date is fluoridation of the community water supply. By fluoridation is meant the adjustment of the fluoride ion content of a given water supply to provide a concentration that will afford maximum protection against caries (reductions in caries of 50% to 70%) without producing undesirable fluorosis of the enamel. The levels range from 0.6 parts per million for warmer climates to 1.2 ppm for colder areas. The optimum level of fluoride adjustment for moderate climates is 1 ppm. Currently in the United States 52% of the population has the benefit of fluoridation.[6] A number of communities have a natural water supply with a fluoride content of at least 0.7 ppm or greater, which is adequate for caries prevention.

Interest in fluoridation was sparked by the investigations of Dr. Frederick McKay relative to brown staining of teeth, which was subsequently named mottled enamel.[7] Today this condition is called dental fluorosis. Dr. McKay noticed that individuals with this staining exhibited significantly lower incidences of dental caries. Later, in 1931, the element fluorine was identified by H.V. Churchill as the causative agent.[7]

Shortly thereafter, Dr. H. Trendly Dean of the U.S. Public Health Service directed a number of studies that supported the finding that optimum fluoride content of the drinking water for prevention of dental caries was 1 ppm.[7] In 1945, research with controlled fluoridation began. Test communities were paired with nonfluoridated control communities, yielding impressive results: in the primary dentition, with fluoridation from birth, a caries reduction of up to 50% occurred. In the permanent dentition, an even greater reduction can be realized, with 60% to 70% fewer carious lesions. Some individuals may even be completely caries-free.[7]

Additional benefits from fluoridation include:

1. Improved aesthetic appearance of teeth.
2. Assistance in normal bone maintenance and improvement of calcium metabolism. This is of particular importance in the prevention of osteoporosis, especially for women.

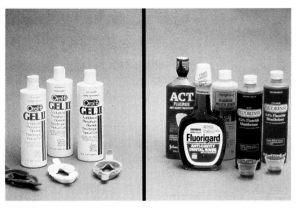

Fig. 12-5 Fluoride products for office and home use. (Courtesy of Oral-B Laboratories.)

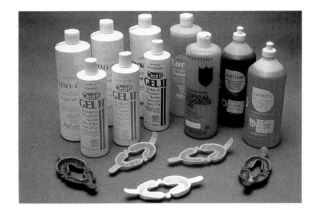

Fig. 12-6 APF gels. (Courtesy of Oral-B Laboratories.)

3. Improved bone density, which affects all bones including alveolar bone.
4. A degree of topical fluoride protection. This is provided during ingestion as the fluoridated water passes over the teeth.
5. The possibility of less malocclusion if fewer teeth are lost to caries.

A second type of fluoridation mechanism employs fluoridation of the school water system. This methodology is of benefit for those children residing in an area with no central water system. Because the children ingest the water for only the portion of each day that they attend school, the fluoride content is increased to a higher level than the optimum for the community. Benefits from this type of program are greater on late-erupting teeth, because they are exposed to the systemic effects.

Other means of providing systemic fluoride have included fluoridation of commonly ingested food products such as milk and salt. To date, such mechanisms have not been shown to provide substantial benefits, primarily because of barriers such as use and practicality.

Fluoridation has been shown to be the most effective, reliable, efficient, cost-effective method discovered for the prevention and control of the insidious, pervasive disease of dental caries. Less than one dollar per child is the total cost per year for the use of such a program.[6] Fluoridation is therefore likely to be among the most beneficial public health care measures ever devised.

External sources of fluoride therapy

Fluoride therapy provided via external sources is generally divided into treatment rendered in the dental office and that provided to the patient for home use (Fig. 12-5).

The types of fluoride therapy that are available in the dental office include topical applications for caries control, iontophoresis and applications of fluoride solutions and pastes for the treatment of hypersensitivity, and subgingival irrigation with fluoride solutions as a component of periodontal therapy. Other modalities that show potential for future use include pit and fissure sealants incorporated with time-released fluoride, fluoride varnish, and time-released fluoride pellets that are bonded directly to one or more teeth in the mouth.

Topical application

The topical application method of fluoride therapy is the most commonly utilized office fluoride mechanism at this time. The dental hygienist is frequently the individual who performs this function in most dental offices. Several different types of fluoride products are currently used for topical application.

APF The agent used most often is acidulated phosphate-fluoride (APF). This is comprised of 1.23% sodium fluoride with 0.1 M orthophosphoric acid. The pH range is between 3.0 and 3.5. Depending upon the manufacturer, the basic formulae may vary.

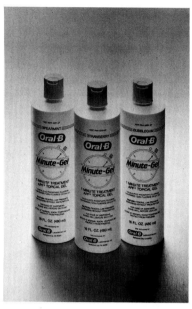

Fig. 12-7 One-minute fluoride gel product. (Courtesy of Oral-B Laboratories.)

APF may be obtained either as a gel, thixotropic agent, or solution (Fig. 12-6). Thixotropic fluoride is a form of gel that flows only under pressure. This feature allows the insertion of the agent into the mouth without leaking or dripping. In addition, it flows interproximally and covers all surfaces. Its consistency then allows the material to cling to all tooth surfaces for complete coverage.

APF uptake on enamel surfaces is equivalent regardless of the form, when all factors such as pH and fluoride content are the same. Caries reduction with the use of APF ranges from 44% to 70%, as demonstrated in a number of clinical studies. Although it appears that the caries-protection ability of the fluoride is obtained regardless of plaque accumulation on the teeth, there seems to be a distinct advantage to application on plaque-free teeth.

The usual frequency of application is every 6 months, in conjunction with recall appointments. The more frequent the application, however, the greater the protection that is afforded the teeth. Patients with high caries rates should have more frequent topical applications, because the promotion of remineralization is facilitated by low concentrations of fluoride at frequent intervals.

Acidulated phosphate-fluoride will not cause tooth staining. It is a stable solution when stored in a poly-ethylene container and has an acceptable taste. Most companies manufacture the fluoride agent in a number of flavors to appeal to patients, especially children. The product is applied and left in place usually for a minimum of 4 minutes.

A given fluoride product's ability to deposit fluoride ions in both sound and decalcified teeth is measured by in-vitro uptake. In order to be anticariogenic, topical fluoride applications should produce a surface enamel fluoride concentration of at least 1,000 ppm. This concentration level represents the Minimum Therapeutic Level (MTL) for topical fluoride applications. Of the wide variety of fluoride products currently available, significant variations exist among those that are intended for professional use. Many brands meet or exceed the MTL when administered via a 4-minute tray application. However, data relating to fluoride uptake for specific brands are generally not available, and acceptance of a product by the American Dental Association is not a reliable guide as to whether a product meets the MTL.

In addition, significant differences exist among commercial brands both in pH and the inclusion of extraneous ingredients. These factors can markedly influence fluoride uptake. Some companies, for example, elevate the pH to anywhere from 4.6 to neutral pH to improve the flavor and lessen the acidic aftertaste. Although such adjustments appeal to patient acceptance, no scientific support exists for clinical efficacy of fluoride uptake. In fact, an APF gel with a pH of 4.5 yields only 23% of the fluoride uptake level of an APF gel with a pH of 3.1. In order to provide optimum uptake, the pH of the product must be low.

One of the major drawbacks of most professional topical fluoride products is the necessity for a full 4-minute application. Although 4 minutes is not an extensive amount of time, it can be problematic for young children, disabled patients, geriatric patients, and others who find it difficult to tolerate a fluoride treatment of this length. Accordingly, the Oral-B Company has developed an improved 1.23% APF gel that requires only a 1-minute treatment time. This product, known as Oral-B Minute-Gel, is now available on the market (Fig. 12-7).

A 1-minute application of Minute-Gel provides 12,000 ppm, which is 12 times the recommended MTL. A traditional 4-minute application with this product yields an uptake of 15,5000 ppm.[8] Therefore, 80% of the fluoride uptake occurs within 1 minute. This product, in addition to a greatly improved fluoride uptake level, is advantageous in the saving of time, especially in practices where topical fluoride treatments are performed routinely for all patients.

Sodium fluoride The second type of fluoride originally used professionally for topical application is sodium fluoride. It is usually utilized as a 2% aqueous solution, with a neutral pH of 7.0. This agent differs from APF in that a series of 4 applications is given, 2 to 7 days apart, at ages 3, 7, 10, and 13 years. These ages were chosen to coincide with average tooth eruption patterns to provide immediate fluoride protection following eruption. Additional single applications are also given at 4- to 6-month intervals between the series of applications in conjunction with regular recall appointments.

Sodium fluoride has been shown to effect a 30% to 40% reduction in caries in primary teeth. It is a stable product when stored in a polyethylene container and has a fairly acceptable, though somewhat salty, taste. The number of appointments needed for the series of applications is a disadvantage for this product, but can be advantageous in that greater contact with the patient can be used to monitor home care procedures.

Stannous fluoride The third agent that may be used for topical application of fluoride therapy is stannous fluoride. The concentration of the solution will indicate its frequency of application: 8% and 10% solutions are administered as single applications over 4- to 6-month intervals; 2% and 4% solutions follow the same timeframe as with the sodium fluoride (four applications, 2 to 7 days apart, at ages 3, 7, 10, and 13 years).

Caries reduction with the use of stannous fluoride ranges between 30% and 40%. Stannous fluoride solution is very unstable and must be mixed in a polyethylene container just prior to each application: to 10.0 ml of distilled water is added the appropriate amount of stannous fluoride powder (1.0 g for 10% solution, 0.8 g for 8%, 0.4 g for 4%, and 0.2 g for 2%). The solution is then applied to clean teeth that have been dried and isolated. Residual solution should be discarded.

Stannous fluoride has the potential to cause deleterious effects to both the gingiva and the teeth. Gingival reactions may vary from a minor irritation with blanching of the tissue to a severe chemical burn-like effect with sloughing. Healing will occur within several days to a week. The extreme reactions generally occur with the higher concentrations and when the solution is inadvertently applied to irritated or inflamed gingival tissues.

Stannous fluoride may also cause brown staining of the teeth, most commonly in hypocalcified and decalcified enamel surfaces, carious lesions, margins of restorations, and developmental pits and fissures. Patients with any of these situations would be more appropriately treated with a different fluoride product.

If stannous fluoride is the product of choice, the clinician should employ several precautionary measures. If the patient exhibits inflammation of the gingiva, a lubricant such as petroleum jelly may be spread over the tissue. The weaker solutions of 2% or 4% should be used. The patient is draped to protect the clothing from accidental spills that may stain the fabric. All radiographs should be taken before a stannous fluoride application is performed to prevent contamination of the film by the stannous ions. Residual ions in the patient's mouth and on the clinician's hands may remain for as long as several hours. The clinician should change rubber gloves after completing the application of the solution.

In addition to the lack of long-term stability and the adverse reactions to the teeth and gingiva, stannous fluoride has a very unpleasant taste, with limited appeal to most patients.

Stannous fluoride is now available in a water-free gel form, making it a more stable product. Flavoring agents have been added to increase patient acceptance and it is more often applied using a rubber prophylaxis cup or toothbrush.

The two most commonly used methods for applying fluoride topically to the teeth are the tray technique and the paint-on (or cotton roll isolation) technique. Basic preparation of the teeth is the same, regardless of the method used. If the teeth are to be polished, a fluoride-containing prophylaxis paste should be used to replace, at least in part, the fluoride content of the tooth surface that is removed during polishing. Plaque may otherwise be removed from tooth surfaces by thorough toothbrushing and flossing by the patient. The patient's mouth should be rinsed to remove residual prophylaxis paste or toothpaste. The armamentarium for application of the fluoride will vary according to the method used (Fig. 12-8).

Tray technique The materials needed for topical fluoride application using trays are:

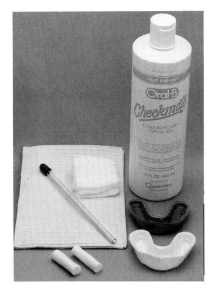

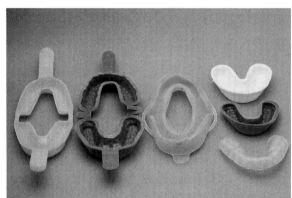

Fig. 12-8 *(left)* Armamentarium for tray technique.

Fig. 12-9 *(below)* Various fluoride trays.

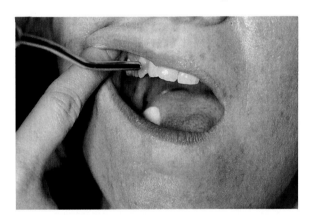

Fig. 12-10 Drying the teeth.

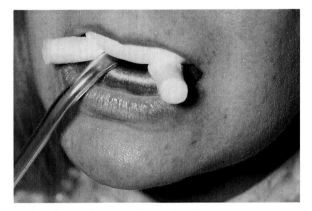

Fig. 12-11 Isolation with cotton rolls.

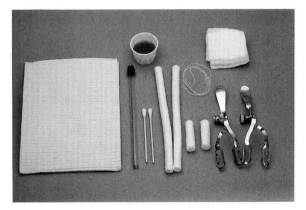

Fig. 12-12 Armamentarium for paint-on technique.

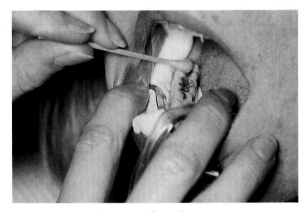

Fig. 12-13 Application of fluoride.

- Maxillary and mandibular trays.
- Saliva ejector.
- Cotton rolls.
- 2 × 2 gauze squares.
- Fluoride gel or thixotropic agent.
- Timer.

A number of companies manufacture disposable fluoride trays made of polyethylene or similar materials. The products vary, having features that attempt to enhance the contact of the fluoride with accessible tooth surfaces (e.g., anatomic contours of the trays, vacuum sealing to prevent moisture contamination, and sponge interiors) (Fig. 12-9). Disposable trays are obtainable as separate, paired trays for maxillary and mandibular arches or as hinged trays having both arch trays together as a single unit. These types of trays are generally cost-effective, comfortable to the patient, and provide optimum ability to control potential disease transmission via their disposability. They are available in several different sizes to fit most patients' mouths.

Other types of trays are available, although used infrequently by comparison. These include wax trays, plastic trays used with disposable sponge inserts, and custom-fitted vinyl trays. Wax trays are advantageous in that they may be contoured to fit the individual patient's mouth, but to do so is somewhat time consuming. Plastic trays pose problems with sterilization and potential disease transmission, while the vinyl trays may present storage difficulties.

For treatment via the tray technique, the patient is seated in an upright position. This will aid in preventing the flow of saliva or excess fluoride to the patient's throat. The fluoride gel is dispensed into the tray and the sides pinched together to distribute the gel evenly around the tray. Some trays have markings to indicate the amount of fluoride needed. It is neither necessary nor desirable to fill the tray with gel to the rim; excess gel will only spill out into the patient's mouth and throat.

Because trays are available either hinged or as separated, paired components, the dental hygienist is able to treat the arches individually or together at the same time. Very young children and patients with an active gag reflex are better handled by placing trays first on one arch, removing that tray, and placing the second tray. The technique employed most often, however, involves applying the fluoride to both arches at once.

The teeth of the maxillary and mandibular arch are dried, with the fingers of the opposite hand used to retract the mucosa (Fig. 12-10). Thorough drying contributes to the effectiveness of the treatment by lessening the dilution of the fluoride. The trays are placed over the maxillary and mandibular teeth and the saliva ejector is inserted. Cotton rolls are placed at the premolar areas and the patient is instructed to close gently (Fig. 12-11). The pressure resulting from this closing action aids in forcing the gel interproximally and into other protected areas. The timer is set for the time required for the particular product.

The trays are removed and the excess gel wiped from all the teeth with gauze squares. The dental hygienist should remove as much of the excess as possible from the teeth to avoid having the patient swallow the gel. The patient may expectorate but should not rinse. Prior to dismissal, the patient (or parent of a young child) should be instructed to avoid rinsing, eating, drinking, or brushing for at least 30 minutes or longer.

Paint-on technique On some occasions, topical fluoride may be applied using cotton rolls to isolate the teeth and a cotton-tipped applicator with which to swab the gel or solution onto the teeth. Examples of patients for whom this technique may be appropriate include very young children, other patients who cannot tolerate fluoride trays, and patients with only a few teeth remaining in an arch. As shown in Fig. 12-12, materials needed to apply topical fluoride using this technique are:

- Cotton rolls.
- Saliva ejector.
- 2 × 2 gauze squares.
- Fluoride gel or solution.
- Cotton-tipped applicators.
- Disposable paper dappen dish or other container not made of glass or metal.
- Timer.
- Garmers or other cotton roll holders (optional).

The patient is seated in an upright position. A small amount of fluoride solution or gel is dispensed into the dappen dish. The teeth on the patient's right side are isolated by cotton rolls placed in the maxillary and mandibular vestibules and on the lingual surface under the tongue. Some clinicians prefer to use special cotton roll holders with which to isolate the teeth.

The saliva ejector is placed in the patient's mouth and the isolated teeth are dried. The applicator is used to moisten all surfaces of the teeth with the fluoride product (Fig. 12-13). Gels or thixotropic agents tend to cling to the tooth surfaces after application, but solutions must be continuously applied throughout the timing period to keep the teeth moist. The timer is set for the appropriate amount of time.

At the end of the treatment, the saliva ejector and cotton rolls are removed and any excess fluoride is wiped from the teeth with gauze squares. Fresh cotton rolls are used when the procedure is repeated on the opposite side of the mouth. At the conclusion of the treatment, the patient may expectorate but should not rinse. Instructions should be given not to rinse, eat, drink, or brush the teeth for a minimum of 30 minutes.

Iontophoresis

A second major type of professionally applied fluoride treatment is known as iontophoresis. Used in dentistry typically for the treatment of hypersensitive teeth, iontophoresis is the impregnation of surface body tissues with ions or ionic drugs using an energy source (e.g., electric current).

The technique of therapeutic ion introduction into body tissues has been used in medicine since 1841 and in dentistry since 1896, when W.J. Morton indicated the cataphoresis of cocaine to anesthetize the dental pulp.[9] Since then, iontophoresis has been used for a variety of dental procedures, ranging from local anesthesia to the treatment of herpes labialis and hypersensitive dentin. It is in the treatment of hypersensitive dentin that iontophoresis is most commonly recognized, using fluoride solutions.

Topical fluoride treatments and pastes containing fluoride have been used somewhat effectively as a mode of therapy for hypersensitivity. It is thought that the fluoride may form a physical barrier on the surface of the dentin, thus shielding it from circumstances that trigger the hypersensitive response. Although some researchers have obtained results showing that high concentrations of fluoride may irritate the odontoblasts, most identify fluoride as an effective therapeutic agent in the treatment of hypersensitivity.

Fluoride iontophoresis has been a treatment choice for hypersensitivity since the mid-1950s. Many of the research studies performed to investigate the efficacy of this method were not well controlled or properly conducted. However, considering the relatively few studies that were appropriately conducted, the technique has been shown to be effective as a desensitizing agent.[9]

The actual means by which fluoride iontophoresis acts as a desensitizer is not known, but several theories have attempted to explain its mode of action. One hypothesis suggests that reparative dentin forms following the application of the electric current, resulting in dead tracts in the primary dentin. These dead tracts could then inhibit the transfer of pain stimuli from the exposed dentin to the pulp tissue. Research on this theory has not been conclusive to date.[9]

The second hypothesis regarding desensitization by iontophoresis suggests that the electric current may cause paresthesia by changing the sensory mechanisms of pain conduction. Whether the electrical current alone produces the long-term desensitizing effect or whether some other mechanism is responsible is not yet clear.[9]

The third theory explaining iontophoretic desensitization proposes that the process causes an increased concentration of fluoride ions in the dentinal tubules, which then may cause microprecipitation of calcium fluoride.[9] This is turn may decrease fluid movement within the tubules that is induced by stimuli. The electric current forces more fluoride ions into the tooth surfaces and to a greater depth than with just a topical application. This increase of fluoride may then be sufficient to precipitate the calcium fluoride crystals that are trapped deeply in the dentinal tubules. This process may also result in enhanced mineralization, forming fluorapatite more deeply within the tooth structure.

Although the mechanism of action is still not clear, fluoride iontophoresis can be a valuable adjunct in the treatment of dentin hypersensitivity.

Specialized equipment necessary to utilize fluoride iontophoresis therapy includes an adequate source of electric power. Units powered by simple dry cell batteries were used most frequently in the past, but these are considered inadequate, because only about 4 to 8 volts can be generated. This low voltage would require a treatment time of 10 minutes or more for desensitization. Because a higher voltage can accomplish the desired results in a much shorter time, a unit that can deliver 25 to 45 volts DC is preferred. The Phoresor* Model PM 600-2 is considered very useful

*Motion Control, Inc., Salt Lake City, Utah.

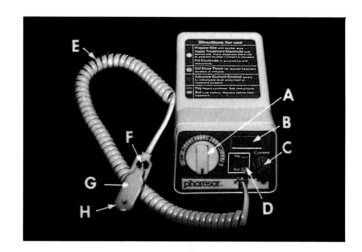

Fig. 12-14 Iontophoresis unit: (A) treatment duration timer; (B) dosage current display; (C) current switch; (D) reject panel; (E) output cable; (F) negative terminal; (G) positive terminal; (H) extension. (From L.P. Gangarosa: *Iontophoresis in Dental Practice,* Quintessence Publ. Co., 1978.)

for fluoride iontophoresis (Fig. 12-14). It is small, operates by a 9V replaceable battery, and has a circuitry design that converts the voltage up to 45 volts DC. Additional features indicate when the battery should be replaced and alert the operator if the battery is placed incorrectly in the unit. A constant current supply feature automatically adjusts for changes in resistance in the external circuit during use.

Other equipment needed includes a set of electrodes (return and active), a series of plastic tips to fit the active (oral) electrode, clip and brush electrodes, 1% sodium nitrate solution, 2% sodium fluoride solution, impression materials and trays (if multiple teeth are to be treated at once), saliva ejector, cotton pellets, cotton rolls, disposable calibrated dappen dishes, alcohol swabs, and 2 × 2 gauze squares. Many of these items are available in kits when the iontophoresis device is purchased.

A detailed instruction manual is provided with most iontophoresis units. The clinician must become thoroughly familiar with the operation of the particular unit being utilized prior to attempting iontophoresis therapy. In general, after assembling all materials and equipment, the clinician makes sure the power supply unit is turned off. The return electrode is then applied to the patient's forearm and connected to the power supply. Depending on the polarity of the drug to be used (e.g., fluoride solution is negative), the appropriate return electrode must be selected. (A positive electrode is used as the return electrode when fluoride is the drug of choice.)

The correct active electrode is selected: the oral electrode with plastic tip, the brush electrode, or the

clip electrode. The plastic tips are available in a variety of shapes and sizes, and are useful in treating facial and lingual surfaces (Fig. 12-15). The brush is used for interproximal, gingival margin, and subgingival areas (Fig. 12-16). Clip electrodes are utilized when the tray technique is employed to desensitize multiple teeth at once (Fig. 12-17).

The fluoride solution is applied to the electrode according to instructions for the given condition to be treated. Cotton soaked with the fluoride solution is used in the plastic tips, while the brush has a small reservoir that is filled with solution. Soft tissues must be insulated during treatment to avoid conducting the current to these areas. The plastic tip will adequately insulate the gingiva during its use. If the tray technique is used, a rubber dam or rubber base impression material in acrylic trays can be used.

The timer switch is turned beyond 5 minutes and the current switch is turned on. The current switch is then turned slowly to elevate the current to the level desired. The mA level is determined by either preset limits or the patient's level of discomfort, whichever is lower.

The timer is set to the appropriate number of minutes for the treatment. The current will start and continue uninterrupted until the desired time has elapsed. The timer will shut off the current at the end of the treatment. When the treatment is completed, the current switch must be turned off and the electrodes removed.

In addition to treatment of hypersensitivity, iontophoresis has been used for surface local anesthesia and treatment of lichen planus, aphthous ulcers, and

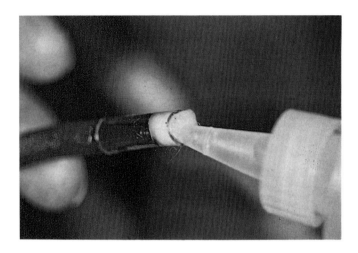

Fig. 12-15 Solution application to plastic tips. (From L.P. Gangarosa: *Iontophoresis in Dental Practice,* Quintessence Publ. Co., 1978.)

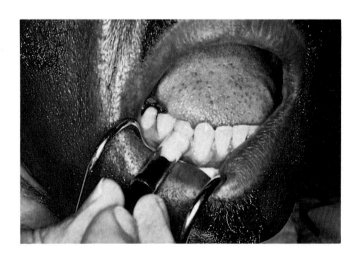

Fig. 12-16 Plastic tip in use. (From L.P. Gangarosa: *Iontophoresis in Dental Practice,* Quintessence Publ. Co., 1978.)

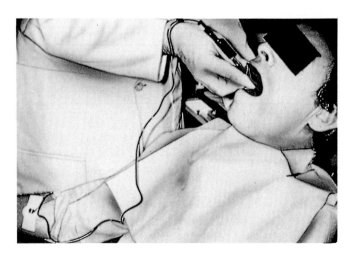

Fig. 12-17 Complete set-up for iontophoresis using clip electrode. (From L.P. Gangarosa: *Iontophoresis in Dental Practice,* Quintessence Publ. Co., 1978.)

oral herpes simplex lesions. Different drugs are used in the therapeutic management of these conditions.

Subgingival irrigation

A third and relatively new method of fluoride therapy involves subgingival irrigation of periodontal pockets with a fluoride solution.[10] The rationale for such treatment lies with the antimicrobial effects of fluoride. Solutions with a high concentration of fluoride are bactericidal, while lower concentration solutions are bacteriostatic. Thus, delivery of the solution directly into the pocket is performed in an attempt to alter the plaque microbiota and chemotherapeutically treat the causative factor of periodontal disease.

Subgingival irrigation is performed either in the dental office using a syringe and large blunt needle or cannula or by the patient using a motorized oral irrigation device. Irrigating agents may include stannous fluoride solution or other antiplaque agents such as sodium hypochloride or chlorhexidine, or aqueous solutions of salt, baking soda, and hydrogen peroxide.

Research studies have shown that simple rinsing of the mouth is not sufficient to deliver solutions into periodontal pockets.[10] Because plaque microbiota found in pockets tends to be very complex in nature, including anaerobic forms, it was hypothesized that introduction of chemotherapeutic agents directly into pockets might have an effect in the treatment of periodontal disease. Preliminary results tend to show that irrigation positively affects plaque microorganisms and periodontal health. One important aspect of many of these studies is the inclusion of thorough scaling and root planing as part of the therapy.

Subgingival irrigation as a component of complete periodontal therapy is presently quite controversial.[10] Many practitioners strongly dispute the contention that irrigation alone can treat or control periodontal disease. As an adjunct to other documented forms of treatment, however, subgingival irrigation appears to be quite promising in the control of periodontal disease.[11] Additional research is necessary to further investigate this modality.

Timed-release fluoride

An additional aspect of fluoride research concerns a mechanism that would provide constant levels of fluoride over long periods of time. The idea of continuous low levels of fluoride providing greater benefits than the traditional approach of a topical application

every 6 months is supported by research on remineralization of existing carious lesions.[1-3,12] As a result, much research effort has been directed toward identifying means by which fluoride may be delivered to the teeth on a consistent basis.[13,14]

Currently, studies are being directed toward the development of a timed-release pellet that can be bonded to a tooth in the patient's mouth. The pellet then slowly releases fluoride after mixing with saliva, maintaining a constant low topical level of fluoride in the mouth. This is still an experimental methodology not available for general public use.

Another type of timed-release fluoride therapy involves pit and fissure sealants that release fluoride slowly into the oral environment. Current research in this area has led to the development of a sealant material that will not only mechanically protect the teeth but will also release fluoride at the interface of the tooth enamel and sealant. Because developmental pits and fissures derive the least benefit from topical and systemic fluoride, this mechanism would provide additional protection to highly caries-susceptible surfaces.

Initial attempts to formulate a fluoride-releasing sealant comprised simple mixing of soluble fluoride salts with the sealant material. The fluoride was released when water dissolved the salt, resulting in rapid loss of the element, too rapid to be of any significant value. In addition, the sealant material became weakened, with an accompanying loss of protection to the teeth.

Dr. H. Ralph Rawls of Louisiana State University School of Dentistry, along with dental students and research associate Barbara Zimmerman, developed a sealant material that released fluoride by the exchange of ions.[15] The sealant itself was left intact, and the fluoride release was accomplished slowly and steadily, over a long term. The mechanism used was molecular binding of an organic fluoride salt into an insoluble polymer structure, called an ion exchange resin. Ions from the saliva replace the fluoride ions in the resin by means of an exchange reaction. Because the fluoride component of the material is quite small and it is being replaced, not totally lost, the sealant itself is not significantly decreased in strength.

The fluoride itself, although released rapidly from the resin particles, disperses slowly through the sealant. Thus, the release of the fluoride is controlled, resulting in a nearly constant fluoride concentration at the sealant-enamel junction.

The National Institute of Dental Research is currently studying timed-release fluorides, with the Rawls project a component of this overall study. In vitro studies were performed preliminarily, with clinical trials planned.[15]

Supplemental mechanisms of fluoride therapy

Fluoride dentifrices

The most commonly used type of fluoride supplementation is a dentifrice containing fluoride. A number of these products are currently available, with several of them carrying acceptance by the American Dental Association as therapeutically effective (Fig. 12-18). Sodium fluoride, sodium monofluorophosphate, and stannous fluoride are the compounds used most frequently in dentifrice formulae. Other ingredients include a compatible abrasive agent and essential dentifrice components.

In general, caries reduction benefits range from 20% to 30%, with newly erupted teeth receiving the greatest benefit. Children raised in fluoridated communities exhibit additional caries reduction, thus indicating the cumulative benefit of a combined fluoride therapy program. Parents should be educated concerning fluoride toxicity (see later section in this chapter).

Dentifrices containing stannous fluoride may cause light staining of the teeth. Such products should not be recommended to patients with exposed cementum.

Fluoride mouthrinses

The regular use of mouthrinses containing fluoride can provide an efficient and effective means of fluoride therapy. Studies have indicated caries reductions between 20% and 50%, depending on the frequency of use (daily, weekly, or bimonthly) and fluoride concentration of the product. This format of therapy is easily incorporated into school health programs because of the ease of administration and low relative cost.

Mouthrinses are now available both over-the-counter and as prescription products (Fig. 12-19). One of the major differences in the two types is the amount of fluoride: over-the-counter products contain concentrations of 0.05% fluoride while prescription products usually contain 0.2% fluoride. (Different products will vary in specific amounts.)

Most products utilize sodium fluoride, although stannous fluoride products are also available. Full listings of available products are given in publications of the American Dental Association's Council on Dental Therapeutics. Mouthrinses with fluoride concentrations of 0.2% at a neutral pH (7.0) are used once per week of every 2 weeks. Products with concentrations of sodium fluoride 0.05% at neutral pH or acidulated phosphate sodium fluoride 0.044% at pH of 4.0 may be used on a daily basis. The patient is instructed to swish 5 ml (1 teaspoon) vigorously for at least 60 seconds, and then swallow or expectorate, depending on directions for the particular product.

Self-applied gels

Some patients are especially prone to dental caries and therefore require a more aggressive approach to home fluoride therapy. Included in this group are patients with xerostomia, overdentures, rampant caries, and extensive gingival recession, and patients undergoing radiation therapy, especially of the head and neck area. For these individuals, a system that utilizes custom trays and a fluoride gel on a daily or weekly basis can be very beneficial in the control of caries. The types of gels used can be either 0.4% stannous fluoride or 0.5% APF with a pH range of 4.5 to 7.0. The technique for application is similar to that of the professional tray fluoride treatment. The patient should first brush and floss to remove all plaque from all tooth surfaces and then swallow several times to remove as much saliva as possible. A small amount of gel is dispensed into the trays. Care should be taken not to dispense so much gel that it overflows once the trays are applied (Fig. 12-20). The patient then inserts the trays into his or her mouth and gently closes the teeth together. The trays should remain in place for 4 minutes. The patient removes the trays, expectorates the remaining gel, and rinses and dries the trays for subsequent use. As with professional applications, the patient should refrain from eating, drinking, and rinsing for 30 minutes.

Dietary supplements

For those individuals who live in areas without fluoridated water, fluoride supplements in the form of pills, drops, chewable tablets, or mouthrinses may be prescribed. Although many foods contain fluoride naturally, the element occurs in such small amounts as to be negligible for the purpose of caries reduction. Consequently, dietary supplementation can be used to provide the optimum level of fluoride.

Any form of dietary fluoride supplement that is chewed or dissolved in the mouth has the potential for topical as well as systemic benefits if mixed with the saliva and the resulting liquid is swished in the mouth prior to swallowing. Some mouthrinses may also be swallowed after the rinsing is completed. As with all forms of fluoride therapy, newly erupted teeth derive the greatest benefits. Patients should be cautioned not to rinse, eat, or drink for 30 minutes after chewing or rinsing.

In order to achieve maximum results, supplemental dietary fluoride should commence as soon after birth as possible and continue until approximately 16 to 18 years of age. Studies have shown caries reductions of up to 80% in primary teeth and up to 40% in permanent teeth.

Dietary fluoride supplements are available by prescription only, and the dosage is regulated by the amount of natural fluoride found in the drinking water. Table 12-1 shows the recommended dosages by age and fluoride concentration.

When fluoride supplements are prescribed, the amount of obtainable fluoride should not exceed 264 mg of sodium fluoride, which is a 4-month supply. This amount is less than the identified toxic and lethal doses, should a child accidentally swallow all the prescribed pills or drops. As with any medication, fluoride supplements should be stored in a location that is inaccessible to children to avoid accidental ingestion.

Fluoride supplements may also be distributed to children as part of the school health program. While such an approach has the disadvantage of beginning usually at the kindergarten level (thus losing the years from birth to age 5), it is still a method of providing some form of fluoride therapy. Regardless of the age at which therapy is instituted, a program requiring daily ingestion of a substance over a period of approximately 15 years is often very difficult to supervise and control on a consistent basis.

Fluoride toxicity

Although fluoride provides documented therapeutic

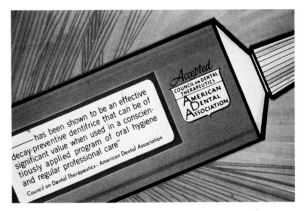

Fig. 12-18   American Dental Association, Council on Dental Therapeutics Seal of Approval.

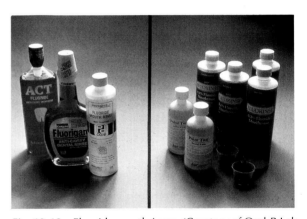

Fig. 12-19   Fluoride mouthrinses. (Courtesy of Oral-B Laboratories.)

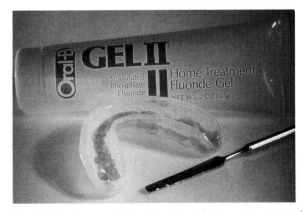

Fig. 12-20   Appropriately filled fluoride tray. (Courtesy of Oral-B Laboratories.)

Table 12-1 Daily dosage of fluoride according to age and fluoride content of water supply

Fluoride in water (ppm)	Birth to 24 months	25 to 36 months	37 months to 13 years
0.3 or less	0.25 mg	0.5 mg	1.0 mg
Greater than 0.3 to 0.7	0.0 mg*	0.25 mg	0.5 mg

*Unless breast-fed; during the period of breast feeding, use 0.125 mg.

Source: J.R. Mellberg and L.W. Ripa. Fluoride in Preventive Dentistry. Chicago: Quintessence Publ. Co., 1983.

benefits, the substance is toxic and requires that knowledgeable health professionals who utilize it be cognizant of the need to manage it with responsibility. It is impossible to consume enough water fluoridated at 1 ppm to provide an acute lethal dose of fluoride to humans. The fluoride content of products used in the dental office pose a potential hazard, however, and products for home use are potentially hazardous for a very small child. The acute lethal dose of fluoride for humans is approximately 30 mg per kilogram of body weight.[16] A large tube of toothpaste, which today may be flavored as bubble gum or may be attractively colored, has enough fluoride to be dangerous to a small child if the entire tube is ingested. Therefore parents should be educated to keep fluoride toothpaste, home gels, and rinses out of the reach of children. Child-sized toothbrushes should be utilized with parents dispensing a small amount of paste.

Usually the ingestion of large amounts of fluoride will induce vomiting, but the dental hygienist must not rely on this occurrence. An application of a topical APF office fluoride treatment involves the use of 123 mg of fluoride. When performed properly, 3 to 5 mg of fluoride are ingested or taken up by the tissues. Care must be employed so as not to place excess amounts of fluoride in the tray and to assure proper evacuation of fluoride that flows into the mouth in order that the ingested amount is negligible.

One death of a 3-year-old boy from a fluoride treatment in a dental office involved swallowing 400 mg of stannous fluoride. That is in excess of the fatal amount. The type of fluoride treatment employed should take into account the maturity of the child. Careful use of trays or a paint-on technique should be utilized for small children for maximum control of the fluoride product.

Assuming that vomiting will occur upon ingestion of potentially dangerous amounts of fluoride and will therefore remove the fluoride is imprudent. The dental hygienist must be aware of the dangers of improper application of fluoride and be prepared to administer calcium-containing products such as milk or, more particularly, 10% to 20% calcium carbonate solution as an antidote. The introduction of calcium changes the fluoride compound to nontoxic calcium fluoride. All members of the dental office professional staff should be knowledgeable about fluoride and be prepared to act in case patients exhibit the symptoms of nausea and vomiting associated with fluoride toxicity.

References

1. Wei, S.H. (ed.) Clinical Uses of Fluorides. Philadelphia: Lea & Febiger, 1985, pp. 153–174.

2. Silverstone, L.M. Remineralization and enamel caries: new concepts. Dental Update 10(4): 1983.

3. Silverstone, L.M., and Featherstone, M.J. The effect of different remineralization regimens on lesion progression in vitro. Caries Res. 15:198, 1981.

4. McDonald, J.L., Schenehorn, B.R., and Stookey, G.K. Influence of fluoride upon plaque and gingivitis in the beagle dog. J. Dent. Res. 57:899, 1978.

5. Mazza, J., Newman, M.G., and Sims, T.N. Clinical and antimicrobial effect of stannous fluoride on periodontitis. J. Clin. Periodontol. 8:203, 1981.

6. Horowitz, A.M., and Thomas, H.B. Conference on dental caries prevention in public health programs. II. J. Public Health Dent. 43:27, 1983.

7. The Fluoride Story (presentation). Redwood City, Calif.: Oral-B Laboratories, 1985.

8. Technical Report on Oral-B Minute-Gel. Redwood City, Calif.: Oral-B Laboratories, 1985.

9. Gangarosa, L.P. Iontophoresis in Dental Practice. Chicago: Quintessence Publ. Co., 1983.

10. Gross, A., and Tinanoff, N. Effect of SnF_2 mouthrinse on initial bacteria colonization of tooth enamel. J. Dent. Res. 56:1179, 1977.

11. Newman, M.G., and Goodman, A.D. (eds.) Guide to Antibiotic Use in Dental Practice. Chicago: Quintessence Publ. Co., 1984.

12. Silverstone, L.M. Personal communication, 1986.

13. Holm, G., Holst, K., and Mejare, I. The caries preventive effect of fluoride varnish in the fissures of the first permanent molar. Acta Odontol. 42(4):193, 1984.

14. Turpin-Mair, J.S., et al. The potential of a self-etching fluoride releasing composite. Quintessence Int. 14:(12): 1257–1272, 1983.

15. Zimmerman, B.F., Rawls, H.R., and Bassett, R.G. Fluoride release and physical properties of an experimental, resin-filled sealant. J. Dent. Res. 63:295, Abstr. 1116, 1984.

16. Whitford, G. Fluorides: mechanism of action, efficacy and safety, pp. 5–17. *In* Dental Caries Prevention in Public Health Programs. Bethesda: U.S. Dept. of Health and Human Services, 1981.

Glossary

Abrasion   The mechanical wearing away of tooth structure by forces other than mastication.

Abscess   A localized collection of pus in a cavity formed by the disintegration of tissue.

Abutment   The anchorage tooth used to support a fixed or removable prosthetic appliance.

Acute   Having a rapid onset, severe symptoms, short duration.

Acute herpetic gingivostomatitis   Viral infection of oral mucous membranes, characterized by formation of vesicles that rupture and form painful ulcers; may occur anywhere in the oral cavity.

Aeration   The exchange of carbon dioxide for oxygen by the blood in the lungs; the charging of a liquid with air or gas.

Aerobe   A microorganism that requires the presence of free oxygen to live and grow.

Ageusia   Absence or impairment of the sense of taste.

AIDS   Acquired immune deficiency syndrome; a breakdown of the immune system that renders the individual vulnerable to a variety of serious opportunistic diseases.

Amalgam   An alloy of silver, tin, copper, mercury, and sometimes zinc, used for dental restoration.

Amelogenesis imperfecta   Imperfect formation of enamel, resulting in brownish coloration and friability of the teeth.

Anaerobe   A microorganism that lives and grows in the absence of oxygen.   **facultative a.,** A microorganism that can live and grow with or without oxygen.   **obligate a.,** A microorganism that can grow only in the complete absence of oxygen.

Analgesia   Absence of sensibility to pain, particularly the relief of pain without loss of consciousness; absence of pain or noxious stimulation.

Anaphylaxis   A sudden, severe, unusual, or exaggerated allergic reaction of an organism to foreign protein or other substances; characterized by sudden shock, collapse, or respiratory and circulatory failure.

Anemia   A reduction below normal in the number or volume of erythrocytes or in the quantity of hemoglobin in the blood.

Anesthesia   Partial or total loss of sensation, with or without loss of consciousness, due to injury or disease, or induced by the administration of a drug.

Angioedema   A condition characterized by the sudden and temporary appearance of large areas of painless swelling in the subcutaneous tissue or submucosa, usually around the face.

Anorexia   Lack or loss of appetite for food; aversion to food.

Antibiotic   A chemical substance produced synthetically or by a microorganism that has the capacity, in dilute solutions, to kill or inhibit the growth of other microorganisms; used in the treatment of infectious diseases.

Antibody   A protein substance produced by the immune system in reaction to an invading microorganism or other cell.

Antigen   A substance that is foreign to the bloodstream or other body tissues and therefore stimulates the formation of specific blood serum antibodies and white cell activity.

Antiseptic   Any substance that inhibits the growth of bacteria.

Apex   The terminal end of the root of the tooth.

Aphthous ulcer   Canker sore; painful ulcer caused by rupture of a vesicle; a depressed spherical ulcer with an elevated border.

Apnea   Temporary cessation of breathing.

Armamentarium   The equipment and instruments utilized during a specific procedure.

Ascites   Abnormal accumulation of fluid within the peritoneal cavity.

Asepsis   Freedom from infection or infectious material; condition in which septic material is absent; absence of microorganisms.

Atrophy   Decrease in size of a normally developed organ or tissue; wasting away.

Attrition   Gradual wearing away of tooth structure as a result of mastication.

Auscultation   Listening for sounds produced within the body, performed with a stethoscope or the unaided ear.

Autoclave   A device for the sterilization of materials by steam under pressure.

Bacteremia   The presence of bacteria in the bloodstream.

Bactericidal   Destructive to bacteria.

Bacteriostatic   Capable of arresting the growth or multiplication of bacteria.

Biocidal   Destructive to living organisms.

Biopsy   Removal and examination, usually microscopic, of tissue from the living body, usually performed to determine whether a tumor is benign or malignant.

Bradycardia   Slowness of the heartbeat, as evidenced by slowing of the pulse rate to less than 60 per minute.

Bronchospasm   Spasmodic contraction of the muscular coat of the smaller divisions of the bronchi, such as occurs in asthma.

Calcification   The deposit of calcium salts in a tissue; process by which organic tissue becomes hardened by deposition of calcium and other inorganic salts within its substance.

Cancer   Any malignant, cellular tumor; neoplastic disease in which normal body cells are transformed into malignant ones.

Candidiasis   Infection by fungi of the genus *Candida*, generally *C. albicans*, most commonly involving the skin, oral mucosa (called thrush), respiratory tract, and vagina.

Canker sore   See *aphthous ulcer*.

Carcinoma   Malignant new growth made up of epithelial cells tending to infiltrate surrounding tissues and to give rise to metastases; a form of cancer.

Caries   See *dental caries*.

Cariogenic   Producing caries; said of certain foods.

Carious   Affected with decay or caries.

Carrier   One who harbors disease organisms in his body without manifest symptoms, thus acting as a carrier or distributor of infection.

Cataphoresis   The transmission of electronegative ions or drugs into body tissues or through a membrane by use of an electric current.

Chancre   The primary lesion of syphilis, occurring at the site of entry of the infection; begins as a papule that breaks down into a reddish ulcer, generally firm and accompanied by little or no pain; heals of its own accord.

Cheilitis   Inflammation of the lips.

Cheilosis   Fissuring and dry scaling of the vermilion surface of the lips and corners of the mouth, a characteristic of riboflavin deficiency.

Chemotherapy   Treatment or prevention of disease by means of chemical substances.

Chromogenic   Producing color or pigment.

Chronic   Persisting for a long time; situation showing little change or extremely slow progression over a long period.

Coagulation   Formation of a clot; change from a soluble into an insoluble protein.

Col   Concave depression of the interdental gingiva between the two peaks formed by the facial and lingual papillae.

Commissure   Angle of the lips or eyelids.

Congenital   Present at and existing from the time of birth.

Contagious   Capable of being transmitted from person to person.

Contamination   The soiling or making impure by mixture or contact, as by the introduction of microorganisms.

Corrosion   Act or process of deterioration, especially by chemical action.

Corticosteroid   Any of the hormones produced by the adrenal cortex; also, their synthetic equivalents. Called also adrenocortical hormone and adrenocorticosteroid.

Curettage   The cleansing of a diseased surface, using an instrument called a curet.

Cuspidor   Small bowl-shaped sink components of some dental units, used by patients for expectoration.

Cyanosis   Bluish discoloration of the skin and mucous membranes due to excessive concentration of reduced hemoglobin in the blood. Adjective: cyanotic.

Decalcification   Loss of or process of removing calcium salts.

Dehiscence   Isolated area in which a root is denuded of bone when the denuded area extends to the margin of the bone.

Dehydration   Removal of water from the body or tissue, or the condition that results from undue loss of water.

Dental caries   Destructive process causing decalcification of the tooth enamel, leading to continued destruction of enamel and denture, and cavitation of the tooth.

Dentinogenesis imperfecta   A hereditary condition marked by imperfect formation and calcification of dentin, giving the teeth a brown or blue opalescent appearance.

Desensitization   Prevention or reduction of sensitivity.

Desquamation   The shedding of epithelial elements in scales or sheets.

Diaphoresis   Perspiration, especially profuse perspiration.

Diastema   A space or cleft; in dentistry, a space between teeth.

Digital   Pertaining to the fingers.

Dilaceration   Abnormal curvature or angulation in the root or crown of a formed tooth.

Disinfection   Destruction of infection-producing organisms; usually refers to chemical substances that are used on inanimate objects.

Diuresis   Increased excretion of urine.

Dorsal   Directed toward or situated on the back surface; opposite of ventral.

Dyspnea   Labored or difficult breathing.

Edema   An abnormal accumulation of fluid in the intercellular spaces of the body.

Edentulous   Without teeth.

Embolism   The sudden blocking of an artery by a clot of foreign material (embolus) that has been brought to its site of lodgment by the blood current. The obstructing material is most often a blood clot, but may be a fat globule, air bubble, clump of bacteria, or piece of tissue.

Endemic   Disease that is present in a group of people or community at all times.

Endocardium   The endothelial lining membrane of the cavities of the heart and the connective tissue bed on which it lies.

Endocarditis   Exudative and proliferative inflammatory alterations of the endocardium, characterized by the presence of vegetations on the surface of the endocardium or in the endocardium itself, and most commonly involving a heart valve; may also affect the inner lining of the cardiac chambers or elsewhere on the endocardium.

Endotoxin   A heat-stable toxin present in the intact bacterial cell but not in cell-free filtrates of cultures of intact bacteria; lipopolysaccharide complexes that occur in the cell wall.

Enzyme   Any protein that acts as a catalyst, increasing the rate at which a chemical reaction occurs.

Erosion   The wasting away or loss of tooth structure by a chemical process that does not involve known bacterial action.

Erythema   Redness of the skin caused by congestion of the capillaries in the lower layers of the skin; occurs with any skin injury, infection, or inflammation.

Etiology   The science that deals with causes of disease.

Exostosis   A bony outgrowth projecting from a bone surface.

Exudate   A fluid with a high content of protein and cellular debris that has escaped from blood vessels and has been deposited in tissues or on tissue surfaces, usually as a result of inflammation.

Fenestration   Isolated area in which a root is denuded of bone when the marginal bone is intact.

Fibrillation   A small, local, involuntary muscular contraction due to spontaneous activation of single muscular cells or muscle fibers; a cardiac arrhythmia marked by rapid randomized contractions of the atrial myocardium, causing a totally irregular, often rapid, ventricular rate.

Fluorosis   A condition due to ingestion of excessive amounts of fluorine or its compounds. Dental fluorosis is an enamel hypoplasia resulting from prolonged ingestion of drinking water containing high levels of fluoride, manifested by a mottled discoloration of the teeth.

Frenum   A small fold of mucous membrane passing between two anatomical structures, one of them more fixed, serving to check undue movement of the movable one.

Furcation   Area lying between and at the base of two or more anatomically divided roots.

Gastrointestinal   Pertaining to the stomach and intestine.

Germicide   An agent that destroys pathogenic organisms.

Gingivectomy   Surgical excision of infected and diseased gingival tissue to eliminate periodontal pockets.

Gingivitis   Inflammation of the gingiva.

Glomerulonephritis   A variety of nephritis characterized by inflammation of the capillary loops in the glomeruli of the kidney. Occurs in acute, subacute, and chronic forms and is usually secondary to an infection, especially with the hemolytic streptococcus.

Glycoprotein   Any of a class of conjugated proteins consisting of a compound of protein with a carbohydrate group.

Grand mal   A major epileptic seizure attended by loss of consciousness and convulsive movements (as distinguished from petit mal, a minor seizure).

Granulation   The formation in wounds of small, rounded masses of tissue during healing; also the mass so formed.

Halitosis   Offensive odor of the breath.

Hemangioma   A benign tumor made up of newly formed blood vessels, clustered together. In most cases, it appears as a network of small blood-filled capillaries near the surface of the skin, forming a reddish or purplish mark.

Hematoma   A localized collection of clotted blood that accumulates in an organ, space, or tissue. Bruises are common examples.

Hemoglobin   The oxygen-bearing protein of red blood cells; it is bright red when saturated with oxygen and purple when it is not carrying oxygen.

Hemophilia   A condition characterized by impaired coagulability of the blood, and a strong tendency to bleed.

Hemorrhage   The escape of the blood from a ruptured vessel; bleeding.

Hepatitis   Inflammation of the liver.

Herpes simplex   An acute viral disease marked by groups of vesicles on the skin, often on the borders of the lips, nose, or genitalia.

Herpes zoster   An acute viral disease characterized by inflammation of spinal ganglia and by a vesicular eruption along the area of distribution of a sensory nerve, caused by the virus of chickenpox; also called shingles.

Hodgkin's disease   A primary lymph node neoplastic disease characterized by painless, progressive enlargement of the lymph nodes, spleen, and lymphoid tissues generally, which often begins in a cervical node on the side of the neck and spreads through the body.

Hyperglycemia   Excess of glucose in the blood.

Hyperparathyroidism   Excessive secretion of parathyroid hormone.

Hyperplasia   Abnormal increase in volume of a tissue or organ caused by the formation and growth of new normal cells.

Hypertension   Persistently high blood pressure.

Hyperthyroidism   Condition caused by excessive production or ingestion of thyroid hormone; the most common symptoms include weight loss, increased appetite, rapid heart rate, tremor, and fatigue.

Hypertonic Pertaining to or characterized by an increased tonicity or tension; having an osmotic pressure greater than that of the solution with which it is compared.

Hypertrophy Increase in volume of a tissue or organ produced entirely by enlargement of existing cells.

Hyperventilation Abnormally prolonged and deep breathing, usually associated with acute anxiety or emotional tension.

Hypoglycemia An abnormally low level of sugar in the blood.

Hypoparathyroidism Condition caused by lack of parathyroid secretion, resulting in reduced plasma calcium level and increased plasma phosphate level.

Hypopituitarism A condition due to abnormally diminished production of anterior pituitary hormones caused by destruction of the pituitary gland; it leads to atrophy of the thyroid and adrenal glands and the gonads.

Hypoplasia Incomplete development or underdevelopment of an organ or tissue.

Hypotension Consistently low blood pressure.

Hypovolemia Abnormally decreased volume of circulating fluid (plasma) in the body.

Hypoxia Diminished availability of oxygen to the body tissues.

Iatrogenic Any adverse or inadvertent diagnosis and/or treatment by a professional.

Idiopathic Self-originated; occurring without known cause.

Immunity The condition of being highly resistant to a disease because of the formation of humoral antibodies or the development of immunologically competent cells, or both, or as a result of some other mechanism (e.g., interferon activities in viral infections).

Immunoglobulin A protein of animal origin with known antibody activity; synthesized by lymphocytes and plasma cells and found in the serum and in other body fluids and tissues.

Incipient Beginning to exist; coming into existence.

Infarct A localized area of ischemic necrosis produced by occlusion of the arterial blood supply or the venous drainage of the part.

Inflammation A localized protective response elicited by injury or destruction of tissues, which serves to destroy, dilute, or wall off both the injurious agent and the injured tissue. Characterized by heat, redness, swelling, pain, and loss of function.

Infrabony Beneath the level of the bone.

Insidious Of gradual and subtle development; coming on imperceptibly.

Insomnia Abnormal wakefulness; an inability to fall asleep easily or to remain asleep throughout the night.

Intramuscular Within the muscular substance; an injection made into the substance of a muscle.

Intravenous Within a vein.

Iontophoresis The introduction of ions of soluble salts into the body by an electric current.

Ischemia Deficiency of blood in a part, due to functional constriction or actual obstruction of a blood vessel.

In vitro In an artificial environment, as in a test tube.

In vivo Within the living body.

Jaundice Yellowness of skin, sclerae, mucous membranes, and excretions resulting from deposition of bile pigments in the blood and skin.

Keratin A protein material formed as a transformation product of the cellular proteins of the flat cells on the surface of the epithelium; a form of protective adaptation to function.

Keratinization Process of formation of a horny protective layer on the surface of stratified squamous epithelium, especially on the epidermis and masticatory oral mucosa.

Laceration A wound produced by the tearing of body tissue.

Lavage To wash out or irrigate.

Lesion Any pathological or traumatic discontinuity of tissue or loss of function of a part.

Leukemia A progressive, malignant disease of the blood-forming organs, marked by distorted proliferation and development of leukocytes and their precursors in the blood and bone marrow.

Leukocyte A white blood corpuscle capable of ameboid movement whose chief function is to protect the body against disease-causing microorganisms; may be classified in two main groups: granular (basophils, eosinophils, neutrophils) and nongranular (lymphocytes, monocytes).

Leukoplakia White patches formed on the oral mucous membranes from surface epithelial cells; a potentially malignant lesion, characterized by hyperkeratosis of the stratified squamous epithelium.

Lumen The cavity or channel within a tube or tubular organ, as a blood vessel or the intestine.

Macroglossia Excessive size of the tongue.

Malaise A feeling of uneasiness or indisposition.

Malignant Tending to become progressively worse and to result in death; having the properties of anaplasia, invasiveness, and metastasis; said of tumors.

Malocclusion Malposition of the teeth resulting in the faulty meeting of the teeth or jaws.

Mandible The horseshoe-shaped bone forming the lower jaw.

Mastication The act of chewing.

Matrix The intercellular substance of a tissue, as bone matrix, or the tissue from which a structure develops.

Maxilla One of two identical bones that form the upper jaw.

Meninges The three membranes covering the brain and spinal cord: the dura mater, arachnoid, and pia mater.

Metastasis The transfer of disease from one organ or part to another not directly connected with it.

Microglossia   Abnormal smallness of the tongue.

Mucositis   Inflammation of mucous membranes.

Myocardium   The middle and thickest layer of the heart wall, composed of cardiac muscle.

Necrosis   Death of tissue within a circumscribed area.

Neoplasm   Any new and abnormal growth, specifically one in which cell multiplication is uncontrolled and progressive; may be benign or malignant.

Nephritis   Inflammation of the kidney.

Nidus   Point of origin of a process.

Obturator   A disk or plate that closes an opening.

Occlusion   The act of closure or state of being closed; an obstruction or a closing off; the relation of the teeth of both jaws when in functional contact during activity of the mandible.

Oropharyngeal   Pertaining to the oropharynx, the part of the pharynx between the soft palate and the upper edge of the epiglottis.

Orthopnea   Ability to breathe easily only in the upright position.

Osseous   Of the nature or quality of bone; bony.

Osteomyelitis   Inflammation of bone.

Osteoporosis   Abnormal loss of density of bone.

Palliative   Affording relief; also, a drug that so acts.

Pallor   Paleness, as of the skin.

Palpation   The act of feeling with the hand; in physical diagnosis, the application of the fingers with light pressure to the surface of the body for the purpose of determining the condition of the parts beneath.

Palpitation   A heartbeat that is unusually rapid, strong, or irregular enough to make a person aware of it, usually over 120 per minute, as compared to the normal 60 to 100.

Parenteral   By means other than the alimentary canal; e.g., by subcutaneous, intramuscular, intrasternal, or intravenous means.

Paresthesia   An abnormal sensation, as burning, tingling, or numbness.

Parotid glands   Largest of the three main pairs of salivary glands, located on either side of the face, just below and in front of the ears.

Patent ductus arteriosus   Abnormal persistence of an open lumen in the ductus arteriosus, between the aorta and the pulmonary artery, after birth.

Pemphigus   Any skin disease characterized by severe blistering.

Pericardium   The fibroserous sac enclosing the heart and the roots of the great vessels.

Pericoronitis   Acute inflammation of the soft tissue adjacent to a partially erupted tooth.

Periodontitis   Inflammation of the periodontium.

Periodontium   The tissues investing and supporting the teeth, including the cementum, alveolar bone, periodontal ligament, and gingiva.

Peritoneum   The serous membrane lining the walls of the abdominal and pelvic cavities (parietal peritoneum) and investing contained viscera (visceral peritoneum), the two layers enclosing a potential space, the peritoneal cavity.

Petechia   A minute, pinpoint, nonraised, perfectly round, purplish red spot caused by intradermal or submucous hemorrhage, which later turns blue or yellow.

Petit mal   A relatively mild epileptic attack (contrasted with grand mal, a major seizure).

Pharynx   The throat; the musculomembranous cavity, about 12.5 cm long, behind the nasal cavities, mouth, and larynx, communicating with them and with the esophagus.

Placebo   A substance given to a patient as medicine or a procedure performed on a patient that has no intrinsic therapeutic value and relieves symptoms or helps the patient in some way only because the patient believes or expects that it will.

Plasma   The fluid portion of the blood in which corpuscles are suspended.

Pneumonitis   Inflammation of lung tissue.

Polymerization   The chemical joining of similar monomers to form a compound of a high molecular weight.

Polyp   Any growth or mass protruding from a mucous membrane.

Polyuria   Excessive excretion of urine.

Pontic   The suspended member of a fixed partial denture, replacing the lost tooth. It restores function and usually occupies the space previously filled by the lost tooth.

Preauricular   In front of the auricle of the ear.

Premedication   Preliminary medication, usually of a drug, administered before an operation is performed, to prevent untoward results as a consequence of the operation.

Prodrome   A symptom indicating the onset of a disease.

Prognosis   A forecast of the probable cause and outcome of an attack of disease and the prospects of recovery as indicated by the nature of the disease and the symptoms of the case.

Prone   Lying face downward.

Prophylaxis   Prevention of disease; preventive treatment.

Pruritus   Itching.

Pseudomembrane   False membrane.

Psychosomatic   Referring to the influence of the mind over the body; specifically, physical symptoms that have an emotional or mental origin.

Pterygomandibular   Pertaining to the pterygoid process and the mandible.

Purpura   A hemorrhagic disease characterized by extravasation of blood into the tissues, under the skin, and through the mucous membranes, and producing spontaneous ecchymoses (bruises) and petechiae (small red patches) on the skin.

Purulent Containing or forming pus.

Pus A protein-rich inflammation product composed of cells (leukocytes), a thin fluid (liquor puris), and cellular debris.

Quadrant One fourth of the circumference of a circle; any one of the four quarters of the dentition, with the dividing line of the maxillary or mandibular teeth at the midline between the central incisors.

Raphe A seam; used in anatomical nomenclature as a general term to designate the line of union of the halves of various symmetrical parts.

Rarefaction The condition of being or becoming less dense.

Recession Gradual drawing away of a tissue or part from its normal position.

Resection Excision or removal of a portion of an organ or other structure.

Resorption Removal of bone or tooth structure by pressure.

Retromolar Behind the molar; the bony area immediately posterior to the terminal posterior tooth.

Rheumatic fever A disease associated with the presence of hemolytic streptococci in the body, so called because two of the commonest symptoms are fever and pain in the joints, similar to that of rheumatism.

Ruga A ridge or fold; palatal rugae are the irregular ridges in the mucous membrane covering the anterior portion of the hard palate.

Sarcoma A tumor, often highly malignant, composed of cells derived from connective tissue such as bone, cartilage, muscle, blood vessel, or lymphoid tissue.

Sclerosis An induration, or hardening; especially hardening of a part from inflammation and in disease of the interstitial substance.

Septum A wall or partition dividing a body space or cavity.

Serous Thin and watery, like serum.

Serum As in blood serum, the clear, straw-colored liquid portion of the plasma that does not contain fibrinogen or blood cells, and remains fluid after clotting of blood.

Slough To shed or cast off.

Slurry A suspension of a solid in a liquid.

Sonic Of or pertaining to sound; noting or pertaining to a speed equal to that of sound in air at the same height above sea level.

Sphygmomanometer An instrument for measuring arterial blood pressure.

Spore A refractile, oval body formed within bacteria, especially Bacillus and Clostridium, which is regarded as a resting stage during the life history of the cell and is characterized by its resistance to environmental changes.

Sporicidal Capable of killing spores.

Stenosis Narrowing or contraction of a body passage or opening.

Stensen's duct Excretory passage for the parotid salivary gland.

Sterilization Process by which all forms of life are destroyed; freedom from all microorganisms and their pathogenic products.

Stomatitis Inflammation of the mucosa of the mouth, of which gingivitis and glossitis are forms.

Subcutaneous Beneath the layers of the skin.

Subgingival Below the margin of the gingiva.

Submental Below the chin.

Sulcus A groove or furrow; the gingival sulcus refers to the groove or space between the surface of the tooth and the epithelium lining the free gingiva.

Suppuration Formation or discharge of pus.

Suprabony Above the level of the bone.

Supragingival Above the margin of the gingiva.

Suture The line of union of adjoining bones of the skull; a stitch or series of stitches made to secure apposition of the edges of a surgical or traumatic wound; used also as a verb to indicate application of such stitches; material used in closing a wound with stitches.

Syncope A temporary suspension of consciousness due to cerebral anemia; fainting.

Syndrome A combination of symptoms resulting from a single cause or so commonly occurring together as to constitute a distinct clinical picture.

Systemic Pertaining to or affecting the body as a whole.

Tachycardia Abnormally rapid heart rate, usually taken to be above 100 beats per minute.

Tactile Pertaining to touch.

Telangiectasia Dilation of a group of capillaries.

Tenacious Adhesive; viscid.

Thrombocytopenia Decrease in number of platelets in circulating blood.

Thrombosis Formation, development, or presence of a thrombus.

Thrombus An aggregation of blood factors, primarily platelets and fibrin with entrapment of cellular elements, frequently causing vascular obstruction at the point of its formation.

Titer The quantity of a substance required to react with or to correspond to a given amount of another substance.

Topography A special description of an anatomic region or a special part.

Torus A swelling or bulging projection.

Toxin A poison, especially a protein or conjugated protein produced by certain animals, some higher plants, and pathogenic bacteria.

Trauma A wound or injury, especially damage produced by external force.

Tremor An involuntary trembling of the body or limbs.

Trismus Motor disturbance of the trigeminal nerve, especially spasm of the masticatory muscles, with difficulty in opening the mouth.

Ulcer   A local defect, or excavation, of the surface of an organ or tissue, produced by sloughing of necrotic inflammatory tissue.

Ultrasonic   Beyond the audible range; relating to sound waves having a frequency of more than 20,000 cycles per second.

Uvula   A pendant, fleshy mass of the soft palate.

Valvulitis   Inflammation of a valve, especially of a valve of the heart.

Vasodilator   Causing dilation of blood vessels.

Ventral   Directed toward or situated on the front surface.

Vesicle   A small bladder or sac containing liquid; a small circumscribed elevation of the epidermis containing a serous fluid; a small blister.

Virulence   The degree of pathogenicity of a microorganism as indicated by case fatality rates and/or its ability to invade the tissues of the host; the competence of any infectious agent to produce pathologic effects.

Whitlow   A purulent infection involving the pulp of the distal phalanx of a finger.

Xerostomia   Dryness of the mouth from lack of normal secretion.

Xiphoid process   The pointed process of cartilage, supported by a core of bone, connected with the lower end of the body of the sternum.

General references

ADA Council on Dental Therapeutics. Accepted Dental Therapeutics. 39th ed. Chicago: American Dental Association, 1982.

Alban, A. An improved Snyder test. J. Dent. Res. 49:641, 1970.

Allen, D.L., McFall, W.T., and Hunter, G.C. Periodontics for the Dental Hygienist, 3rd ed. Philadelphia: Lea & Febiger, 1980.

American College of Surgeons. Early Care of the Injured Patient, 3rd ed. Philadelphia: W.B. Saunders Co., 1983.

Ball, R.O., Zucker, S.B., and Fretwell, L.D. Teaching preventive dentistry to patients with impaired vision. J. Dent. Handicap. 4(1):23–25, 1978.

Baran, S. The camera is a valuable dental tool. J. Am. Dent. Assoc. 104(1):410, 1981.

Berkow, R. (ed.) The Merck Manual. Vol I. General Medicine, 14th ed. Rahway, N.J.: Merck & Co., 1982.

Bickley, H.C. Practical Concepts in Human Disease, 2nd ed. Baltimore: Williams & Wilkins Co., 1980.

Blair, D.M., and Contrell, J.R. Symposium on medical emergencies in the dental office. Dent. Clin. North America. 26(1): 1982.

Braun, R.J. Dentist's Manual of Emergency Medical Treatment. Reston, Va.: Reston Publ. Co., 1979.

Cain, H.D. Flint's Emergency Treatment and Management, 7th ed. Philadelphia: W.B. Saunders Co., 1984.

Castano, F.A., and Alden, B.A. (eds.) Handbook of Clinical Dental Auxiliary Practice, 3rd ed. Philadelphia: J.B. Lippincott Co., 1980.

Christen, A.G., and Harris, N.O. Primary Preventive Dentistry. Reston, Va.: Reston Publ. Co., 1982.

Enlow, D.H. A Handbook of Facial Growth, 2nd ed. Philadelphia: W.B. Saunders Co., 1982.

Ericksen, H.M., et al. Chemical plaque control and extrinsic tooth discoloration. J. Clin. Periodontol. 12:343–350, 1985.

Fitch, M.A., and Moxley, R.A. Changing Patient Behavior: a Behavioral Modification Manual for Dental Professionals, 2nd ed. Lakewood, Colo.: RAM Press, 1984.

Freehe, C.L. Photography in dentistry: equipment and technique. Dent. Clin. North Am. 27(1):3–73, 1983.

Geboy, M.J. Communication and Behavior Management in Dentistry. Baltimore: Williams & Wilkins Co., 1985.

Glickman, I. Clinical Periodontology, 6th ed. Philadelphia: W.B. Saunders Co., 1984.

Goerig, A.C., and Mathias, J.H. A practical approach to clinical photography. Quintessence Int. 13(5):581–584, 1982.

Goerig, A.C., and Mathias, J.H. A practical approach to clinical photography. II. Quintessence Int. 13(6):679–684, 1982.

Goerig, A.C., and Mathias, J.H. A practical approach to clinical photography. III. Quintessence Int. 13(7):783–686, 1982.

Goldman, H.M., Shuman, A.M., and Isenberg, G.A. An Atlas of the Surgical Management of Periodontal Disease. Chicago: Quintessence Publ. Co., 1982.

Grant, D.A., Stern, I.B., and Everett, F.G. Periodontics in the Tradition of Orban and Gottlieb, 5th ed. St. Louis: C.V. Mosby Co., 1979.

Horowitz, A.M., and Thomas, H.B. (eds.) Dental Caries Prevention in Public Health Programs. Bethesda: U.S. Dept. of Health and Human Services, 1981.

Horowitz, A.M., and Wei, S.H. Fluoride: An Update for the Dental Practice. New York: Medcom, Inc., 1976.

Huff, B.B. (ed.) Physicians' Desk Reference, 40th ed. Oradell, N.J.: Medical Economics Co., 1986.

Huntley, D.E., and Ralston, B.J. A plaque control program for blind patients. J. Dent. Handicap. 3(1):23–26, 1977.

Illinois Department of Public Health, Division of Dental Health. A Guide To Oral Hygiene For Long Term Care Facilities, 1979.

Judd, R.L., and Ponsell, D.D. The First Responder: The Critical First Minutes. St. Louis: C.V. Mosby Co., 1982.

Kerr, D.A., and Ash, M.M., Jr. Oral Pathology: An Introduction to General and Oral Pathology for Hygienists, 4th ed. Philadelphia: Lea & Febiger, 1978.

Krasse, B. Caries Risk: A Practical Guide for Assessment

and Control. Chicago: Quintessence Publ. Co., 1985.

Lange, B.M., Entwistle, B.M., and Lipson, L.F. Dental Management of the Handicapped: Approaches for Dental Auxiliaries. Philadelphia: Lea & Febiger, 1983.

Ligh, R.Q. The visually handicapped patients in dental practice. the J. Dent. Handicap. 4(2):38–40, 1979.

Little, J.W., and Falace, D.A. Dental Management of the Medically Compromised Patient, 2nd ed. St. Louis: C.V. Mosby Co., 1982.

McDonald, R.E., and Avery, D.R. Dentistry for the Child and Adolescent, 4th ed. St. Louis: C.V. Mosby Co., 1983.

Menaker, L. (ed.) Biological Basis of Dental Caries: an Oral Biology Textbook. Philadelphia: J.B. Lippincott Co. (Harper Medical), 1980.

Miller, B.F., and Keane, C.B. Encyclopedia and Dictionary of Medicine, Nursing and Allied Health, 3rd ed. Philadelphia: W.B. Saunders Co., 1983.

Mueller, K., and Grant, D. Communicating with the deaf patient. J. Dent. Handicap. 3(2):22, 1978.

Nanda, S.K. The Developmental Basis of Occlusion and Malocclusion. Chicago: Quintessence Publ. Co., 1983.

Nelson, L.C. Photography in the dental office. Dent. Clin. North Am. 27(1):178–190, 1983.

Newbrun, E. Cariology, 2nd ed. Baltimore: Williams & Wilkins Co., 1983.

Nield, J.S., and O'Connor, G.H. Fundamentals of Dental Hygiene Instrumentation. Philadelphia: W.B. Saunders Co., 1983.

Nizel, A.E. Nutrition in Preventive Dentistry, 2nd ed. Philadelphia: W.B. Saunders Co., 1980.

Nowak, A.J. Dentistry For The Handicapped Patient. St. Louis: C.V. Mosby Co., 1976.

Page, R.C. Oral health status in the United States: prevalence of inflammatory periodontal diseases. J. Dent. Educ. 49(6):354–363, 1985.

Palmer, C., Cassidy, M., and Larsen, C. Nutrition, Diet and Dental Health: Concepts and Methods. Chicago: American Dental Hygienists Association, 1981.

Pattison, G.L., and Pattison, A.M. Periodontal Instrumentation: a Clinical Manual. Reston, Va.: Reston Publ. Co., 1979.

Pawlak, E.A., and Hoag, P.M. Essentials of Periodontics, 3rd ed. St. Louis: C.V. Mosby Co., 1984.

Phagan, P.A. Preventive Dentistry: a Manual for the Dental Hygienist. Milan: Dental Science and Technique International, 1985.

Phagan, P.A. Practical clinical applications of current concepts of disease prevention. 11th Asia Pacific Dental Congress Newsletter, Nov., 1984.

Pollack, R.L., and Kravitz, E. (eds.) Nutrition in Oral Health and Disease. Philadelphia: Lea & Febiger, 1985.

Ramfjord, S.P., and Ash, M.M., Jr. Periodontology and Periodontics. Philadelphia: W.B. Saunders Co., 1979.

Randolph, P.M., and Dennison, C.D. Diet, Nutrition and Dentistry. St. Louis: C.V. Mosby Co., 1981.

Robbins, S.L., Cotran, R., and Kumar, V. Pathologic Basis of Disease, 3rd ed. Philadelphia: W. B. Saunders Co., 1984.

Rose, L.F., and Kaye, D. (eds.) Internal Medicine for Dentistry. St. Louis: C.V. Mosby Co., 1983.

Shafer, W.G., Hine, M.K., and Levy, B.M. A Textbook of Oral Pathology, 4th ed. Philadephia: W.B. Saunders Co., 1983.

Silverstone, L.M. Fluorides and remineralization, pp. 153–175. In Wei, S.H. (ed.) Clinical Uses of Fluorides: a State of the Art Conference on the Uses of Fluorides in Clinical Dentistry. Philadelphia: Lea & Febiger, 1985.

Silverstone, L. Preventive Dentistry. London: Update Books, 1978.

Simon, R.R., and Brenner, B.E. Procedures and Techniques in Emergency Medicine. Baltimore: Williams & Wilkins Co., 1982.

Sims, W. The interpretation and use of Snyder's tests and lactobacillus counts. J. Am. Dent. Assoc. 80:1315, 1970.

Sonis, S.T., Fazio, R.C., and Fang, L. Principles and Practice of Oral Medicine. Philadelphia: W.B. Saunders Co., 1984.

Special Report: National Preventive Dentistry Demonstration Program. Princeton: Robert Wood Johnson Foundation, 1983.

Tepe, J.H., et al. The long term effect of chlorhexidine on plaque, gingivitis, sulcus depth, gingival recession and loss of attachment in beagle dogs. J. Periodont. Res. 18(6):452–458, 1983.

The Camera Book. New York: American Photographic Book Publ. Co., 1985.

Thomas, C.L. (ed.) Taber's Cyclopedic Medical Dictionary, 15th ed. Philadelphia: F.A. Davis Co., 1985.

Walsh, M.M., and Robertson, P.B. Professional mechanical oral hygiene practice and control of periodontal diseases. Calif. Dent. Assoc. J. 12:58–62, 1985.

Wander, D. Photography. I. Uses in general dental practice. Dental Update 10(5):297–304, 1983.

Wander, D. Photography. II. Close-ups: principles and equipment. Dental Update 10(6):357–364, 1983.

Wander, D. Photography. III. Obtaining results. Dental Update 10(6):417–429, 1983.

Ward, H.L., and Simring, M.R. Manual of Clinical Periodontics, 2nd ed. St. Louis: C.V. Mosby Co., 1978.

Wei, S.H., et al. Caries activity tests. I.A.D.R. abstract no. 839, 1973.

Weinstein, P., Getz, T., and Milgram, P. Oral Self Care: Strategies for Preventive Dentistry. Reston, Va.: Reston Publishing Co., 1985.

Wessels, K.E. (ed.) Dentistry for the Handicapped Patient. Littleton, Mass.: John Wright-PSG, 1978.

Wilkins, E.M. Clinical Practice of the Dental Hygienist, 5th ed. Philadelphia: Lea & Febiger, 1983.
Wilkins, E.W., Jr. MGH Textbook of Emergency Medicine, 2nd ed. Baltimore: Williams & Wilkins, 1983.
Williams, S.R. Nutrition and Diet Therapy, 5th ed. St. Louis: Times Mirror/Mosby, 1985.

Wood, N.K., and Goaz, P.W. Differential Diagnosis of Oral Lesions, 2nd ed. St. Louis: C.V. Mosby Co., 1975.
Woodall, I.R., et al. Comprehensive Dental Hygiene Care, 2nd ed. St. Louis: C.V. Mosby Co., 1985.
Zwemer, T.J. (ed.) Boucher's Clinical Dental Terminology, 3rd ed. St. Louis: C.V. Mosby Co., 1982.

Other resources

Abbott Laboratories HTLV-III EIA
Blood Screening Test
800-323-9100

AIDS

AIDS Bibliography
National Institute of Allergy and Infectious Disease
Office of Scientific Director
Building 5 Room 135
National Institutes of Health
9000 Rockville Pike
Bethesda, Md. 20205

"Facts about AIDS"
U.S. Public Health Service
Office of Public Affairs
Room 7210
200 Independence Ave. S.W.
Washington, D.C. 20201

U.S. Public Health Service—Hot Line
800-342-AIDS

Associations and government agencies

American Association for Cancer Education
100 Bergen St.
Newark, N.J. 07103

American Cancer Society
90 Park Ave.
New York, N.Y. 10016

American Cancer Society
37 S. Wabash Ave.
Chicago, Ill. 60603

American Dental Association
Council on Dental Materials, Instruments and Equipment
211 East Chicago Ave.
Chicago, Ill. 60611
(312) 440-2500

American Diabetes Association
2 Park Ave.
New York, N.Y. 10016

American Epilepsy Society
179 Allyn St.
Suite 304
Hartford, Conn. 06103

American Heart Association
7320 Greenville Ave.
Dallas, Tex. 75231

American Public Health Association
1015 15th St. N.W.
Washington, D.C. 20009

American Society of Hematology
6900 Grove Rd.
Thorofare, N.J. 08086

American Society of Maxillofacial Surgeons
120 Oak Brook Center Mall
Suite 722
Oak Brook, Ill. 60521

Baby Bottle Tooth Decay
Centers for Disease Control
Dental Disease Prevention Activity
Center For Preventive Services
Atlanta, Ga. 30333
(404) 329-1830

National Cancer Institute
U.S. Department of Health and Human Services
Public Health Services
National Institutes of Health
Bethesda, Md. 20205

National Foundation of Dentistry for the Handicapped
1250 14th St. Suite 610
Denver, Colo. 80202

Publications

Close Up Photography and Photomacrography
Publication N-12
Eastman Kodak
Rochester, N.Y.

Fluoride and Dental Health Pamphlet
Dental Disease Prevention Activity
Center for Prevention Services
Centers for Disease Control
Atlanta, Ga. 30333
(404) 329-1830

Handbook for Scientific Photography
Alfred A. Blaker
W.H. Freeman and Co.
San Francisco, California

Manual of Close-Up Photography
Lester Lefkowitz
AM Photo
Garden City, New Jersey

Nutrition (pamphlet):
NIH Publication 81-2079
National Institutes of Health
9000 Rockville Pike
Bethesda, Md. 20205

Radiation, Chemotherapy and
  Dental Health (pamphlet):
NIH Publication 81-2090
National Institutes of Health
9000 Rockville Pike
Bethesda, Md. 20205

Water Fluoridation Course
Homestudy Services Branch
Center for Professional Development
  and Training
Centers for Disease Control
Atlanta, Ga. 30333

Index

A

AIDS	24, 25
Acquired immune deficiency syndrome. See AIDS.	
Airway obstruction	76, 78, 80, 81, 86
Alcoholism	115, 116
American Dental Association, Council on Dental Therapeutics,	15
Seal of Approval	203
American Heart Association	76, 81
American Joint Committee on Cancer	45
American Red Cross	76
Anesthetics, local	85
Angina pectoris	84
Antibiotics,	
plaque control by	181
premedication indications	31
regimen summary	34
Antimicrobials	182
Antiseptics	182
Anxiety	70
Aphthae	22
Asthma	86

B

Balsa wood wedge	175, 176
Basic life support	76, 77, 78, 79, 80, 81
Bite, wax	89
Blood pressure	35, 36, 37
Body temperature	36

C

Calculus	127, 128, 129
Cancer,	
chemotherapy management	113
nutrition counseling	112
oral changes with chemotherapy	113
oral changes with radiation	111
oral changes with surgery	111
posttreatment phase	114
pretreatment phase	111
radiation management	113
surgical management	113
treatment phase	113
treatment planning	110–114
xerostomia	111, 112
Cancer, oral,	
clinical staging	45
cytology	94, 95
detection	45
Carcinoma,	
adeno-	46
adenoid cystic	47
squamous cell	46
Cardiac arrest	84
Cardiopulmonary resuscitation (CPR),	
for children	80
procedures	76, 77, 78, 79, 80, 81
Caries,	
etiology	160
fluoride storage by	190
fluoride therapy	190, 191
nursing bottle	163

remineralization   190, 191
   zones of   190, 191
Caries Activity Tests   161
Cerebral vascular accident   80
Charting. *See* Dental record.
Consciousness, altered state   80, 82, 83
Crossbite   61

D

Dental deposits, composition   124–129
Dental disease, control   160–189
Dental floss,
   adjuncts for   170, 171
   Superfloss®   172, 174
   use procedures   168, 169
Dental hygiene,
   efficiency optimization   118–123
   motions   119
   procedures   118–123
   sequencing   118
   therapy phase   116
Dental hygienist,
   as periodontal co-therapist 130–146
   patient education by   163
   positioning   119, 120, 121, 122, 123
   tooth polishing effects   154
Dental Plaque Index   57
Dental record,
   dentition abnormalities   65, 66, 67, 68
   of emergency care   76
   periodontal probing   53
   photography for   96–103
   plaque control   56
   tooth numbering   64
Dentifrices   183, 202
Dentition,
   abnormalities   65, 66, 67, 68
   clinical examination   62, 63, 65, 66
   existing restorations   65
Denture cleansers   177
Diabetes   82, 109
Disease transmission, control of   12–30
Disinfection methods   16, 17

E

Emergencies,
   action plan   71

cardiovascular   84, 85
causes   70
drug list   74, 75
equipment for   72, 73, 74, 75
local anesthetic   85
medico-legal aspects   76
office manual   71, 72
oxygen-delivering systems   72, 73
preparation for   70–87, 71
specific   80, 82, 83, 84, 85, 86, 87
team approach   71
Epilepsy   87, 110
Examination, clinical,   40
   armamentarium   40, 130–146
   cytology   94, 95
   dentition   62, 63, 65, 66
   extraoral   40, 41, 42
   gingiva   49, 52, 53, 54, 55
   intraoral   40, 41, 42
   lips   42, 43
   occlusion   58, 59, 60, 61
   palate   43
   supplemental components   88–103
   tongue   44
   vestibule   42, 43

F

Fear   70
Fluoridation   192, 204
Fluoride therapy,   190–205
   acidulated phosphate-fluoride (APF)   193, 194
   dentifrices   202
   dietary supplement   202
   iontophoresis   198, 199, 200
   mouthrinse   202, 203
   paint-on technique   196, 197
   self-applied gel   202
   sodium fluoride   195
   stannous fluoride   195
   subgingival irrigation   201
   systemic   192
   timed-release fluoride   201
   topical   193
   toxicity   203
   tray technique   195, 196, 197, 203
Fluorides,
   daily dosage   204
   water supply content   204

Food debris 125
Food diary 162
Food guide, basic-four 162
Foreign body 80, 81, 85

G

Gauze strip 170, 171
Gingiva,
    clinical examination 49, 52, 53, 54, 55
    stimulation 172, 175, 176
Gingival Index 57
Gingivitis Index (GI) 57
Gingivostomatitis, herpetic 21
Gonorrhea 26

H

Health assessment 31–69
Health hazards 12–30
Heart failure, acute congestive 84
Heimlich maneuver 80, 81
Hematological disorders 108, 109
Hepatitis 17
Hepatitis A 17, 18
Hepatitis B 18, 19, 20
Hepatitis, non-A, non-B 20
Herpes simplex, 21, 23
    Type I oral herpes 21
    Type II venereal herpes 22
Hormonal imbalance 114, 115
Hyperglycemic hyperosmolar nonketotic
    coma (HHNK) 82
Hypersensitivity control 150
Hypertension 85
Hyperventilation 86
Hypoglycemia 82

I

Impressions,
    cast separation 91, 92
    pouring 90
    procedures for taking 88, 89, 90
Instruments,
    gingival curettage 140–145
    hand 130–146
    root planing 139, 140, 141

subgingival debridement 134, 135
supragingival debridement 132, 133
Interocclusal record 89
Iontophoresis 198, 199, 200

L

Lactobacillus acidophilus count 161
Lichen planus 114, 115
Life support 76, 77, 78, 79, 80, 81
Lighting 123
Lips, clinical examination 42, 43
Lupus erythematosus 114, 115
Lymphoma 46, 47

M

Materia alba 125
Medical consult form 38, 39
Medical history, 31, 32, 33, 69
    form 32, 33
    past dental treatment 38
Medications, prescribed 34
Melanoma 47, 48
Mercury poisoning 27, 28
Monitored Modulated Therapy 144
Mouthrinse, fluoride 202, 203
Myocardial infarction, acute 84

N

Nutrition 112, 161

O

Occlusion, clinical examination 58, 59, 60, 61
Office Emergency Procedures—
    Self-Study Course 72
O'Leary's Local Irritant Index 56, 57
Operating zone 121, 122
Operatory, preparation of 12
Oral health, maintenance 159–205
Oral hygiene, for disabled 178, 179, 180, 181
Oral Hygiene Index (OHI) 57
Oral lesions, benign 48
Orthostatic hypotension 83
Overbite 61
Overjet 61

P

Palate, clinical examination 43
Patient,
  positioning 99, 101, 102, 103, 119
  postsurgical, treatment 147–152
  tooth polishing effects 154
Patient education,
  for disabled 178, 179, 180, 181
  for hearing impaired 181
  for visually impaired 179
  hygienist's role 163
Pellicle, acquired 124
Perio-Aid® 172, 174
Periodontal diseases,
  antibiotics for 182
  etiology 182
  fluoride therapy 190, 191
  treatment planning 115
Periodontal dressing 147, 148
Periodontal probing 50, 51, 52, 53
Periodontium, clinical examination 50, 51, 52
Photography,
  equipment 96, 97, 98, 99
  for dental record 96–103
  guidelines 99–103
  patient positioning 99, 101, 102, 103
Physicians' Desk Reference 34
Pit and fissure sealants, 183–187
  longevity 187
  placement procedures 185, 186, 187
  protection by 184
Plaque,
  composition 124, 125, 160
  control 165–172, 175–177, 181–183
  formation 125
Preventive dentistry 159–205
Procedures, preliminary 11–105
Proximal cleaning 170, 171, 172, 173
Pulp test 92, 93, 94
Pulse rate 35

R

Radiation injuries 27
Respiration rate 38

S

Shock,
  cardiogenic 83
  hypovolemic 83
  insulin 82
Silness & Löe Plaque Index (PI-1) 57
Simplified Oral Hygiene Index (OHI-S) 57
Snyder test 161
Stains 126
Sterilization methods 13–15
Stress 70
Stroke 80
Study models, 88–93
  armamentarium for 88
  preparation for 88, 89, 90
Suture removal 148, 149, 150, 151
Syncope, vasodepressor 83
Syphilis 26

T

Temporomandibular joint, clinical examination 40
Throat culture 96
Tongue, clinical examination 44
Tooth mobility 54
Tooth numbering systems 63, 64
Tooth polishing,
  agents 155
  air 156
  contraindications 154
  indications 154
  manual 157
  mechanisms 153–158
  methods 155, 156, 157
  motor-driven 155, 156
  procedure effects 153, 154
  proximal surface 157, 158
Toothbrush,
  automatic 168
  denture 176, 177
  interproximal 172, 173
  manual 164, 165
  partial clasp 176, 177
Toothbrushing, 165–168
  Bass (sulcular brushing) method 166
  Charters' method 167
  circular method 168
  modified Stillman's method 165, 166
  of orthodontic appliances 167
  rolling stroke method 165, 166
Treatment planning, 107–158
  cancer 110–114
  diabetes 109

epilepsy   110
hematological disorders   108, 109
individualization   108–116
systemic disorders   108–116
Tuberculosis   25, 26

V

Vestibule, clinical examination   42, 43
Vital signs   35

W

Wound, open   86

X

Xerostomia   111, 112